Perioperative Pain Management for Orthopedic and Spine Surgery

T0177503

PERIOPERATIVE PAIN MANAGEMENT FOR ORTHOPEDIC AND SPINE SURGERY

Edited by
John S. Reach, Jr.
James J. Yue
Deepak Narayan
Alan D. Kaye
Nalini Vadivelu

OXFORD
UNIVERSITY PRESS

Oxford University Press is a department of the University of Oxford. It furthers
the University's objective of excellence in research, scholarship, and education
by publishing worldwide. Oxford is a registered trade mark of Oxford University
Press in the UK and certain other countries.

Published in the United States of America by Oxford University Press
198 Madison Avenue, New York, NY 10016, United States of America.

© Oxford University Press 2019

Library of Congress Cataloging-in-Publication Data
Names: Reach, John S., Jr., editor. | Yue, James J., editor. | Narayan, Deepak, editor. |
Kaye, Alan D., editor. | Vadivelu, Nalini, editor.
Title: Perioperative pain management for orthopedic and spine surgery /
edited by John S. Reach, Jr., James J. Yue, Deepak Narayan, Alan D. Kaye, and Nalini Vadivelu.
Description: New York, NY : Oxford University Press, 2019. | Includes bibliographical references.
Identifiers: LCCN 2018025977 | ISBN 9780190626761 (paperback)
Subjects: | MESH: Pain Management—methods | Orthopedic Procedures—methods |
Perioperative Care | Spine—surgery
Classification: LCC RD768 | NLM WE 168 | DDC 617.4/71—dc23
LC record available at https://lccn.loc.gov/2018025977

9 8 7 6 5 4 3 2 1

Printed by Webcom, Inc., Canada

Contents

Preface

Orthopedic and spine surgeries are among the top procedures triggering pain of the greatest intensity in the post-surgical period. With the recent, immense advancements of pain medications and techniques in the field of orthopedic and spine surgery, there is a growing interest from practicing surgeons of these specialties to update their understandings of the physiologic basis of pain and pain assessment in the post-operative period, and to study the different facets of current therapies engaged for pain relief in the post-operative period following orthopedic and spine surgeries.

Perioperative Pain Management in Orthopedic and Spine Surgery contains all the essential topics required for the trainee and practitioner in the field of orthopedic and spine surgery to quickly assess the patient with pain, to diagnose pain and painful conditions, determine the feasibility and safety of surgical procedure needed, and arrange for advanced pain management consults and care if needed. This book is also useful for medical practitioners of non-surgical specialties to understand the evidence and surgical clinical experiences behind decision-making in these specialties. The chapters in this book have drawn upon the extensive experience of their authors, whom have presented their work with lucidness, pragmatism, and as much relevance to current day practice as possible. We thank each of them for their pertinent efforts.

We wish to thank Oxford University Press, especially the editorial staff, Andrea Knobloch and Tiffany Lu, for their help. We extend our special thanks to our colleagues and families for their motivation.

We hope you find *Perioperative Pain Management in Orthopedic and Spine Surgery* a handy and practical tool to extend unsurpassed patient care.

John S. Reach, Jr.
James J. Yue
Deepak Narayan
Alan D. Kaye
Nalini Vadivelu

Contributors

Salahadin Abdi, MD, PhD, CBA
Department of Pain Medicine
Division of Anesthesiology, Critical
    Care, and Pain Medicine
University of Texas MD Anderson
    Cancer Center
Houston, TX

Paula Trigo Blanco, MD
Resident in Anesthesiology
Yale-New Haven Hospital
New Haven, CT

Mark V. Boswell, MD, PhD
Lolita S. and Samuel D. Weakley
    Endowed Research Chair
Department of Anesthesiology and
    Perioperative Medicine
University of Louisville School of
    Medicine
Louisville, KY

Raysa Cabrejo, BS
Medical Student
Yale School of Medicine
New Haven, CT

Kenneth D. Candido, MD
Chairman, Department of
    Anesthesiology
Advocate Illinois Masonic
    Medical Center
Clinical Professor of Anesthesiology
Clinical Professor Surgery
Department of Anesthesiology
University of Illinois Chicago
Chicago, IL

Hector J. Cases, MD
Neurologist and Pain Specialist
Tampa Pain Relief Centers – Brandon
Brandon, FL

Charles Chang, MD
Yale Department of Orthopaedics and
    Rehabilitation
New Haven, CT

Richard Cleveland Sims, MD
Anesthesiology Resident
Department of Anesthesiology
University of Florida
Gainesville, FL

Sabrina DaCosta, MD
Department of Anesthesiology
Yale Unversity
New Haven, CT

Sudhir A. Diwan, MD
Professor, Program Director, and Chair
Department of Anesthesia
Louisiana State University Health
 Science Center
New Orleans, LA
Executive Director
Manhattan Spine and Pain Medicine
New York, NY

S. Gabriel Farkas, MD
Resident
Department of Anesthesiology
Westchester Medical Center
Valhalla, NY

Kenneth Fomberstein, MD
Department of Anesthesiology
Westchester Medical Center
Valhalla, NY

Raj J. Gala, MD
Department of Orthopaedics and
 Rehabilitation
Yale School of Medicine
New Haven, CT

J. H. Gan
Registrar, Department of Anaesthesia
Epsom and St Helier University
 Hospitals NHS Trust
Carshalton, United Kingdom

Jay S. Grider, DO, PhD, MBA
Chief, Division of Pain and Regional
 Anesthesia
Medical Director
University of Kentucky HealthCare
 Pain Services
Lexington, KY

Abhishek Gupta, MD
Department of Anesthesiology
Westchester Medical Center
Valhalla, NY

Graham R. Hadley, MD
Resident
Department of Anesthesiology,
 Perioperative Care, and Pain Medicine
New York University
New York, NY

Michael E. Harned, MD
Associate Professor of Anesthesiology
University of Kentucky HealthCare
 Pain Services
Lexington, KY

Mark R. Jones, MD
Resident
Department of Anesthesiology, Critical
 Care, and Pain Medicine
Beth Israel Deaconess Medical Center
Harvard Medical School
Boston, MA

Alice Kai, MD
Department of Internal Medicine
New York University Winthrop Hospital
Mineola, NY

Alan D. Kaye, MD, PhD
Professor, Program Director, and Chair,
 Department of Anesthesia
LSU Health Science Center
New Orleans, LA

Chang-Yeon Kim, MD
Othopaedic Resident
University Hospitals Cleveland
 Medical Center
Cleveland, OH

Daniel Krashin, MD
Departments of Psychiatry and Pain
    Medicine & Anesthesia
University of Washington
Seattle, WA

Sree Kunnumpurath, MS
Pain Management Consultant
North Downs Hospital
Caterham, UK

Teresa M. Kusper, DO, MBS
Resident Physician
Department of Anesthesiology
Advocate Illinois Masonic
    Medical Center
Chicago, IL

Kay Lee, MD
Assistant Professor
Department of Anesthesiology
Montefiore Medical Center
Albert Einstein College of Medicine
Bronx, NY

Zachariah Mirsky, MD
Resident Physician
Department of Anesthesiology
Yale New Haven Hospital
New Haven, CT

Natalia Murinova, MD, MHA
Director
University of Washington Medicine
    Headache Center
Seattle, WA

Vital Nagar, MD, PhD
St. Croix Regional Medical Center
St. Croix Falls, WI

Deepak Narayan, MD
Professor of Surgery
Yale University School of Medicine
New Haven, CT

Anh L. Ngo, MD, MBA
Instructor in Anaesthesia
Beth Israel Deaconess Medical Center
Chief Medical Officer
Chief Technology Officer
Incubator for Patient Safety and
    Outcomes
Boston, MA

Matthew Novitch, BS
Medical Student
Medical College of Wisconsin
Wausau, WI

Vwaire Orhurhu, MD
Clinical Fellow in Anaesthesia
Beth Israel Deaconess Medical Center
Harvard Medical School
Boston, MA

William Park, MD
Pulmonary and Sleep Disorder Clinic
Valley Medical Center
Renton, WA

Dipan Patel, MD
Assistant Professor of Surgery, Trauma/
    Surgical Critical Care
Grady Memorial Hospital
Associate Program Director, Acute
    Care Surgery Fellowship
Department of Surgery
Emory University School of Medicine
Atlanta, GA

Clara Pau, MD
Resident
Department of Anesthesiology
Yale School of Medicine
New Haven, CT

Bruce A. Piszel, MD
Pain Medicine Specialist
Tampa Pain Relief Centers – Brandon
Brandon, FL

Rene Przkora, MD, PhD
Chief, Pain Medicine Division
Department of Anesthesiology
University of Florida
Gainesville, FL

Muhammad Asad Qureshi, FCPS, FRCSEd
Professor and Head
Department of Spine Surgery
Combined Military Hospital
Rawalpindi, Pakistan

Maunak V. Rana, MD
Director of Pain Management,
 Clinical Associate Professor of
 Anesthesiology and Surgery
Department of Anesthesiology
Advocate Illinois Masonic Medical Center
Chicago, IL

Hassan Rayaz, MD
Department of Anesthesiology
Yale Unversity
New Haven, CT

John S. Reach, Jr., MSc, MD
Director and Chief of Orthopedic Foot
 and Ankle Surgery
Associate Professor
Department of Orthopedic Surgery
Yale University School of Medicine
New Haven, CT

Maricarmen Roche Rodriguez, MD
Resident in Anesthesiology
Yale-New Haven Hospital
New Haven, CT

Marissa Rubin, MD
Department of Anesthesiology
Westchester Medical Center
Valhalla, NY

Michael Rubin, MD
Department of Anesthesiology
Westchester Medical Center
Valhalla, NY

John-Paul Sara, MD
Department of Anesthesiology
Westchester Medical Center
Valhalla, NY

Chirag D. Shah, MD, JD
Chief Resident Physician, Department
 of Physical Medicine &
 Rehabilitation
Rush University Medical Center
Chicago, IL

Siddarth Thakur, MD
Pain Medicine Fellow
University of Texas MD Anderson
 Cancer Center
Houston, TX

Donna-Ann Thomas, MD
Assistant Professor of Anesthesiology
Division Chief, Pain Medicine
Yale School of Medicine
New Haven, CT

Andrea Trescot, MD, DABIPP, FIPP
Chair, Education Committee of World
 Institute of Pain
Director, Florida Society of
 Interventional Pain Physicians
President, Alaska Society of
 Interventional Pain Physicians
Wasilla, AR

Ivona Truszkowska, MD
Department of Anesthesiology
Westchester Medical Center
Valhalla, NY

Nalini Vadivelu, MD
Professor Department of Anesthesiology
Yale University School of Medicine
New Haven, CT

James J. Yue, MD
Associate Professor
Department of Orthopedic Surgery
Yale University School of Medicine
New Haven, CT

1 Pathophysiology of Pain and Pain Pathways

Paula Trigo Blanco, Maricarmen
Roche Rodriguez, and Nalini Vadivelu

INTRODUCTION: CLASSIFICATION OF PAIN

Pain is a complex phenomenon that originates from real or potential tissue injury or damage. Pain is experienced by each individual in a unique manner. *Nociception* is the detection, transduction, and transmission of noxious impulses caused by mechanical, thermal, and chemical tissue damage.

Pain can be classified according to its duration:

- *Acute pain*: Pain of less than 6 months' duration. Biologically, it has a protective function because it informs the individual about a condition that can be detrimental to the body.
- *Chronic pain*: Persistent or intermittent pain, usually lasting longer than 6 months. It is often accompanied by behavioral changes, such as depression, anxiety, sleeping disorders, fear, or hopelessness.
- *Acute-on-chronic pain*: Acute pain exacerbation in a patient with preexisting chronic pain.

Pain can be categorized into two major types based on pathophysiology. These are *nociceptive pain* and *neuropathic pain*. Frequently, both types are concomitantly present in the same patient.

The nociceptive pathway represents the normal physiologic response to a noxious insult or tissue injury. It is usually described as well-localized pain. Nociceptive pain can be further divided into:

- *Somatic pain*: Superficial pain, such as cutaneous or musculoskeletal pain.
- *Visceral pain*: Originates in hollow organs, abdomen (acute pancreatitis, prostatic pain, nephrolytiatic pain), chest (angina pectoris, myocardial infarction), and smooth muscle. The receptors are unmyelinated C fibers. Visceral pain is

characterized by dull, deep, not well-defined pain, and it commonly induces pronounced autonomic symptoms (sweating, arterial pressure and heart rate changes, vasomotor phenomena). It is also known as *referred pain* because it presents in an area distant from the original location but is supplied by nerves from the same spinal segment as the actual site of pain.

As a result of tissue injury, multiple and diverse inflammatory mediators are released locally. These include cytokines (interleukin-1 [IL-1], IL-6, tumor necrosis factor-α [TNF-α]), vasoactive amines, and other factors released by leukocytes, mast cells, or vascular endothelial cells.

Neuropathic pain is a complex, chronic pain that occurs as a result of tissue injury and results in damage or dysfunction of nerve fibers, which send distorted signals to superior pain centers in the central and peripheral nervous system [1]. The symptoms of neuropathic pain include tingling, numbness, and shooting and burning pain. Examples of neuropathic pain include *phantom limb syndrome*, an unusual condition habitually seen after limb amputations in which the patient's brain continues to receive pain signals from the nerves that originally transmitted impulses from the missing extremity. Other medical conditions commonly associated with neuropathic pain are diabetic neuropathy, postherpetic neuralgia, spinal cord injury pain, post-stroke central pain, alcoholism, human immunodeficiency virus (HIV) infection, acquired immunodeficiency syndrome (AIDS), multiple sclerosis (MS), chemotherapy, and facial nerve problems. However, neuropathic pain frequently has no obvious cause.

The diagnosis of neuropathic pain is essentially clinical, based on a thorough history with detailed documentation of the symptoms reported by the patient and a physical exam (neurological and musculoskeletal). Additional testing such as blood tests, imaging studies (X-rays, magnetic resonance imaging [MRI]), and electrodiagnostic testing can be performed.

Effective therapeutic management of neuropathic pain can be challenging. Treatment and optimization of the underlying condition may help in alleviating the pain and preventing further nerve damage. Some patients respond well to nonsteroidal anti-inflammatory drugs (NSAIDs), such as ibuprofen, indomethacin, or naproxen. Other groups of patients require opioid medications (morphine, hydromorphone, fentanyl), with variable response. Anticonvulsants (gabapentin, pregabalin) and antidepressant drugs have been widely used with good effect in most patients [2,3].

In refractory cases, invasive therapies, such as the implantation of electrical stimulator devices, are offered to the patient in order to control the pain symptoms. Other adjuvant treatments that can help are physical therapy, cognitive behavioral therapy, aquatherapy, relaxation, meditation, and acupuncture.

As mentioned earlier, neuropathic pain does not respond well to conventional pain treatments and may worsen and become disabling. Therefore, a multidisciplinary approach that combines therapies can be the most effective way to offer pain relief and improve the quality of life to this group of patients already suffering from a chronic and debilitating condition.

PAIN PATHWAYS: NEUROANATOMY OF PAIN

The areas of the central and peripheral nervous systems responsible for the transmission and perception of pain may be divided into afferent and efferent pathways.

Table 1.1 Nociceptors

Receptor class	Type	Body area	Modality
Mechanoreceptors	Free nerve endings	Skin	Touch
	Golgi-Mazzoni endings	Skin	Pressure
	Hair follicle	Hairy skin	Touch
	Meissner's corpuscle	Glabrous skin	Touch, vibration
	Merkel's disk	Skin	Touch
	Pacinian corpuscle	Skin	Pressure, vibration
	Ruffini's endings	Hairy skin	Pressure
Nociceptors	Mechanical	Skin	Mechanical impulse
	Thermal	Skin	Hot/cold stimulus
	Polymodal (free nerve endings)	Skin	Mechanical/thermal/ chemical
Thermoreceptors	Krause's end bulbs (cold)	Skin	Cold
	Ruffini's endings (heat)	Skin	Heat

Afferent Pathways

Nociceptors

The afferent pathway originates in the *nociceptors* (pain receptors). The nociceptors are free nerve endings located in epidermis (high concentration), subcutaneous tissue, muscles, tendons, and visceral organs. There are two types of nociceptors: *exteroceptors* (in skin) and *interoceptors* (located in viscera). In addition, other specialized somatosensory receptors, sensitive to other forms of impulses, can be found in high proportions in the skin (Table 1.1).

Every sensory unit is composed of an end-organ receptor, an axon, a dorsal root ganglion, and axon terminals in the spinal cord.

Peripheral Nerve Afferent Fibers

Nerve fibers are classified into three types (A, B, C) based on their size, speed of conduction, degree of myelination, and distribution (Table 1.2).

Table 1.2 Nerve fibers

Nerve fiber class	Diameter (μm)	Conduction rate (m/sec)	Myelin	Location
Aα	11–16	60–80	Myelinated	Efferent to muscles
Aβ	6–11	30–60	Myelinated	Afferent from skin and joints
Aγ	1–6	2–30	Myelinated	Efferent to muscle spindles
Aδ	1–6	2–30	Myelinated	Afferent sensory nerves
B	3	3–15	Myelinated	Preganglionic sympathetic
C	0.5–1.5	0.25–1.5	Nonmyelinated	Postganglionic sympathetic

A fibers may be divided into four subtypes (α, β, γ, δ).

- *A fibers*: These neurons have a large diameter (1–0 μm), are myelinated, exhibit a low threshold for activation, and transmit impulses at the highest conduction velocity of all the neurons in the body (5–100 m/sec).
  - Subclass Aα fibers (afferent or efferent fibers) transmit motor and proprioceptive signals.
  - Subclass Aβ (afferent or efferent fibers) and Aγ fibers (efferent fibers) carry pressure and cutaneous touch impulses. They also regulate muscle spindle reflexes.
  - Subclass Aδ (afferent fibers) mediate pain sensation.
- *B fibers*: Nerve fibers type B, such as preganglionic fibers of the autonomic nervous system and the postganglionic sympathetic and visceral afferents, are medium-sized (diameter of <3 μm) myelinated fibers with a low conduction velocity (ranging from 3 to 14 m/sec). They have intermediate excitability (higher threshold than A fibers but lower than C fibers).
- *C fibers*: Unmyelinated or lightly myelinated nerve fibers; their conduction velocities are low, in the range of 0.25–1.5 m/sec. These fibers include the preganglionic fibers in the autonomic nervous system and nerve fibers at the dorsal roots (which carry pain, temperature, touch, and pressure information).

The small unmyelinated fibers (C fibers that transmit diffuse burning and aching pain) and the large myelinated afferent neurons (Aδ fibers, with faster transmission than C fibers; responsible for well localized sharp pain) are activated by mechanical, chemical, and thermal tissue damage, and they travel to the dorsal horn of the spinal cord to form a *synapsis* (peripheral afferent neuron). The peripheral afferent neuron or *first-order neuron* has its cell body (or somata, portion of a neuron containing the cell nucleus) in the dorsal root ganglion and emits axonal projections into the dorsal horn and other areas of the spinal cord.

Spinal Cord Network

The spinal cord network is formed where a first-order neuron forms a synapse with a *second-order neuron*. Based on the afferent input received, the second-order neuron can be a nociceptive-specific (high-threshold mechanoreceptor neurons) or a wide dynamic range neuron (polymodal-nociceptive neurons).

The nociceptive-specific neurons are excited only by noxious cutaneous and/ or visceral stimuli, and they release glutamate and different neuropeptides to activate the dorsal horn neurons. The wide dynamic range nociceptive neurons are excited by both noxious and non-noxious cutaneous and/or visceral stimuli. They are activated by a variety of noxious stimuli (mechanical, thermal, chemical) and respond incrementally to increasing intensity of stimuli. Similar to the first-order neuron and second-order synapse, other synaptic communications take place between first-order and regulatory internuncial neurons and also with the cell bodies of the sympathetic nervous system.

The cell body of the second-order neuron is in the dorsal horn of the spinal cord. Their axons cross to the contralateral side of the spinal cord, ascending in the lateral spinothalamic tract to synapse in the thalamus. These ascending pathways mediating pain consist of three different tracts: the neospinothalamic tract, the paleospinothalamic tract, and the archispinothalamic tract. Each pain tract originates in different areas of the spinal cord, and they all ascend to terminate in different regions of the central nervous system (CNS).

In the CNS, the thalamus, hypothalamus, and cerebral sensory cortex perceive, describe, and localize the pain. The connection between the limbic system and the reticular formation control the affective and emotional component in the response to pain. The perception of pain is associated with an autonomic response due to the connection between the cortex, the thalamus, and the brainstem with the autonomic nervous system.

The *neospinothalamic tract* constitutes the classical lateral spinothalamic tract (LST). It has a few synapses, and it carries information to the midbrain, thalamus, and postcentral gyrus (perception of pain). The first-order nociceptive neurons in the dorsal root ganglion make synaptic connections in Rexed layer I neurons (marginal zone). Axons from layer I neurons decussate in the anterior white commissure, then enter the cord and ascend in the contralateral anterolateral quadrant.

The majority of the pain fibers of the lower extremities, chest, and abdomen terminate in the ventroposterolateral (VPL) nucleus (related to discriminatory functions) and ventroposteroinferior (VPI) nucleus of the thalamus, which sends the signals to the primary sensory cortex.

The first-order nociceptive neurons from above the neck have somata in the trigeminal ganglion. Trigeminal fibers travel to the pons, descend to the medulla, and form synapses in the spinal trigeminal nucleus, then cross the midline and ascend as trigeminal lemniscus.

All of the neospinothalamic fibers ending in VPL and ventroposteromedial (VPM) are somatotopically oriented. They send axons that synapse on the primary somatosensory cortex (Brodmann's areas 1 and 2), and they provide the perception of the painful sensation as well as the location of the painful stimulus.

The other division of the spinothalamic tract, the *paleospinothalamic tract*, forms more synapses, and it sends information mainly to the reticular formation, pons, limbic system, and midbrain. In the thalamus, the second-order neurons synapse with third-order neurons, which send axonal projections into the sensory cortex [9].

Sometimes non-noxious stimuli activate neurons that usually respond only to impulses transmitting pain, causing *hypersensitivity* (increased sensitivity of the system involved in the pain processing), hyperalgesia, and allodynia. Hyperalgesia and allodynia are commonly seen in various peripheral neuropathies and central pain disorders [4].

Hyperalgesia is an increased perception of pain from a stimulus that normally causes pain. Peripheral and/or central sensitization may be involved. Hyperalgesia differs from allodynia in that hyperalgesia is an increased sensitivity to pain due to a decrease in the nociceptor's threshold for pain by either peripheral or central mechanisms, whereas allodynia is a perception of pain from stimuli that are not painful. Hyperalgesia can be classified as primary (peripheral) and secondary (central).

Primary hyperalgesia takes place at the site of the injury when the nociceptive fiber is stimulated by chemical agents released by the injured tissue. Substances such as bradykinin, histamine, prostaglandins, leukotrienes, acetylcholine, serotonin, and substance P lower nociceptors' threshold for activation and therefore increase the nociceptive input into the CNS. Subsequent tissue damage provokes the nociceptor to respond with a greater number of action potentials (defined as the change in electrical potential associated with the passage of an impulse along the membrane of a muscle cell or nerve cell) to the same stimulus given before the injury occurred.

Secondary hyperalgesia occurs after severe or persistent injury secondary to repeated firing of the C fibers and release of excitatory neurotransmitters (e.g., glutamate) and neuropeptides, with a consequent increase in the firing of neurons in the dorsal horn of the spinal cord, a phenomenon called "wind-up." This results in long-term changes in the excitability and sensitivity of the dorsal horn neurons (central sensitization), which can lead to spontaneous pain, diminish the threshold for nociception, and create a "memory" for the C fiber input [5].

Unlike hyperalgesia, *allodynia* is pain caused by normally non-noxious stimuli. Mechanical impulses (e.g., light touch) activate Aβ fibers to produce the sensation of touch. However, in patients with allodynia, activation of these systems produces pain. One mechanism for allodynia is a result of *central sensitization* that reflects a greater excitability and a decrease in the threshold for activation of neurons in the central CNS.

"Central sensitization" is a commonly used term that denotes an enhancement in the function of neurons and pain impulses in nociceptive pathways; it is originated by membrane excitability augmentation and synaptic efficacy as well as reduced inhibition. Sensitization is a manifestation of the extraordinary plasticity of the somatosensory nervous system in response to inflammation and neural damage [5,6].

This complex interaction between the central and peripheral nervous systems was examined in 1965, when psychologist Ronald Melzack and physiologist Patrick Wall published the *gate control theory* [7]. This theory postulates that the information coming in over C fibers is modulated through presynaptic inhibition from incoming Aβ fibers in the substantia gelatinosa in the dorsal horn of the spinal cord. According to the gate control theory, pain signals are not transmitted to the brain as soon as they are initiated at the injured tissues. They need to encounter certain "neurological gates" at the spinal cord level, and these gates determine whether the pain signals should reach the brain or not (open or close the gate). In other words, pain is perceived when the gate gives way to the pain signals, and it is less intense or not at all perceived when the gate closes and the signals cannot pass through. This theory explains how pain seems to be lessened when the painful area is rubbed or massaged because activation of non-nociceptive fibers inhibits the firing of nociceptive ones in the laminae. The cells in the substantia gelatinosa act as a gate, stimulating or inhibiting the transmission of impulses to CNS. gate control theory has visualized the mechanism of pain perception in a new dimension, and it has paved the way for various pain management strategies.

Efferent Pathways

Efferent pathways are the nerve fibers connecting the reticular formation, midbrain, and substantia gelatinosa. Pain afferents stimulates the neurons in the periaqueductal gray matter (PAG) in the midbrain, activating descending anti-nociceptive pathways that travel from the midbrain to the dorsal horn of the spinal cord, where they block the transmission of nociceptive signals. They are responsible for pain sensation modulation and inhibition of afferent pain stimulus. In terms of the gate control theory, these efferent pathways may open or close the gate (partially or completely). As a matter of fact, they play a significant role in cognitive behavioral therapy's modulation of pain perception.

MODULATION OF PAIN: NEUROPLASTICITY

Endorphins may block the transmission of painful impulses attaching to opioid receptors on the plasma membrane of the afferent neuron, resulting in inhibition of releasing of the neurotransmitter. [5,8]

Neuroplasticity is the ability of the nervous system to adjust its structure and function. Negative changes in these pathways occur via sensitization and long-term potentiation (LTP). *Sensitization* refers to a repeated stimulus that results in amplification of a response and occurs from injury to neurons. This leads to alterations in pain modulation and the excitability of the neurons participating in the transmission of nociceptive signals. Peripheral sensitization can occur, such as from chronic muscle pain, which then contributes to a central sensitization. Central sensitization represents neuronal function and is caused by the increase in membrane excitability and reduced inhibition in response to neuronal injury. Neuroplasticity can also occur by physical changes in the nervous system and pain pathways or by cognitive and emotional processes that alter the response to these pain pathways. These changes can cause an increase in the intensity of pain. These changes are noted in phantom pain, chronic back pain, and fibromyalgia. Successful treatment can be achieved by creating new LTPs due to the plasticity of these neurons, as well as by dampening the transmission of the sensitized inputs [5].

REFERENCES

1. Woolf CJ. Dissecting out mechanisms responsible for peripheral neuropathic pain: implications for diagnosis and therapy. *Life Sci.* 2004;74:2605–2610.
2. Allegri M, Baron R, Hans G, Correa-Illanes G, Mayoral Rojals V, Mick G, Serpell M. A pharmacological treatment algorithm for localized neuropathic pain. *Curr Med Res Opin.* 2016 Feb;32(2):377–384.
3. Attal N, Cruccu G, Baron R, Haanpää M, Hansson P, Jensen TS, Nurmikko T. EFNS guidelines on the pharmacological treatment of neuropathic pain: 2010 revision. European Federation of Neurological Societies. *Eur J Neurol.* 2010 Sep;17(9):1113–1123.
4. Jensen TS, Finnerup NB. Allodynia and hyperalgesia in neuropathic pain: clinical manifestations and mechanisms. *Lancet Neurol.* 2014 Sep;13(9):924–935.
5. Latremoliere A, Woolf CJ. Central sensitization: a generator of pain hypersensitivity by central neural plasticity. *J Pain.* 2009 Sep;10(9):895–926.
6. Abbadie C, Trafton J, Liu H, Mantyh PW, Basbaum AI. Inflammation increases the distribution of dorsal horn neurons that internalize the neurokinin-1 receptor in response to noxious and non-noxious stimulation. *J Neurosci.* 1997 Oct 15;17(20):8049–8060.
7. Melzack R, Wall PD. Pain mechanisms: a new theory. *Science* 1965;150:971–979.
8. Lubenow T, Ivankovich A, Barkin R. Management of acute postoperative pain. In Barash P, ed. *Clinical Anesthesia.* 5th ed. Philadelphia, PA: Lippincot Williams & Wilkins; 2006:1405–1440.
9. Fu X, Froicu D, Sinatra R. Anatomic and physiologic principles of pain. In Vadivelu N, Urman R, Hines R, eds. *Essentials of Pain Management.* New York: Springer; 2011:31–44.

2 Preventive Analgesia for the Management of General Surgical Pain

M. A. Qureshi, J. H. Gan,
S. Kunnumpurath, Clara Pau, Alice Kai,
Zachariah Mirsky, William Park,
and Nalini Vadivelu

INTRODUCTION

Pain created by surgery has the ability to produce both structural and functional changes in pain pathways. These changes may be reduced if timely and adequate pain relief is delivered to the patient. Poor control of pain can result in remodeling of the "hardwired" pathways involved in pain transmission, which can result in central sensitization and hyperalgesia (Figure 2.1). Furthermore, poorly controlled pain and delay in its recognition may lead to a chronic pain state, further complicating the patient's recovery and quality of life [1].

MOLECULAR MECHANISMS

Crile originally observed the phenomenon of central sensitization in postoperative patients in 1916 [2]. He saw a relationship between tissue damage during an operation, the intensification of acute pain immediately postoperatively, and the development of long-term postop pain. Subsequently, Woolf demonstrated the same phenomenon in an animal model in 1983 [3, 22]. He showed that a thermal injury in the periphery caused an amplification of painful stimuli evoked activity and an augmentation of the flexion reflex response.

Tissue damage releases local inflammatory factors (e.g., prostaglandin, bradykinins, substance P) from neurons and extraneuronal sources, which leads to peripheral sensitization of the nociceptors. This results in altered transduction and increased conduction

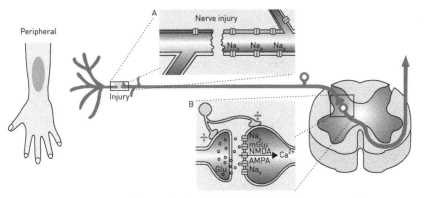

FIGURE 2.1 Cascade of events after peripheral nervous system lesion resulting in central sensitization. Reprinted by permission from Macmillan Publishers Ltd, copyright 2006.

of nociceptive impulses toward the central nervous system (CNS). The barrage of pain signals from the nociceptors onto the neurons in the dorsal horn causes an alteration in the responsiveness of these neurons. Signals from Aδ and C fibers may be amplified, causing hyperalgesia, while activity in Aβ fibers are interpreted not as touch but as pain. This central sensitization may outlast the stimuli and become a "pain memory."

PERIOPERATIVE PAIN MANAGEMENT STRATEGIES

Preemptive analgesia was also first described by Crile in 1916, following his observation of central sensitization [2]. It was further developed by Wall and Woolf in an attempt to manage perioperative pain and prevent central sensitization from occurring [4,5]. *Preemptive analgesia* is the delivery of an analgesic intervention before the surgical procedure has begun. It is important to emphasize that the delivery of analgesia has to occur before the onset of tissue damage and the resulting altered processing of afferent input. Early observations and animal studies have shown a reduction in pain if analgesia was administered before the noxious stimuli. However, subsequent clinical studies of preemptive analgesia comparing anti-nociceptive interventions before incision versus after incision yielded contradictory results. This is understandable when one considers that both preincisional and postincisional noxious inputs contribute to postoperative sensitization, pain, and analgesic consumption. The most likely conclusion, therefore, is that for a certain proportion of studies of preemptive analgesia, the postincision or postsurgical administration condition is as beneficial in reducing central sensitization as is the preoperative condition. In addition, the lack of a control group in studies of preemptive analgesia confounds interpretation of the results and has contributed to the premature and erroneous conclusion that there is no clinical benefit to preoperative nociceptive blockade.

Preventive analgesia encompasses multimodal anti-nociceptive interventions that are started preoperatively and given for an increased duration during the postoperative period. It was found to be more effective in terms of decreasing postoperative pain and reducing analgesic consumption compared to preemptive analgesia in the postoperative period. The focus of preventive analgesia is not on the timing of analgesia or anesthetic intervention but on attenuating the impact of a barrage of noxious stimuli on the central nociceptors that may result in peripheral and central sensitization.

Consequently, the delivery of pain relief throughout the perioperative course results in an effective analgesic duration of action greater than that expected for the particular intervention. The components of preventive analgesia include a combination of opioids, N-methyl-D-aspartate (NMDA) receptor antagonist, α_2 receptor agonists, gabapentinoids, and local anesthetics delivered through a variety of routes.

CHRONIC POSTSURGICAL PAIN

A common chronic pain state following surgery is *chronic postsurgical pain* (CPSP). Nerve injury during surgery has been implicated in the development of CPSP. Inflammatory and immune reactions after damage to axons result in release of neurotransmitters that act locally and in the spinal cord to produce hypersensitivity and ectopic neural activity. This results in central sensitization and development of CPSP. For CPSP to be correctly identified, it must be pain that develops after a surgical procedure and which has been present following the surgery for at least 2 months. The diagnosis requires that other potential causes have been excluded such as malignancy and infection. Finally, it must be emphasized that if a preexisting pain problem was present, it should be excluded as the potential cause following the surgical procedure.

This chapter will explore the various modalities available to provide preemptive and preventive analgesia and the evidence for its use. It is important to recognize that poorly treated perioperative pain can lead to emotional and psychological distress and develop into a chronic pain state.

SUBSTANCES AND INTERVENTIONS USED FOR PREVENTIVE ANALGESIA

Paracetamol (Acetaminophen)

Paracetamol is the baseline drug of analgesia given to patients undergoing multiple different types procedures in a surgical setting. It is most effective in adults given as a regular 4- to 6-hour interval dose with a maximum of 4 g in a 24-hour period. It is can be delivered via multiple routes including oral, intravenous, and rectal. It exhibits both analgesic and antipyretic effects.

Despite its common use, the exact mechanism of action of paracetamol is unclear. It is thought to exert its analgesic activity by inhibiting the synthesis of prostaglandins acting centrally on the CNS and peripherally by blocking pain impulse generation [6]. The use of intravenous paracetamol results in a faster speed of onset and more reliable pharmacokinetics than that of rectal or oral administration.

The delivery of paracetamol via the intravenous route avoids first-pass hepatic exposure and metabolism via portal circulation; this reduces the burden on the liver and may reduce the potential for hepatic injury. The incidences of hepatic injury following dosing guidelines of up to 4 g daily are rarely associated with hepatotoxicity [7].

Intravenous paracetamol has also been showed to be very effective when given preemptively. A randomized controlled trial of 300 patients who underwent laparoscopic cholecystectomy showed that patient who had intravenous paracetamol preemptively required less opiate rescue postoperatively and had lower visual analogue scores (VAS) [8]. Intravenous paracetamol has been given prophylactically as a component of multimodal treatment. It is regularly part of the analgesic plans for patients undergoing fast-track surgical procedures. A large study of bariatric patients who were given intravenous paracetamol, parecoxib, and surgical site infiltration before fast-track surgery described a significant reduction in hospital stays from 3 to 2 days [9].

Paracetamol has shown good efficacy, safety, and lack of the adverse effects associated with other analgesics. The use of paracetamol as part of a multimodal approach in dealing with perioperative pain is an attractive option for patients undergoing surgical procedures.

Nonsteroidal Anti-inflammatory Drugs (NSAIDs)

NSAIDs have been used in the perioperative period for many years to relieve pain, reduce inflammation, and for its antipyretic properties. They work through the inhibition of cyclooxygenase (COX) enzyme. COX enzymes are responsible for the production of prostaglandins, prostacyclin, and thromboxanes from arachidonic acid. Prostaglandins themselves do not cause pain but instead sensitize peripheral nociceptors to a variety of neurochemicals (e.g., substance P and bradykinin). In addition to their role in mediating the inflammatory process, COX enzymes are also responsible for maintaining clotting and renal hemostasis and gastrointestinal protection. There are two subtypes of COX enzymes, COX-1 and COX-2. COX 1 is a constitutive enzyme because it is produced by a cell under all types of physiological conditions, while COX-2 is an inducible enzyme that is only produced under certain specific conditions like inflammation. Prostaglandins are central in the inflammatory process, and reducing their effect on nociceptors will result in analgesia.

There are two main types of NSAIDs, those that unselectively inhibit COX-1 and COX-2 and those that selectively inhibit COX-2 only. Selective COX-2 inhibition is thought to improve the side-effect profile of NSAIDs because constitutively expressed COX-1 is not affected by the drug, hence limiting the risk of bleeding and renal failure. Unfortunately, this has not been found to be true in clinical practice. Selective COX-2 inhibitors have no effect in reducing the risk of renal injury or bleeding but do reduce the risk of gastrointestinal bleeding through the reduction of peptic ulceration. In addition, there is evidence that COX-2 inhibitors increase the risk of heart attack, thrombosis, and stroke through an increase of thromboxane production unbalanced by prostacyclin (which is reduced by COX-2 inhibition).

NSAIDs have been used in numerous studies to examine their role as a preventive analgesia. In a review done by Katz et al. [10] they found 14 studies that examined the preemptive and preventive effects of NSAID administration in the perioperative period. Of the six studies that reported preventive effects, four reported positive findings, and, of these Rueben et al. [11]. demonstrated significant long-term benefits at 1 month and 1 year after surgery, respectively. Buvanendran et al. found that a 2-week perioperative regimen of rofecoxib in total knee arthroplasty patients improved range of motion in comparison to controls at a 1-month follow-up. Reuben et al. administered celecoxib or placebo for 5 days to patients scheduled for spinal fusion, beginning 1 hour before surgery. The incidence of chronic donor-site pain was significantly lower in the celecoxib group. Patients who had celecoxib were found to have a 74% lower risk for developing chronic pain than placebo-treated patients at 1 year. In summary, there is convincing evidence that NSAIDs have a definite role as a preemptive and preventive analgesia with a success rate of 70%. They may even have a prolonged effect far longer than the duration of the drug due to its anti-inflammatory properties.

Despite the evidence, the use of NSAIDs should be undertaken with caution due to a number of side effects. They should be avoided in those who have renal impairment as this may worsen following administration. They may exacerbate and worsen bronchospasms in patients with history of asthma and should be completely avoided in patients with a history of duodenal ulcers and gastric bleeding. Fundamentally, the decision to administer NSAIDs should lie with the clinician after balancing its definite analgesia benefits against all possible side effects.

Opioids

Opioids are one of the commonest and oldest groups of drugs. They act on three principal classes of opioid receptors: µ, κ, and δ, which can be found in the brain, spinal cord, and digestive tract. Opioid receptors are G-protein coupled receptors which are activated by endogenous ligands such as dynorphins, enkephalins, endorphins, endomorphins, and nociceptin. Activation of opioid receptors results not only in analgesia but also in sedation, meiosis, euphoria, and reduction of GI motility depending on the subset of receptor activated. Opioids can be delivered via multiple routes and offer a great deal of flexibility in their use as preemptive analgesia.

Early studies by Woolf and Wall showed that less morphine was required to prevent the development of spinal hyperexcitability following noxious stimuli than to reverse it after it was well established. Animal studies have also demonstrated that the application of µ-opiate receptor agonists preempt development of hyperalgesia and allodynia following a noxious insult. However, pretreatment with opioid in more recent human trials is less convincing in decreasing central hyperalgesia and allodynia. Several studies have demonstrated that preoperative opioid administration reduces postoperative pain and consumption of analgesics when compared with postoperative administration, [12,13] while others did not show any benefit [14]. In recent year, there has also been some evidence to suggest that some opioids under the right circumstances may facilitate central hyperalgesia and allodynia [15]. While the exact mechanism that causes central hyperalgesia is still unclear, it is thought that NMDA receptor activation and increased excitatory neuropeptide transmitter such as cholecystokinin (CCK) may play a role. Despite this, opioids continue to have a significant role in pain management during the perioperative period.

Due to the prevalence of opioid receptors throughout the body, there are quite a few side effects associated with opioid use. Opioid use commonly results in constipation and nausea, which fortunately can be avoided with the concomitant use of laxatives and antiemetics. Other side effects such as fatigue, dizziness, and somnolence are often present at the start of treatment but subside after a short while. The use of a strong opioid requires careful monitoring of patients in the postoperative period for complications such as respiratory depression, somnolence, and urinary retention. Acute overdose of an opioid can be reversed by an opioid receptor antagonist, naloxone. It should be remembered that the half-life of naloxone is usually shorter than the half-life of the opioid, and repeat doses of naloxone are frequently required. Rare side effects such as reduction in bone density and immune system suppression are usually only seen after prolonged opioid use.

In an attempt to improve the side-effect profile of opioids, synthetic opioids have been manufactured to selectively activate only certain opioid receptors, improve their bioavailability, and limit of their duration of action. Some more recently released opioids such as tapentadol have a dual mode of action as an agonist of the μ-opioid receptor and as a norepinephrine reuptake inhibitor. Tapentadol has a better gastro-intestinal side-effect profile compared to opiates, which leads to less discontinuation of the medication. A recent prospective double-blinded study showed that tapentadol was effective as a preemptive analgesic [16]. Patients undergoing laparoscopic cho-lecystectomy who had tapentadol preoperatively required significantly less analgesia peri- and postoperatively compared to patients in the placebo group. Further research is required to clarify the ideal choice of synthetic opioids as a preemptive analgesia due to the sheer number of choices currently available.

NMDA Receptor Antagonists

The NMDA receptor is a glutamate receptor and ion channel protein found in nerve cells. It is activated when glutamate and glycine binds to it. Despite ligand binding, current flow through the ion channel is voltage-dependent, and extracellular magne-sium (Mg^{2+}) and zinc (Zn^{2+}) ions can bind to specific sites on the receptor and block the passage of other cations.

The role of NMDA receptors in pain was first described in the 1980s by two groups demonstrating that spinal delivery of NMDA receptor antagonists inhibits the hyperexcitability of spinal cord nociceptive neurons induced by C fiber stimulation. C fiber stimulation by noxious stimuli causes the excitatory synaptic release of glutamate. Glutamate activates peripheral and spinal NMDA receptors that are involved in the transduction of the pain signal and also in descending inhibitory impulses. Activation of NMDA receptors causes the spinal cord neuron to become more responsive to all of its inputs, resulting in central sensitization. In addition, activation of NMDA receptors not only increases the response to noxious stimuli but blunts the neuronal sensitivity to opioid agonist.

Ketamine is a NMDA receptor antagonist that exhibits analgesic properties and can also be used as an anesthetic induction agent. Ketamine may reduce hyperalgesia, wind-up, and central sensitization, and therefore the development of CPSP. In clinical practice, ketamine delivered at low doses (0.15 mg/kg) and given before surgical inci-sion has been shown to reduce the postoperative morphine requirement in the first 24 hours after cholecystectomy [17]. Similar findings are also seen when ketamine is used as a preemptive analgesia in thoracotomy patient [18] and in those requiring an ampu-tation [19]. Perioperative intravenous ketamine has been used successfully in patients with chronic pain who are on high opioid doses. These patients are particularly diffi-cult to manage due to opioid tolerance, and use of ketamine has resulted in reduced opioid consumption and pain intensity after back surgery [20]. A number of studies carried out looking into the role of ketamine in the perioperative period have shown that it exhibits preventive effect and not necessarily a preemptive analgesic effect [21].

The use of ketamine should be done with caution in patients with a history of is-chemic heart disease or abnormal heart rhythms as these may be worsened. Ketamine should be avoided in patients with high intracranial pressure as this will be worsened. It can cause a number of psychomimetic effects such as hallucinations and nightmares, which should be monitored for in the postoperative period. Despite these cautions, ke-tamine is a useful adjuvant in patients with a complex pain history and offers options as a preventive analgesic agent.

Magnesium is a physiological antagonist to the NMDA receptor. It not only blocks the NMDA receptor but is also postulated to reduce catecholamine release during sympathetic stimulation. Small-scale randomized trials have produced mixed results. A recent meta-analysis of 25 trials comparing magnesium versus placebo has shown that perioperative magnesium reduced cumulative intravenous morphine consumption by 24.4% at 24 hours postoperatively [22]. Numeric pain scores at rest and on movement at 24 hours postoperatively were reduced by 4.2 ($p < 0.0001$) and 9.2 ($p = 0.009$) out of 100, respectively. The majority of trials used a bolus dose of magnesium in the perioperative period ranging from 30 to 50 mg/kg. Magnesium has a very good safety profile, with only a slightly higher incidence of bradycardia but not hypotension, sedation, or symptomatic hypermagnesemia.

Regional Anesthesia

Regional anesthesia is the use of local anesthetics to block sensations of pain. It allows for distinct body areas such as the abdomen, arm, or leg to be anesthetized and allows surgery to take place with or without a general anesthetic. This form of anesthesia is divided broadly into two types:

- *Central neural axial block*: Examples include epidural and spinal anesthesia. The local anesthetic is delivered close to the spinal cord, and the nerves are blocked at their origin in the spine. This allows for large regions of the body to be blocked to sensation.
- *Peripheral nerve blocks*: A local anesthetic is injected near a specific nerve or groups of nerves to block sensations of pain from the area of the body supplied by that nerve. Nerve blocks are most commonly used for surgery on the arms, hands, legs, and feet.

Regional analgesia has demonstrated some promising results as a preventive analgesia in the perioperative period. Epidural analgesia when commenced before laparotomy and thoracotomy surgery and continued into the postoperative period has been shown to reduces the incidence of CPSP in patients undergoing surgery. In one study, delivery of paravertebral blocks initiated before incision and continued into the postoperative period reduced the incidence of CPSP in thoracic and breast cancer surgery patients [23]. The delivery of a successful block before the surgical incision and continuing this well into the postoperative period may have a role in reducing the nociceptive pain transmissions that result in central sensitization.

As a form of preemptive analgesia, regional anesthesia was examined in a meta-analysis of preemptive epidural compared with epidural commenced after completion of thoracic surgery. This showed that it did not affect development of CPSP, although it was very effective at ameliorating acute pain. Regional analgesia delivered before the surgical incision with the aim of being more effective than the same treatment started after surgery has been delivered and has shown little benefit for preventing CPSP [24].

The use of a regional blockade by itself is often suboptimal, and therefore a multimodal approach utilizing regional anesthesia (central/peripheral) with other analgesic drugs for neuropathic pain and opioids is the solution to achieving an adequate level of pain relief in the perioperative period.

Local Anesthetics

As membrane-stabilizing drugs, local anesthetics prevent the generation of action potentials along nerve axons. They achieve this by inhibiting the voltage-gated sodium channels, preventing the influx of sodium and inhibiting transmission of pain sensation. Local anesthetics can be administered via wound infiltration, nerve blocks, and centrally either in the epidural or arachnoid space. They are commonly delivered with an opioid to improve the quality of analgesia.

There are many different types of local anesthetic, broadly divided into either an amide or an ester. Each individual agent is designed to have a different speed of onset, duration, and potency depending on their pharmacokinetic profile. An awareness of maximum doses and signs and symptoms of toxicity help in the safe delivery of these drugs. For example, lignocaine has a fast onset, lasts 1–3 hours, and has a toxic dose of 3 mg/kg while bupivacaine has a slower onset but lasts 2–8 hours and has a toxic dose of 2 mg/kg.

Intravenous lignocaine was traditionally used as a Class 1 antiarrhythmic due to its sodium channel blocking properties. Recent trials have found a new role for lignocaine due to opioid sparing and anti-inflammatory abilities when used as a preventive analgesia. This delivery of lignocaine has shown that it is useful in patients undergoing abdominal procedures such as laparoscopic colectomy. Lauwick et al. found a bolus dose of lignocaine followed by an infusion reduces opioid consumption postoperatively in patients undergoing laparoscopic cholecystectomy [25]. Koppert et al. found similar results in patients undergoing major abdominal surgery after a bolus and infusion of lignocaine, where the lignocaine group required nearly 60% less morphine than placebo [26]. The opiate-sparing was greatest at day 3 postop, which may represent a true preventive analgesia effect. Patients receiving intravenous lidocaine were found to have improved bowel function and reduced hospital stay [27]. The use of these infusions in non–abdominal surgery is still unproven, but there has been some evidence that it may have a preventive effect following breast and abdominal surgery [26,28].

α_2 Adrenoreceptor Agonists

The α_2 adrenoreceptors are present in both the peripheral and central nervous systems. α-Adrenoceptors are found in vascular smooth muscle and sympathetic nerve terminals. In smooth muscle, α_2 adrenoceptors are linked to G_i-proteins. Binding of an α-agonist to these receptors decreases intracellular cyclic adenosine monophosphate (cAMP), causing smooth muscle contraction. In nerve terminals, activation of α_2 adrenoceptors results in a fall of cAMP. This allows potassium efflux through calcium-activated channels, which prevents calcium ions from entering the nerve terminal, leading to a suppression of neural firing. This suppression inhibits norepinephrine release and reduces the activity of the ascending noradrenergic pathways located on the sympathetic nerve terminals. This is also the feedback mechanism by which norepinephrine release is modulated. In addition, stimulation of α_2 receptors in the dorsal horn of the spinal column inhibits nociceptive neurons and reduces the release of substance P. Although there is some evidence for supraspinal and peripheral sites of action, it is thought that the spinal mechanism produces most of the α_2 agonist drugs' analgesic action [29,30].

Commonly used drugs for analgesia in this class are clonidine and dexmedetomidine. While both drugs are α_2 agonists, dexmedetomidine is 800 times more selective for α_2 compared to α_1 resulting in lesser side effects (e.g., hypotension and bradycardia). A trial comparing dexmedetomidine versus placebo given preoperatively has shown a reduction of postop opiate consumption after abdominal surgery [31]. While α_2-agonists have been shown to reduce postopiate requirement, their role as a preventive analgesia in reducing hyperalgesia and chronic pain is rather lacking. A meta-analysis on α_2 agonist use confirmed that although it does decrease postoperative opioid consumption, pain intensity, and nausea, it is of uncertain efficacy in preventing hyperalgesia or development of chronic pain [32].

The beneficial effects of these drugs have to be balanced with the possibility of developing hypotension from the clonidine and bradycardia from the dexmedetomidine. In comparison to other classes, the analgesic effects of α_2 adrenoceptor agonists are considered better than paracetamol but not as effective as NSAIDs and ketamine [32].

Gabapentinoids

Gabapentinoids are derivatives of the inhibitory neurotransmitter γ-aminobutyric acid (GABA). They were originally developed for the management of patients with epilepsy. However, they have been shown also useful in the treatment of neuropathic pain, restless leg syndrome, and anxiety. Gabapentinoids cause their effect by blocking the $\alpha_2\delta$-subunit on voltage-gated calcium channels. This action on the presynaptic membrane inhibits calcium influx, resulting in a reduction in excitatory neurotransmitters release. Gabapentin has been described as an anti-hyperalgesic drug that selectively affects the nociceptive process involving central sensitization. In volunteers, oral gabapentin profoundly suppressed established cutaneous hyperalgesia after heat-capsaicin sensitization and was able to prevent the development of cutaneous sensitization.

Evidence for the use of gabapentinoids as single agents in pain modification in the perioperative period is limited. However, when used as part of a multimodal analgesia, gabapentinoids significantly reduce pain and postoperative opioid consumption in multiple types of surgical procedures [33,34].

Gabapentin is one of the older gabapentinoid agents. There have been multiple studies examining the preemptive and preventive analgesic effects of perioperative gabapentin. The use of gabapentin as a preventive analgesia has demonstrated impressive preventive effects through the reduction of postoperative opioid requirements, reduction in the incidence of pain at the surgical incision site 1 month after surgery, and a reduction in neuropathic pain 3 months after surgery [35,36]. In addition, when used in conjunction with local anesthetics, perioperative gabapentin reduced the incidence of chronic pain in breast cancer surgery patients. Only one study evaluated the preemptive effects of gabapentin. Pandey and colleagues compared preincisional versus immediate postincisional administration of gabapentin with a placebo in donor nephrectomy patients and no found no preemptive effect [37]. The absence of preemptive effect was thought to be due to too early administration of postincisional gabapentin in the postincisional group.

Pregabalin was developed as a successor to gabapentin. It has a higher potency, is longer acting, and has a more favorable side-effect profile and better oral bioavailability compared to gabapentin. The use of pregabalin has shown some promise when used as preventive analgesia against developing CPSP. This was demonstrated in a meta-analysis comprising patients undergoing cardiac surgery, lumbar discectomies, and knee surgery. However, there have been methodological issues with the meta-analysis excluding negative industry-conducted studies which may have led to publication bias and a falsely positive signal [38].

Common side effects of gabapentinoids include drowsiness, dizziness, fatigue, and muscle tremor. Most of these side effects are mild, self-limiting, and usually more evident when starting the medication or after dose escalation. Less common side effects include vision disturbances and indigestion

CONCLUSION

Because pain in the perioperative period is likely to be multifactorial, large-scale, multicenter, randomized studies are urgently needed to aid better understanding of CPSP and the value of various analgesic agents as preemptive or preventive analgesics. Currently, NSAIDS have the strongest evidence as a preventive analgesia, while the role of other drugs as preventive agents is still unclear. The development of CPSP is common, although the exact mechanism is complex. Considering the multifactorial pathogenesis of chronic pain, it is unlikely that a single agent will be effective in preventing chronic pain. Instead, a multimodal approach taking into account psychosocial aspects of the patient is more likely to ameliorate the development of CPSP.

REFERENCES

1. Woolf CJ, Chong MS. Preemptive analgesia: treating postoperative pain by preventing the establishment of central sensitisation. *Anesth Analg.* 1993;77:362–379.
2. Crile GW. In: Man AA, ed. *An Adaptive Mechanism. Association.* New York: The Macmillan Company; 1916:242–260.
3. Woolf CJ. Evidence for a central component of post-injury pain hypersensitivity. *Nature.* 1983;306(5944):686–688.
4. Wall PD. The prevention of postoperative pain. *Pain.* 1988;33:289–290.
5. Woolf CJ. Central mechanisms of acute pain. In Bond MR, Charlton JE, Woolf CJ, eds. *Proc. 1991, 6th World Congr on Pain.* Amsterdam, The Netherlands: Elsevier; 1991:25–34.
6. Aronoff DM, Oates JA, Boutaud O. New insights into the mechanism of action of acetaminophen: its clinical pharmacologic characteristics reflect its inhibition of the two prostaglandin H2 synthases. *Clin Pharmacol Ther.* 2006;79(1):9–19.
7. Benson GD, Koff RS, Tolman KG. The therapeutic use of acetaminophen in patients with liver disease. *Am J Ther.* 2005;12(2);133–141.
8. Mustafa A, Bahadır C, Ramazan Ç, Hülya K, et al. Comparing the efficacy of preemptive intravenous paracetamol on the reducing effect of opioid usage in cholecystectomy. *J Res Med Sci.* 2013;18(3):172–177.
9. Bergland A, Gislason H, Raeder J. Fast-track surgery for bariatric laparoscopic gastric bypass with focus on anaesthesia and peri-operative care. Experience with 500 cases. *Acta Anaesthesiol Scand.* 2008;52(10):1394–1399.
10. Katz J, Clarke H. Preventive analgesia and beyond: current status, evidence, and future directions. In: Macintyre PE, Walker SM, Rowbotham DJ, eds. *Clinical Pain Management: Acute Pain.* 2nd ed. London: Hodder Arnold Ltd.; 2008:154–198.

11. Reuben SS, Bhopatkar S, Maciolek H, et al. The preemptive analgesic effect of rofecoxib after ambulatory arthroscopic knee surgery. *Anesth Analg.* Jan 2002;94(1):55–59.

12. Reuben SS, Sklar J, EI-Mansouri M. The preemptive analgesic effect of intraarticular bupivacaine and morphine after ambulatory arthroscopic knee surgery. *Anesth Analg.* 2001;92:923–926.

13. Mavioglu O, Ozkardesler S, Tasdogen A, et al. Effect of analgesia administration timing on early post-operative period characteristics: a randomized, double-blind, controlled study. *J Int Med Res.* 2005;33:483–489.

14. McCarty EC, Spindler KP, Tingstad E, et al. Does intraarticular morphine improve pain control with femoral nerve block after anterior cruciate ligament reconstruction? *Am J Sports Med.* 2001;29:327–332.

15. Lee HJ, Yeomans DC. Opioid induced hyperalgesia in anesthetic settings. *Korean J Anesthesiol.* 2014;67(5):299–304.

16. Yadav G, Jain G, Samprathi A, et al. Role of preemptive tapentadol in reduction of post-operative analgesic requirements after laparoscopic cholecystectomy. *J Anaesthesiol Clin Pharmacol.* 2016:32(4);492–496.

17. Roytblat L, Korotkorucko A, Katz J, et al. Postoperative pain: the effect of low dose ketamine in addition to general anesthesia. *Anesth Analg.* 1993;77:1161–1168.

18. Fiorelli A, Mazzella A, Passavanti B, et al. Is pre-emptive administration of ketamine a significant adjunction to intravenous morphine analgesia for controlling postoperative pain? A randomized, double-blind, placebo-controlled clinical trial. *Interact Cardiovasc Thorac Surg.* Sep 2015;21(3):284–290.

19. Wilson JA, Nimmo AF, Fleetwood-Walker SM, et al. A randomised double blind trial of the effect of pre-emptive epidural ketamine on persistent pain after lower limb amputation. *Pain.* Mar 2008;135(1-2):108–118.

20. Loftus RW, Yeager MP, Clark JA et al. Intraoperative ketamine reduces perioperative opiates consumption in opiate dependent patients with chronic back pain undergoing back surgery. *Anesthesiology.* 2010;113:639–646.

21. Macintyre PE, Shug SA, Scott DA, Visser EJ, Walker SM. APM: SE Working Group of the Australian and New Zealand College of Anaesthetist and Faculty of Pain Medicine. *Acute Pain Management: Scientific Evidence.* 3rd ed. Melbourne: ANZCA & FPM; 2010.

22. Albrecht E, Kirkham KR, Liu SS, et al. Peri-operative intravenous administration of magnesium sulphate and postoperative pain: a meta-analysis. *Anaesthesia.* Jan 2013;68(1):79–90.

23. Searle RD, Simpson KH. Chronic post surgical pain. *Contin Educ Anaesth Crit Care Pain.* 2010;10(1):12–14.

24. Bong CL, Samuel M, Ng JM, et al. Effects of preemptive epidural analgesia on post-thoracotomy pain. *J Cardiothorac Vasc Anesth.* 2005;19:786–793.

25. Lauwick S, Kim DJ, Michelagnoli G, et al. Intraoperative infusion of lidocaine reduces postoperative fentanyl requirements in patients undergoing laparoscopic cholecystectomy. *Can J Anaesth.* Nov 2008;55(11):754–760.

26. Koppert W, Weigand M. Neumann F, et al. Perioperative intravenous lidocaine has preventative effects on post-operative pain and morphine consumption after major abdominal surgery. *Anesth Analg.* 2004;98:1050–1055.

27. McCarthy GC, Megalla SA, Habib AS. Impact of intravenous lidocaine infusion on postoperative analgesia and recovery from surgery a systematic review of randomized control trials. *Drugs.* 2010;70:1149–1163.

28. Grigoras A, Lee P, Sattar F, et al. Perioperative intravenous lidocaine decreases the incidence of persistent pain after breast surgery. *Clin J Pain.* 2012;16:1312–1322.

29. Virtanen R, Savola JM, Saano V, et al. Characterization of the selectivity, specificity and potency of medetomidine as an a2-adrenoceptor agonist. *Eur J Pharmacol.* 1988;150:9–14.

30. Jaakola ML, Salonen M, Lehtinen R, et al. The analgesic action of dexmedetomidine—a novel alpha2-adrenoceptor agonist in healthy volunteers. *Pain.* 1991;46:281–285.

31. Unlugenc H, Gunduz M, Guler T, Yagmur O, Isik G. The effect of pre-anaesthetic administration of intravenous dexmedetomidine on postoperative pain in patients receiving patient-controlled morphine. *Eur J Anaesthesiol.* May 2005;22(5):386–391.

32. Blaudszun G, Lysakowski C, Ella N, et al. Effect of perioperative systemic alpha 2 on postoperative morphine consumption and pain intensity systematic review and meta analysis of RCT. *Anesthesiology.* 2012;116:1312–1322.

33. Dierking G, Duedahl TH, Rasmussen ML, et al. Effects of gabapentin on postoperative morphine consumption and pain after abdominal hysterectomy: a randomized, double-blind trial. *Acta Anaesthesiol Scand.* 2004;48:322–327.

34. Fassoulaki A, Patris K, Sarantopoulos C, et al. The analgesic effect of gabapentin and mexiletine after breast surgery for cancer. *Anesth Analg.* 2002;95:985–991.

35. Menigaux C, Adam F, Guignard B, et al. Preoperative gabapentin decreases anxiety and improves early functional recovery from knee surgery. *Anesth Analg.* 2005;100:1394–1399.

36. Fassoulaki A, Stamatakis E, Petropoulos G, et al. Gabapentin attenuates late but not acute pain after abdominal hysterectomy. *Eur J Anaesthesiol.* 2006;23:136–141.

37. Pandey CK, Singhal V, Kumar M, et al. Gabapentin provides effective postoperative analgesia whether administered pre-emptively or post-incision. *Can J Anaesth.* 2005;52:827–831.

38. Bonin RP, Orser BA, Englesakis M, et al. The prevention of chronic postsurgical pain using gabapentin pregabalin: a combined systematic review and meta analysis. *Anesth Analg.* 2012;115:428–442.

3 Perioperative Nonopioid Analgesics of Use in Pain Management for Spine Surgery

Kenneth Fomberstein, Michael Rubin,
Dipan Patel, Ivona Truszkowska,
and S. Gabriel Farkas

INTRODUCTION

Numerous factors contribute to a patient's experience of pain in the perioperative period. First and foremost, the degree of pain any practitioner might expect to encounter in this setting is directly related to the type of surgery performed, the size of the surgical incision, and the tissues that were invaded during the procedure [1]. Furthermore, there are different types of pain, whether nociceptive, neuropathic, or some combination of the two, depending on the tissue trauma involved. These factors often have implications for whether acute pain following surgery may transition into chronic pain, one that may manifest as a long-lasting and debilitating condition [2].

Spine surgery in particular is associated with some of the most intense pain in the acute postoperative setting, making the approach to treating pain crucial [3]. Adequate analgesic control is paramount in the postoperative setting as it can drastically decrease comorbidities, improve patient satisfaction, and lead to faster recovery as well as decreased hospital stays [4]. When assessing pain severity and management, it is important to consider that a patient's pain experience is complicated and that each case represents a complex individual who brings with him or her a unique set of past experiences, emotions, and internal physiology. Many factors may contribute to the overall experience of pain, for example, a history of preoperative pain, age, gender, weight, anxiety or depression, psychological distress, and even genetics [5]. Furthermore, patients requiring spine surgery often have histories of chronic pain and opioid tolerance. This can make controlling postoperative pain more challenging.

It is imperative to find the best method for controlling postoperative pain, one that maximizes comfort, helps patients recover faster, and has the least impact on healthcare expenditures.

Given the complex nature of the pain experience, as well as the various physiological mechanisms responsible for the transmission and subsequent perception of pain, there is an equally complicated approach to treating perioperative pain. The underlying goal for any treatment regimen is to maximize pain relief while minimizing adverse side effects. Although opioid analgesia is extensively used in the perioperative setting due to its high efficacy for pain relief, opioids are not the ideal choice for a treatment regimen. There is a wide dosing range for opioid requirements between patients due to differences in individual pharmacokinetics and tolerance in past use [6]. Additionally, there are numerous adverse side effects associated with opioid use. Among these unwanted effects are respiratory depression, sedation, pruritus, urinary retention, and constipation [7]. Also, there is always the fear of addiction among opioid users, particularly in patients who progress to chronic pain, which is common following spine surgery.

The concept of multimodal analgesia attempts to address the issues inherent with opioid use. It involves using different classes of medications that target specific parts of the pain transmission pathway, whether by acting centrally or peripherally [8]. By pinpointing various parts of the pathway, an added benefit from these medications arises: the tendency to have additive or synergistic effects, which in turn lowers the dosage requirements of other medications like opioids [9]. By lowering opioid requirements in the postoperative period, patients experience fewer adverse side effects while also receiving adequate analgesia [3]. This is particularly important in spine surgery, in which patients often present at the time of surgery with some degree of preexisting opioid tolerance, only compounding the challenge of prescribing adequate pain coverage [10]. Multimodal analgesia also takes into consideration the timing of drug administration. When given medication preemptively, patients are found to have an increased pain threshold, have reduced opioid requirements, and improved outcomes [11–13].

Preemptive analgesia is a treatment modality focused on reducing sensitization of peripheral and central pain pathways by initiating treatment prior to the surgical procedure. This sensitization is the result of the transmission of pain signals in response to tissue damage [14]. Preemptive analgesia can be defined as treatment that (1) is initiated prior to the start of surgery, (2) prevents the establishment of central sensitization secondary to surgical injury, and (3) prevents the establishment of central sensitization secondary to surgical and inflammatory injury [15]. Central sensitization or "wind-up" is the process through which neurons of the dorsal horn become sensitized by noxious stimuli [16]. Preemptive analgesia seeks to reduce immediate postoperative pain and prevent the development of chronic pain. Centered on the core concept of a multimodal approach to manage postoperative pain, this strategy aims to be more effective than simply initiating treatment after surgery.

Nociceptive signals are transmitted via peripheral and central neurons as a response to noxious stimuli [16]. Nociceptors are subdivided based on their location in tissues and response to different stimuli. Myelinated Aδ nociceptors produce a rapid sharp pain response and specialize in detecting mechanical and thermal injury. The unmyelinated C nociceptors mediate a delayed burning response and respond to mechanical, thermal, or chemical stimuli. The dorsal horn transmits the nociceptive signals via mediators such as aspartate, glutamate, and substance P [14]. Subsequent stimuli lead to an increased response by the somatosensory system even to painless sensations (allodynia), as well as an amplification of pain (hyperalgesia) [16]. By administering analgesics prior to the surgery and thus prior to procedure-related tissue damage, the physiological response to nociceptive transmission is reduced.

Painful stimuli that result in tissue damage lead to responses via both the central and peripheral pain pathways. Tissue damage leads to local inflammatory responses, with the release of pain-promoting substances from peripheral nerve endings as well as mediators such as substance P, prostaglandins, serotonin, bradykinin, and histamine. These mediators alter transduction and increase conduction of stimuli toward the central pathway, which impact the responsiveness of the neurons in the dorsal horn [14]. It is possible that the central sensitization may outlast the inciting stimuli that triggered the alterations. Hence, preemptive analgesia seeks to prevent the neurophysiological and biochemical consequences of a noxious stimulus rather than to initiate treatment after these consequences have already been established.

Various analgesic interventions have been investigated, including the use of nonsteroidal anti-inflammatory drugs (NSAIDs), opioids, ketamine, dextromethorphan, peripheral local anesthetics, and neuraxial analgesics. Multiple sites along the pain pathway can be targeted using a variety of interventions to provide analgesia.

The overall conclusion is that preemptive analgesia in surgical patients has not proved to confer major benefits in terms of immediate postoperative pain relief or reduced need for supplemental analgesics. Studies comparing pre- versus postincisional treatment have failed to provide conclusive evidence in support of preemptive analgesia [15]. Evaluation of clinical trials of preemptive analgesia demonstrate that it is essential to consider the ability of the intervention to prevent central sensitization, as well as the duration and intensity of perioperative pain to hide the benefits of preemptive analgesia [16]. Ultimately, multimodal approaches and optimal intraoperative analgesia are still recommended to blunt the surgical stress response and prevent central sensitization.

DEXAMETHASONE

Glucocorticoids are commonly employed to reduce inflammation that can lead to scar tissue and contribute to pain following surgery [7,17]. Although commonly considered as an adjuvant in preventing postoperative nausea and vomiting (PONV), dexamethasone has been demonstrated as a possible analgesic adjuvant. In a meta-analysis performed by De Oliveira et al., dexamethasone given at intermediate doses of 0.1–0.2 mg/kg preoperatively reduced postoperative pain and opioid consumption [18]. In another study, preoperative administration of intravenous dexamethasone 16 mg along with paracetamol, ibuprofen, and morphine significantly reduced pain during mobilization and vomiting after lumbar disk surgery, but no significant effects on pain at rest, morphine consumption, and sustained postoperative pain were demonstrated [19].

NONSELECTIVE NSAIDs

NSAIDs are medications commonly used to alleviate pain and minimize the acute inflammatory response by inhibiting the production of its key mediators, mainly prostaglandins. Most NSAIDs are nonselective competitive inhibitors of both the cyclooxygenase (COX) isoenzymes, COX-1 and COX-2. The COX-2 isoenzyme plays a main role in the production of prostaglandin synthesis. Therefore inhibition of COX-2 and prostaglandin synthesis is largely responsible for the analgesic, anti-inflammatory, and antipyretic effects of NSAIDs [20].

Pain from tissue trauma following surgery can be partially attributed to the local production of various prostaglandins and thromboxanes that contribute to the sensitization of peripheral pain receptors [21]. NSAIDs diminish the sensation of pain by inhibiting the synthesis of prostaglandins in the spinal cord and periphery. The drugs act to increase central sensitization and subsequently reduce the pain threshold at the surgical site and surrounding tissues [22].

According to a recent review, Devin et al. found fair evidence that NSAIDs not only reduce the requirements for opioid analgesia, but improve pain control when used with opioids compared to opioid analgesia used alone [3,23]. They are also known to increase patient ambulation following spine surgery [7]. At one time, spine surgeons were wary of the use of NSAIDs during spinal fusions due to its effects on bone metabolism secondary to its inhibition of osteoblast cell production; however, there has since been evidence to suggest that acute NSAID use in a postoperative setting would have little long-term effect on bone metabolism [24,25], although consumption of ketorolac greater than 120 mg/day orally for longer than 14 days has been associated with significant nonunion rates [26]. However, for patients undergoing laminectomy or discectomy, NSAIDs appear both safe and effective in reducing postoperative pain and opioid requirements. Studies have shown that adding an NSAID alongside opioids in a postoperative pain regimen reduced the daily requirements of opioids 20–30% [21]. Ketorolac is currently one of the main intravenous NSAIDs for use in acute perioperative pain. Standard dose is 30 mg for patients under 65 with normal kidney function and 15 mg for patients older than 65 with normal kidney function. Onset peaks within 10 minutes and lasts for roughly 4 hours.

COX-2 SELECTIVE INHIBITORS

Chronic inhibition of the COX-1 isoenzyme is associated with the well-known gastrointestinal adverse side effects associated with nonselective NSAIDs. However, more important is the consideration of increased risk for bleeding in the acute postoperative setting due to their antiplatelet effects [27,28]. Additional concerns with the use of nonselective NSAIDs include risk of bleeding, gastric ulceration, and renal damage.

As a result, selective COX-2 inhibitors are utilized in efforts to isolate the analgesic and anti-inflammatory effects of the COX-2 isoenzyme while simultaneously avoiding the undesirable side effects from COX-1 inhibition [7]. These medications are generally used when coagulopathy is a concern. Reuben et al. shows that celecoxib given preemptively 1 hour before induction and then again postoperatively every 12 hours for 5 days will see significant reduction in opioid requirements and pain scores following spinal fusion surgery [25]. For general NSAID dosing guidelines, see Table 3.1.

Table 3.1 NSAID dosing and characteristics

Medication	Dose	Facts + Indications	Side effects + Contraindications
Ketorolac	15–30 mg (IV/PO)	Short-term acute pain	Advanced renal disease; coagulopathy
Ibuprofen	300–800 mg (IV/PO)	Moderate–severe pain, antipyretic	Advanced renal disease (CrCl < 30 mL/min)
Diclofenac	50–100 mg (IV/PO)	Postop pain (orthopedic, gynecologic, oral)	Potential increase in cardiovascular thrombotic events (MI, stroke), hypertension; pain treatment following CABG surgery
Naproxen	250–500 mg (PO)	CYP drug interactions; acute pain treatment, fever, osteoarthritis	Potential increase in cardiovascular thrombotic events (MI, stroke), hypertension; pain treatment following CABG surgery
Celecoxib	200–400 mg (PO)	Selective COX-2	Sulfonamide allergy
Parecoxib	20–40 mg (IV)	Prodrug; selective COX-2; short-term pain treatment	Sulfonamide allergy

References 26–28.

CABG, coronary artery bypass graft surgery; MI, myocardial infarction.

ACETAMINOPHEN

Acetaminophen, when given intravenously, is now well-recognized as a safe, effective, and affordable drug therapy for treating postoperative pain. Also known as paracetamol, it has become a staple for pain control whether given intraoperatively or postoperatively due to its rapid onset of action and ability to be given parenterally. It is generally given to patients who are unable to consume NSAIDs due to the adverse side-effect profile of this medication class [7]. The mechanism of action for acetaminophen is not fully understood. It is believed that one mechanism may involve the inhibition of prostaglandin synthesis both centrally and peripherally [7]. Others suggest a role in activating cannabinoid receptors, in the inhibition of descending serotonergic pathways, and a potential role in the modulation of substance P [26]. Though largely speculative, it is established that acetaminophen is not considered in the same class as NSAIDs due to its lack of anti-inflammatory properties.

As a well-established perioperative analgesic, acetaminophen has largely been looked at for its potential to reduce the burden of opioid requirements in the postoperative period. Notably, acetaminophen is generally considered to be insufficient when used as a sole analgesic for spine surgery. Yilmaz et al. assessed the effects of 1 g of acetaminophen given intravenously with 1.5 mg/kg of tramadol and determined that acetaminophen is not as effective when given alone [29]. Shahid et al. compared intravenous acetaminophen to tramadol and determined that acetaminophen is a safer choice in the postoperative period, producing less postop nausea and vomiting and reducing the length of hospital stay [30].

As acetaminophen is primarily metabolized in the liver via conjugation with glucuronide and sulfate and then oxidized by cytochrome P450 (CYP450) enzymes, it should be used cautiously in patients with hepatic impairment [26]. In such scenarios, acetaminophen should be limited to 2 g/day in patients with mild to moderate hepatic impairment [31]. In severe impairment, acetaminophen should be avoided. Though evidence of acetaminophen therapy in spine surgery is limited, it is generally accepted that a 1 g intravenous dose given perioperatively is an effective adjunct analgesic, may reduce opioid requirements, and is well tolerated in adults [7]. The drug can be given intraoperatively or postoperatively and is generally infused over a 15-minute period. The maximum dose in 24 hours is 4 g; however, it is important to consider whether the patient is already taking a narcotic that contains acetaminophen, such as Percocet, when determining a dosing schedule [32].

α_2 ADRENERGIC AGONISTS

The first α2 adrenergic receptor agonists were synthesized in the 1960s and were initially used for nasal decongestion. Early use of clonidine soon became associated with unwanted side effects such as sedation and cardiovascular depression [33]. The development of dexmedetomidine first stems from its use by veterinarians who used xylazine—a clonidine analogue—and detomidine for analgesia and sedation. After an initial evaluation of intubated ICU patients, the US Food and Drug Administration (FDA) approved intravenous dexmedetomidine for use as a short term (<24 hours) sedative and in diagnostic and therapeutic procedures under monitored anesthesia care (MAC) [34].

There are three α_2 subtypes—a, b, and c—all of which have unique physiological response and are distributed broadly in the central nervous system (CNS) and periphery. When presynaptic receptors are stimulated, they reduce norepinephrine release; when postsynaptic receptors are activated, they hyperpolarize neuronal membranes. In the spinal cord, α_2 receptors are located in the dorsal horn, and, when stimulated, they inhibit nociceptive signal transmission. In the periphery, they are located on vascular smooth muscle cells and cause vasoconstriction when activated. Analgesic effect stems from activation of the α_2 receptor subtype c located in the spinal cord through attenuation of nociceptive signal transmission to brain centers [35].

Dexmedetomidine is a highly selective α_2 receptor agonist that works by activating the α_2 adrenergic receptors in the CNS located in locus ceruleus [36]. It is an active S-enantiomer of medetomidine, a water-soluble compound. Compared to clonidine, dexmedetomidine is more specific and selective for α_2 receptors and has a shorter half-life [35]. Dexmedetomidine causes a dose-dependent decrease in arterial blood pressure and heart rate likely due to the associated decrease in norepinephrine levels [37].

Dexmedetomidine undergoes almost complete biotransformation via glucuronidation and CYP450-mediated metabolism with very little unchanged primary drug in the urine and feces; the terminal elimination half-life is approximately 2 hours. It should be used with caution in patients with renal impairment (CrCl <30 mL/

h), and, since the mean clearance values are lower in patients with hepatic impairment, dosing should be adjusted accordingly.

When choosing an appropriate anesthetic plan for both spine or intracranial neurosurgery, the anesthetic agent of choice should possess multiple beneficial characteristics including the ability to maintain hemodynamic stability throughout the operative period, comply with neurophysiological monitoring, and, in the case of spinal surgery, increase perfusion to the spinal cord [35]. The benefits of dexmedetomidine include analgesia, anxiolysis, sedation, and sympatholysis without causing respiratory depression [38]. These are all characteristics that make α_2 agonists an attractive adjuvant to neuroanesthesia and critical care [39]. Dexmedetomidine produces similar preoperative sedation and anxiolysis in comparison to midazolam but has an increased incidence of intraoperative hypotension and bradycardia, especially when given as a bolus [34]. Currently, dexmedetomidine is used as an adjuvant to propofol and remifentanil during spine surgery due to its ability to blunt the hemodynamic response to intubation and its ability to decrease both opioid and volatile agent requirements during surgery. Adverse effects of α_2 agonists include hypertension, hypotension, bradycardia, decreased cardiac output, and increases in systemic and pulmonary vascular resistance [39]. The recommended dose is 1 μg/kg loading dose over 10 minutes followed by a maintenance infusion of 0.2–0.7 μg/kg/h [40].

According to Hwang et al., compared to remifentanil as a propofol adjuvant during neurological surgery, dexmedetomidine led to better postoperative pain control after posterior lumbar instrumentation fusion, exemplified by less patient-controlled epidural analgesia (PCEA) use by patients postoperatively [41]. A study performed by Bekker et al. examined the effect of dexmedetomidine infusion on the stress response of major spinal surgery as well as the quality of recovery of the patients. The results showed that dexmedetomidine use led to lower cortisol and interleukin-10 (IL-10) levels immediately after surgery, which could potentially lead to better overall outcomes for patients, although there was no difference in inflammatory response [42]. Dexmedetomidine is a versatile drug that can be used during spine surgery, neuraxial anesthesia, regional anesthesia, ICU sedation, and MAC procedures. It provides good perioperative hemodynamic stability with decreased opioid requirements, making it a great addition to a short list of currently available sedatives [37].

GABAPENTINOIDS

The gabapentinoids have traditionally been used as anticonvulsants and in the treatment of chronic neuropathic pain. In recent years, however, growing evidence has supported their use as preemptive anxiolytics, in the treatment of postoperative pain, and in the prevention of chronic pain following surgery [43]. As analogues of the inhibitory neurotransmitter, γ-aminobutyric acid (GABA), these agents principally exert their effect by binding to the α2δ subunits of voltage-dependent calcium ion channels and inhibiting the influx of calcium into neurons. The result is a reduction in the release of excitatory neurotransmitters from afferent nerve fibers and a blunting of the normal hyperalgesic state following tissue trauma from surgery [44,45].

Numerous work has been done assessing the role of gabapentinoids in their role in postoperative analgesia and reducing opioid requirements. Rivkin et al. looked at outcomes following lumbar discectomy and showed evidence that the administration of pregabalin diminishes the perception of pain and results in increased functional outcome 3 months following the procedure [26]. Khurana et al. compared the effects of oral gabapentinoids to control on the duration of postoperative pain when given preemptively. In this case, evidence showed that the group receiving pregabalin 150 mg had the greatest reduction in total duration of analgesia, followed by the group receiving gabapentin 600 mg, followed by the control [46]. Pregabalin has a greater affinity for the α2δ calcium channel than does gabapentin, suggesting a mechanism for its greater role in pain reduction following surgery [26].

There is variability in agreement about a standard regimen for treating perioperative pain with gabapentinoids. Some suggest that the use of pregabalin doses greater than 300 mg/day may significantly reduce opioid requirements in the acute postoperative period. Similarly, high doses of gabapentin, 300–900 mg/day, may also result in diminished opioid requirements [26,47]. Others suggest one might expect to find as great as an 80% reduction in the need for opioids in the postoperative period following a single preemptive dose of greater than 1 g of gabapentin [48]. A large randomized controlled trial assessed postoperative pain following lumbar laminectomy. Results suggest that gabapentin 900 or 1200 mg, whether given preemptively or intraoperatively, are effective doses for managing postoperative pain (Table 3.2) [49].

The general consensus appears to be that gabapentinoids have the greatest effect when given preemptively and when continued in the immediate postoperative period [26]. Although there is variability in what constitutes an effective dose and frequency for reduced opioid requirements, one must also consider the adverse side effects associated with higher dosages of these drugs. Side effects for these medications tend to occur at higher doses (>900 mg gabapentin, >300 mg pregabalin) and include dizziness, nausea, and somnolence. Evidence shows that gabapentinoids may prove efficacious in a number of spine surgeries, including discectomies, laminectomies, and fusions [26,50–58].

NMDA ANTAGONISTS (KETAMINE, DEXTROMETHORPHAN)

The N-methyl-D-aspartate NMDA receptor plays a central role in the regulation of processes underlying memory, learning, and neuroplasticity as well as a key role in the mechanisms underlying pain sensitization. When antagonized, flow through the ionotropic channel is diminished, underlying the profound clinical effects and analgesic properties of ketamine (see Box 3.1) [59].

Ketamine is a noncompetitive NMDA antagonist that prevents nociceptive pathway sensitization within the CNS [3]. The exact mechanism underlying its effect is complicated but involves multiple pathways including central and peripheral opiate receptors (μ, δ, and κ receptors) as well as numerous other receptors involved in neurotransmission [26]. When antagonized, there is a decrease in the presynaptic release of glutamate and decreased activation of NDMA receptors by glutamate. Ketamine is a derivative of phencyclidine and is highly lipid soluble, which explains its rapid onset of action. The form available in the United States is composed of a racemic mixture of its two stereoisomers (S(+) the more potent form and R(−) isomer) [36].

Table 3.2 Recommended analgesic doses for reduced postoperative pain

Medication	Dose	Setting	Side effects
Dexamethasone	0.1–0.2 mg/kg (IV) or 8–16 mg	Preop; intraop	Hyperglycemia (rare)
Ketorolac	15–30 mg (IV)	Intraop	Bleeding, gastric ulceration/bleed, renal damage
Celecoxib	200–400 mg (PO)	Preop; postop	Sulfonamide allergy
Acetaminophen	1g (IV) (max 4g/day)	Preop; intraop; postop	GI upset, sweating, hepatotoxicity
Clonidine	0.15–0.30 (IV)	Preop; intraop; postop	Hypotension, bradycardia
Dexmedetomidine	0.5–1 mcg/kg (IV) bolus *Add on:* 0.2–0.7 µg/kg/h	Preop; intraop; postop	Hypotension, bradycardia
Pregabalin	300–1,200 mg (PO)	Preop; postop	Dizziness, nausea, somnolence
Gabapentin	75–300 mg (PO)	Preop; postop	Dizziness, nausea, drowsiness
Ketamine	0.5–1 mg/kg (IV)*Add on: 2–10 µg/kg/min*	Intraop	Hypertension, hallucinations, nystagmusDysphoria, sedation, nausea
Dextromethorphan	40–120 mg (IV)	Preop; intraop	Hypertension
Magnesium	30–50 mg/kg (IV) bolus *Add on: 8–15 mg/kg/h*	Preop; intraop	Drowsiness, bradycardia, prolonged neuromuscular blockade
Esmolol	0.5 mg/kg (IV)*Add on: 0.05 mg/kg/min*	Intraop	Bradycardia, hypotension
Lidocaine	1.5–2 mg/kg (IV) bolus *Add on: 1.5–3 mg/kg/hr*	Intraop	Arrhythmias, allergy, residual motor weakness
Caffeine	100 mg (PO)	Postop	Headache, tachycardia

References 9, 26, 78, 94.

Traditionally, ketamine has been used sparingly as an anesthetic due to its propensity for causing psychomimetic side effects including hallucinations and vivid sensory sensations. Its use is also associated with dysphoria, sedation, diplopia, salivation, and nausea [7,60]. In addition to the well-known psychomimetic effects of ketamine, there are well-known cardiovascular and cerebral effects. These include an increase in systemic blood pressure, heart rate, and systemic vascular resistance. Ketamine also causes cerebral vasodilation resulting in increased cerebral blood flow and an increase

Box 3.1 NMDA Receptor Antagonists

Ketamine

- Associated with increase in systemic BP, HR, SVR, and cerebral vasodilation
- Unwanted side effects: hallucinations, vivid sensory sensations, dysphoria, sedation, diplopia, salivation, and nausea
- Good option in chronic pain patients with established opioid tolerance
- *Dosing: 0.5–1 mg/kg (intravenous) followed by 2–10 µg/kg/min*

Dextromethorphan

- Noncompetitive antagonism of NMDA receptors located in the dorsal horn
- Reduces excitatory transmission of primary afferents along spinothalamic tract
- Similar dissociative properties as ketamine, but less potent
- Very low incidence of side effects and a high safety profile
- *Dosing: 40–120 mg (IV)*

Magnesium (Mg)

- Analgesic effects from noncompetitive NMDA receptor antagonism and repletion of Mg levels
- Mg use may prolong the neuromuscular blockade
- Mg toxicity occurs at serum concentrations of 2.5–5 mmol/L
- *Dosing: 30–50 mg/kg (IV) followed by 8–15 mg/kg/h*

References 9, 26, 51, 54, 55, 57, 58, 63, 68, 71, 74.

in cerebral oxygen consumption [36]. Notably, however, there is no concern for respiratory depression with the use of this agent.

One of the clear benefits of ketamine is its ability to produce significant analgesia and its clear role in a multimodal pain management approach. When given preemptively, there is evidence that ketamine is able to prevent the development of acute and chronic pain due to its inherent ability to interfere with neuronal circuitry [26]. Though it is generally agreed upon to be an effective analgesic, there is conflicting data with respect to the analgesic properties of ketamine as well as its ability to lower opioid requirements in patients undergoing spinal surgery. One potential reason for variability within the evidence likely involves the differences in study size, dose quantity, frequency, and route of ketamine administration used in different studies [26].

Aveline et al. assessed pain scores and narcotic dependency following lumbar microdiscectomy. The results suggested that an adjunct 0.15 mg/kg dose of ketamine along with morphine was superior at reducing pain scores and opioid requirements by 57% up to 24 hours postoperatively compared to morphine alone [61]. Subramaniam et al. reviewed the effectiveness of ketamine adjunct when used as a single intravenous dose, as a continuous infusion, as patient-controlled analgesia, and in epidural preparations. They found that when used as a one-time dose and as a continuous infusion ketamine can produce significant reductions in postoperative opioid requirements [62].

Another important consideration before utilizing ketamine for its analgesic properties is whether the patient is opioid-naïve or not. Patients with chronic pain who undergo surgery need to be managed carefully due to the increased risk of inadequate postoperative pain management [60]. Excessive pain in the postoperative setting can lead to adverse health complications as well as an increased hospital stay; therefore, there are many implications for effectively managing postoperative pain in such susceptible patients.

NMDA receptors contribute to opioid tolerance and the development of hyperalgesia [7]. This fact underlies the belief that agents like ketamine are able to reverse opioid tolerance in patients known to be chronic opioid users. In an effort to address the role of ketamine in patients with chronic pain, Loftus et al. assessed the use of intraoperative ketamine and its effect on the duration and need for opioids in the acute postoperative setting in patients undergoing elective lumbar back surgery with known chronic back pain [60]. They utilized 0.5 mg/kg intravenous ketamine on induction and 10 μg/kg/min for continuous maintenance infusion compared to a matched saline control group. In the postoperative setting, they assessed the need for morphine after 48 hours and found that the ketamine group not only had lower pain intensity scores but also required less postoperative opioid analgesic after 48 hours. They demonstrated they were able to reduce opiate consumption by nearly 37% in chronic pain patients with an established opiate dependency [60].

Though there is variability in recommended doses, it is believed that subanalgesic doses of ketamine (3–5 mg/kg/min), both intraoperatively or in the early postoperative period, can effectively manage acute pain and decrease the need for opioids in the postoperative period [63].

DEXTROMETHORPHAN

Dextromethorphan is another NMDA antagonist that has been assessed for its role as an analgesic and its ability to reduce opioid requirements in the postoperative setting. It has been suggested to effectively contribute to the multimodal approach to pain and improve the patient experience postoperatively [64]. One of the benefits of using dextromethorphan is due to its ability to diminish acute postoperative pain without the unwanted side effects associated with ketamine [65].

Dextromethorphan, a codeine analogue, was initially synthesized by Hoffmann-la Roche in 1954 as an antitussive agent but has since been shown to have analgesic properties as well. Dextromethorphan modulates pain sensation via noncompetitive antagonism of NMDA receptors located in the dorsal horn of the spinal column, the area responsible for relaying, modulating, and transmitting pain [66]. Clinical trials involving the use of dextromethorphan as an analgesic adjunct in spine surgery are sparse, but studies have shown its effectiveness in other perioperative settings. A meta-analyses of 21 published trials showed that preoperative administration of dextromethorphan significantly decreased pain and opioid use in the 24–48 hour postoperative period [67].

Dextromethorphan, the main ingredient in most cough medications, works as an antitussive by increasing the cough threshold by acting at the level of the medulla oblongata [68]. The anti-nociceptive properties of dextromethorphan stem from its dissociative properties, similar in action to ketamine and phencyclidine, but less potent. It has equal antitussive effects as codeine but does not possess addictive properties at normal therapeutic doses. Dextromethorphan modulates pain sensation by reducing the excitatory transmission of the primary afferent pathways along the spinothalamic tract. This process occurs in the dorsal horn of the spinal cord, where dextromethorphan blocks NMDA receptors, reducing the threshold for pain transmission via the Aδ and sensory C fibers [68]. Dextromethorphan is believed to act as a preemptive analgesic by quelling NMDA-mediated calcium current and subsequent modulation of nociception in spinal pain fiber and the CNS. This in turn prevents a pain phenomenon known as "wind-up" that results in amplified subsequent responses to painful stimuli and poorer responses to opioids [67].

The major metabolite of dextromethorphan, dextrorphan, reaches peak plasma concentrations at 1.6–1.7 hours following ingestion. Its metabolites undergo renal elimination, with less than 0.1% of the drug being eliminated in the feces; the half-life of the parent compound is approximately 2–4 hours in individuals with normal metabolism. Due to dextromethorphan's metabolism by cytochrome CYP2D6, any inhibitors of that enzymatic pathway, including monoamine oxidase inhibitors (MAOIs), fluoxetine, paroxetine, and haloperidol, all increase dextromethorphan levels [68].

There is variability in the effectiveness of dextromethorphan as an effective analgesic, and there has been minimal evidence to support its use specifically following spine surgery. Choi et al. failed to show any benefit following the addition of dextromethorphan when given 60 mg orally 1 hour preoperatively then again 6 and 12 hours postoperatively [65]. However, Ilkjaer et al. showed that dextromethorphan when given 150 mg orally could reduce opioid requirements in the acute postoperative setting following abdominal hysterectomy but did not provide prolonged benefits with time [69].

If dextromethorphan is administered at higher doses (35–45 mg) than typically prescribed for treatment of cough, it may be useful in the management of pain in cancer patients. Dextromethorphan is rapidly absorbed by the GI tract; it has an onset time of around 15–30 minutes and a duration of action around 5–6 hours [68]. Dextromethorphan is not a direct antinociceptive drug, but a noncompetitive NMDA receptor antagonist that may suppress central sensitization of the dorsal horn neurons in the spinal cord triggered by nociceptive afferent input from the periphery. The general consensus seems to agree that dextromethorphan reduces the wind-up phenomenon, thus increasing the threshold of subsequent painful stimuli. Patients undergoing spine surgery often have a history of chronic pain which is acutely exacerbated by therapeutic surgery, and dextromethorphan has the potential to blunt this nociceptive surge.

Dextromethorphan administered preoperatively to tonsillectomy patients showed to be effective in reducing postop pain as well as a decreased pain score 7 days postop [70]. According to a double-blind randomized control trial, patients undergoing orthopedic malignancy surgeries who received 60 or 90 mg of dextromethorphan preoperatively and then 2 consecutive days postop, consumed 30–50% less of their PCEA compared to the control group, and they also rated their postop pain to be at least half of what their control group did, although time to ambulation and discharge was unchanged [71]. All studies reviewed demonstrated that dextromethorphan has a very low incidence of side effects and a high safety profile, making it an ideal perioperative analgesic for spine surgery. Appropriate dosing and timing of administration should be left to the clinical judgment of the anesthesia provider.

MAGNESIUM

Magnesium is a cation that plays an important role in a number of physiologic processes, whether it be neurotransmission and signaling, the activation of enzymes, or the regulation of vasomotor tone [72]. Over the past few decades, magnesium has been used increasingly clinically, and, in 1996, it was used in the first randomized clinical trial to improve postoperative analgesia [73]. Although it is not considered a primary analgesic, magnesium is used as an adjuvant to enhance the actions of other analgesics [74], much like caffeine is used to enhance the effects of ibuprofen (see Caffeine section).

While the mechanism of action for magnesium as an analgesic adjuvant is not completely understood, there is much that is known about its physiological effects. For one, magnesium is a noncompetitive NMDA receptor antagonist, blocking glutamate and aspartate from binding to the receptor, thereby preventing the entry of extracellular calcium into the cell [75]. The net result of this is magnesium's ability to produce meaningful clinical effects such as bronchodilation, vasodilation, uterine relaxation (explaining its role in the treatment of eclampsia), and postoperative analgesia [76]. NMDA receptors are found in the dorsal horn of the spinal cord, an area known to be important in the transmission of pain signals [77]. By blocking these receptors, magnesium is able to attenuate central sensitization and help blunt some of the noxious stimuli following surgical trauma.

One of the implications for using magnesium to enhance perioperative pain control is related to episodes of hypomagnesemia that have been known to occur following surgery [78]. The normal physiologic range of magnesium is 0.7–1.1 mmol/L or 1.4–2.2 mEq/L, and it has been reported that the incidence of hypomagnesemia is as high as 71% following cardiac surgery [78]. There are a number of consequences to hypomagnesemia in the perioperative setting, including but not limited to CNS hyperexcitability, increased neuromediators, and an increase in the production of inflammatory mediators [79]. As a result, it appears that the analgesic effects of perioperative dosing of magnesium may be a combination of both NMDA receptor antagonism and the repletion of magnesium levels.

The role of magnesium as a perioperative analgesia adjuvant has since been investigated by a number of authors. A recent meta-analysis by Guo et al. was performed to determine the efficacy and safety of magnesium on postoperative pain [80]. Twenty-seven randomized control trials with more than 1,500 participants were studied and evaluated. The analysis primarily looked at pain scores and total analgesic consumption grouped by the type of surgery. They found evidence that magnesium significantly lowered pain scores at rest up to 24 hours after the surgery and significantly reduced total analgesic use. Notably, this analysis did not include participants having undergone spine surgery.

Levaux et al. investigated the effects of magnesium on pain and overall patient comfort following lumbar surgery [77]. Participants either received an intraoperative infusion of 50 mg/kg of magnesium or an equivalent volume of saline. Investigators found that participants in the magnesium group had a reduction in opioid requirements and pain scores in the postoperative period. They also found that these participants had relatively better sleep in the first 24 hours and overall greater satisfaction compared to participants who received saline controls. Jabbour et al. performed a prospective randomized control trial that assessed the effects of ketamine combined with magnesium on postoperative opioid requirements after scoliosis surgery [81]. Twenty-five patients received an intravenous bolus of ketamine 0.2 mg/kg and magnesium 50 mg/kg, followed by 0.15 mg/kg/h and 8 mg/kg/h infusions respectively compared to matched controls who received saline instead of magnesium. After 48 hours in the postoperative period, the magnesium group had a reduction in opioid consumption, better pain scores, and fewer side effects compared to the control.

There is a wide variation in what is considered an ideal or standard dose of magnesium for significant analgesic effect. It appears that a 50 mg/kg intravenous bolus may have beneficial clinical effects. Yet there are some important considerations to make when using magnesium for pain management. Magnesium toxicity is generally considered to occur at a serum concentrations of 2.5–5 mmol/L [82]. Though rare, hypermagnesemia can have deleterious effects such as sedation, diarrhea, respiratory depression, and prolongation of the neuromuscular blockade [83]. Gupta et al. have reported that 30 mg/kg bolus followed by 10 mg/kg/h infusion of magnesium significantly prolonged the neuromuscular block following 0.5 mg/kg of rocuronium bromide [84]. This could be due to magnesium's ability to reduce the release of acetylcholine in the neuromuscular junction.

β-BLOCKADE (ESMOLOL)

Esmolol is a cardioselective, fast-acting β-blocker that has been used to blunt the sympathetic response to intubation and sensory stimuli from surgery in efforts to diminish the effects of catecholamines produced during the stress response. The use of β-blockers, particularly esmolol, is popular not only due to its rapid clinical onset, but also due to its ability to reduce perioperative adverse events such as cardiovascular complications that may arise due to hemodynamic instability in some susceptible patients [9]. Due to its reliable onset of action, short half-life, and, perhaps most importantly, its clinically underutilized opioid-sparing effects, esmolol may prove to be an important adjunct in the multimodal model of perioperative pain management following spine surgery [85].

Though the study of its use following spine surgery is limited, evidence suggests that an intraoperative infusion of esmolol may dramatically lower opioid requirements in the postoperative period. Collard et al. compared whether intraoperative dosing of esmolol, fentanyl, and remifentanil would reduce opioid requirements in the postoperative period [86]. One study group received an initial 1 mg/kg of esmolol, followed by a continuous infusion of 5–15 µg/kg/min. The second group received an initial 1 µg/kg of fentanyl, followed by a 50 µg bolus every 30 minutes. The third group received an initial 1 µg/kg of remifentanil followed by a continuous infusion of 0.1–0.5 µg/kg/min. At the conclusion of the study, they found that the intraoperative infusion of esmolol resulted in a significant reduction in postoperative opioid requirements, reduced postoperative PONV prophylaxis, and an earlier discharge compared to the groups in which esmolol was not administered [86].

In a second study, Bhawna et al. compared the effects of 0.5 mg/kg esmolol followed by a 0.5 mg/kg/min infusion with a control group receiving an equivalent volume of saline on postoperative pain and postoperative opioid requirements. They found that esmolol was successfully able to decrease postoperative pain compared to the control confusion and that postoperative morphine consumption was also reduced [87]. Shukla et al. similarly sought to assess whether esmolol could reduce postoperative opioid requirements. Their study group received esmolol 0.5 mg/kg followed by an infusion of 0.05 mg/kg/min compared to an equivalent volume of normal saline. By the end of the study, they successfully determined that the group receiving esmolol had a significantly lower incidence of postoperative pain as well as a reduced opioid requirement. They also found that the esmolol group experienced a shorter hospital course compared to the control group [88]. In addition to the opioid-sparing effects, studies have found intraoperative β-blockers to have additional benefit and be associated with decreased anesthetic requirement, PONV anaphylaxis, and hospital stay [86,89,90].

There is clear evidence that intraoperative esmolol has a beneficial effect on postoperative opioid requirements, as well as its other beneficial side-effect profiles previously mentioned; however, little research has shed light on the role of esmolol in spine surgery. Furthermore, the mechanism of action behind the opioid-sparing effects of esmolol is not fully understood, particularly if the effect is a result of central or peripheral action [85]. There has been speculation that esmolol may modulate G-protein coupled receptors involved in the pain pathway thereby producing its central analgesic effect [88], as well as speculation that the blunted cardiovascular response from esmolol may subsequently lower liver metabolism and its metabolism of opioids [91]. More work must be done, particularly in the context of spine surgery, to elucidate the true mechanism behind the opioid-sparing effects of esmolol.

LIDOCAINE

It has been determined that intravenous lidocaine infusion has analgesic properties, making it an additional agent that can successfully contribute to the multimodal model of postoperative pain management [9]. It is a local anesthetic that blocks voltage-gated sodium channels and can be infused to help prevent inflammatory, neuropathic, or hyperalgesic pain [92]. With a very short half-life (1.5 hours after bolus injection or infusions lasting up to 12 hours) and a good safety profile, it has become a common anesthetic for continuous intravenous administration [93,94].

A proposed mechanism of action of systemic lidocaine as an analgesic stems from its ability to inhibit spontaneous nerve impulses in peripheral nerves that sustain surgical trauma and to inhibit the dorsal root ganglions proximal to the damaged nerves [95]. There are additional proposed mechanisms that account for its anti-inflammatory and anti-hyperalgesic effects, but those will not be discussed here [96,97].

In one study assessing the effects of lidocaine following spine surgery, Kim et al. demonstrated that intraoperative intravenous infusion of lidocaine significantly reduced postoperative pain for up to 48 hours and reduced opioid consumption up to 24 hours in patients undergoing lumbar microdiscectomy [98]. The study group was given an intravenous bolus injection of 1.5 mg/kg lidocaine followed by a continuous infusion of 2 mg/kg/h, whereas the control received an equivalent volume of normal saline. Farag et al. also assessed the effects of perioperative intravenous lidocaine on pain reduction, opioid requirements in the first 48 hours, and quality of life following spine surgery [99]. They randomized 116 participants into a study group that received intravenous lidocaine 2 mg/kg/h at induction through up to 8 hours after recovery in the PACU versus a placebo group that received a similar equivalent of saline. The group receiving lidocaine had a significantly better reduction in pain scores as well as a trend for lower opioid requirements; however, there was not a significant reduction in morphine dosing. There was also no significant difference in PONV. Despite these findings, there is still implications for lidocaine use in the perioperative setting as an intervention that may contribute to improvement in pain scores and overall hospital course.

In a Kranke et al. review of continuous intravenous perioperative lidocaine infusion, the effects of lidocaine on pain reduction, opioid requirements, PONV, and length of hospital stay was assessed in more than 1,200 cases [93]. They found that, following intravenous lidocaine infusion, pain relief was maximized in the first 4 hours following surgery; however, pain after 48 hours was not significantly reduced. They also determined that those who received lidocaine experienced less PONV, likely secondary to an accompanying reduction in opioid requirements. Finally, in a number of the studies that were reviewed, they determined that participants experienced a reduction in the total length of stay after using lidocaine infusion [93]. Notably, the data from the review of these studies were acquired from procedures other than spine surgeries.

The ideal dose to maximize the analgesic properties of lidocaine is to give an intravenous bolus of 100 mg or 1.5–2 mg/kg, followed by a continuous infusion of 1.5–3 mg/kg/h [9]. One safety concern to keep in mind when utilizing intravenous lidocaine is in patients with hepatic or renal insufficiency. As this is the primary route for the drug's elimination, impairment of these systems could result in dangerous accumulation of lidocaine. In these cases, another perioperative pain regimen should be considered [93].

CAFFEINE

Caffeine is a naturally occurring compound found in plants, and it has a long history of human consumption in various forms. It is almost completely absorbed in the GI tract, and, owing to its lipophilicity, it is rapidly absorbed in the brain within 6–8 minutes [100]. Due to its rapid absorption and distribution, it has become known as an adjuvant painkiller, most commonly sold over-the-counter to treat migraine headaches [101]. It is commonly combined with a second agent, such as ibuprofen, as the two drugs will exhibit an additive effect when compared to using either drug alone [102]. This concept has been applied clinically to treat acute pain in the postoperative period. By adding caffeine to analgesics, it may be possible to achieve better pain management, possibly reduce postoperative opioid requirements, and improve postoperative recovery and outcomes.

Derry et al. conducted a review of four randomized, double-blind studies assessing the effects of caffeine combined with oral ibuprofen on acute postoperative pain [103]. There were 334 total participants across the four studies. There was evidence that ibuprofen 200 mg taken with caffeine 100 mg could produce the best reduction in moderate to severe postoperative pain in 59% of participants compared to 11% of participants taking placebo alone. Although there is no commonly prescribed formulation that contains ibuprofen 200 mg + caffeine 100 mg, the authors concluded that this regimen could be sufficiently met with a single 200 mg ibuprofen tablet combined with a strong cup of coffee. In a Cochrane review, there was evidence for an increased

---

Box 3.2 Analgesics that Can Be Given Orally

Celecoxib

- COX-2 selective inhibitor; isolates analgesic + anti-inflammatory effects while avoiding undesirable side effects from COX-1 inhibition
- Used when coagulopathy is a concern
- If given preemptively 1 hour before induction and again postoperatively every 12 hours for 5 days, may see significant reduction in opioid requirements
- *Dosing: 200–400 mg (PO)*

Gabapentinoids

- Inhibits voltage-dependent Ca^{++} channels causing decreased release of excitatory neurotransmitters from afferent nerve fibers → blunting hyperalgesic state following surgery
- Pregabalin has greater affinity for α2δ Ca^{++} channels than gabapentin; may have greater role in pain reduction following surgery
- Greatest effect seen when given preemptively and continued in immediate postop period
- Side effects (doses >900 mg gabapentin, >300 mg pregabalin): dizziness, nausea, and somnolence
- *Dosing: Pregabalin 300–1,200 mg (PO); gabapentin 75–300 mg (PO)*

Caffeine

- Adjuvant analgesic, not a primary analgesic

References 9, 17, 22, 23, 45, 46, 90, 93, 94.

---

number of participants experiencing pain relief when given 100 mg caffeine compared to a standard dose of paracetamol and ibuprofen alone [104].

Little is known about the benefits of caffeine in modulating pain following spine surgery. Furthermore, the mechanism of action for how caffeine may contribute as an analgesic is not well understood. It is believed to have some role as a competitive antagonist of adenosine receptors. [105] (For a summary of analgesics that can be administered orally, see Box 3.2.)

CAPSAICIN

Capsaicin is an alkaloid derived from chili peppers and is used as a topical treatment, with concentrations ranging from as low as 0.025% patches to as high as 8% creams [106]. It causes activation of the TRPV1 channel, a thermoreceptor, triggering release of neuropeptides in the nerve terminal of C and Aδ fibers [107]. This includes, but is not limited to, substance P. Depletion of neurotransmitters on these nociceptive fibers leads to decrease in conducted pain signals [108].

Capsaicin is FDA approved for postherpetic neuralgia, but it has also been used as treatment for HIV neuropathy, diabetic neuropathy, osteoarthritis, rheumatic arthritis, itching, psoriasis, cluster headache, and migraines [109,110]. In one study, capsaicin coadministration with topical amitriptyline led to prolonged cutaneous analgesia in rat sciatic nerve compared to amitriptyline alone [111]. It has also been studied in postsurgical pain in both topical and injectable forms. Instillation into the wound after total knee arthroplasty leads to an opioid-sparing effect, earlier gains in active range of motion, and higher patient satisfaction [112,113]. Finally, capsaicin has been shown to hasten recovery from ileus after abdominal surgery with intraperitoneal pretreatment [114].

Extensive training and precautions must be taken with the high-concentration treatment, which may only be administered by a trained clinician, with significant debilitating side effects in case of contamination [106]. This lack of qualified individuals and lack of awareness of availability may be the cause for the current lack of utilization of capsaicin. It is clear, however, that this adjunct should be beneficial to reduce pain and opioid burden if employed postoperatively.

REFERENCES

1. Power I. Recent advances in postoperative pain therapy. *Br J Anaesth.* 2005;95(1):43–51.

2. Corke P. Postoperative pain management. *Aust Prescr.* 2013;36:202–205.

3. Devin CJ, McGirt MJ. Best evidence in multimodal pain management in spine surgery and means of assessing postoperative pain and functional outcomes. *J Clin Neurosci.* 2015;22(6):930–938.

4. Ceyhan D, Güleç MS. Is postoperative pain only a nociceptive pain? [in Turkish]. *Agri.* 2010;22(2):47–52.

5. Sommer M, de Rijke JM, van Kleef M, et al. Predictors of acute postoperative pain after elective surgery. *Clin J Pain.* 2010;26(2):87–94.

6. Fung D Postoperative pain. In: *The Pain Management Handbook*, Gershwin ME, Hamilton ME, eds. Totowa, NJ: Springer Science & Business Media; 1998:239–259.

7. Bajwa SJ, Haldar R. Pain management following spinal surgeries: an appraisal of the available options. *J Craniovertebr Junction Spine.* 2015;6(3):105–110.

8. Lee BH, Park JO, Suk KS, et al. Pre-emptive and multi-modal perioperative pain management may improve quality of life in patients undergoing spinal surgery. *Pain Physician.* 2013;16(3):E217–E226.

9. Carli F, Baldini G. Perioperative pain management & enhanced outcomes. In: Butterworth JF, Mackey DC, Wasnick JD, eds. *Morgan & Mikhail's Clinical Anesthesiology.* 5th ed. New York: McGraw Hill; 2013:1098–1102.

10. Puvanesarajah V, Liauw JA, Lo SF, et al. Analgesic therapy for major spine surgery. *Neurosurg Rev.* 2015;38(3):407–18; discussion 419.

11. Goodwin SA. A review of preemptive analgesia. *J Perianesth Nurs.* 1998;13(2):109–114.

12. Møiniche S, Kehlet H, Dahl JB. A qualitative and quantitative systematic review of preemptive analgesia for postoperative pain relief: the role of timing of analgesia. *Anesthesiology.* 2002;96(3):725–741.

13. Duellman TJ, et al. Multi-modal, pre-emptive analgesia decreases the length of hospital stay following total joint arthroplasty. *Orthopedics.* 2009;32(3):167.

14. Dahl JB, Moiniche S. Pre-emptive analgesia. *Br Med Bull.* 2004;71:13–27.

15. Kissin I. Preemptive analgesia. *Anesthesiology.* 2000;93(4):1138–1143.

16. Gottschalk A, Smith DS. New concepts in acute pain therapy: preemptive analgesia. *Am Fam Physician.* 2001;63(10):1979–1984.

17. Salerno A, Hermann R. Efficacy and safety of steroid use for postoperative pain relief. Update and review of the medical literature. *J Bone Joint Surg Am.* 2006;88(6):1361–1372.

18. De Oliveira GS Jr, Almeida MD, Benzon HT, McCarthy RJ. Perioperative single dose systemic dexamethasone for postoperative pain: a meta-analysis of randomized controlled trials. *Anesthesiology.* 2011;115(3):575–588.

19. Nielsen RV, Siegel H, Fomsgaard JS, et al. Preoperative dexamethasone reduces acute but not sustained pain after lumbar disk surgery: a randomized, blinded, placebo-controlled trial. *Pain.* 2015;156(12):2538–2544.

20. Reuben SS, Ablett D, Kaye R. High dose nonsteroidal anti-inflammatory drugs compromise spinal fusion. *Can J Anaesth.* 2005;52(5):506–512.

21. Dahl V, Raeder JC. Non-opioid postoperative analgesia. *Acta Anaesthesiol Scand.* 2000;44(10):1191–1203.

22. Buvanendran A, Kroin JS. Multimodal analgesia for controlling acute postoperative pain. *Curr Opin Anaesthesiol.* 2009;22(5):588–593.

23. Jirarattanaphochai K, Jung S. Nonsteroidal antiinflammatory drugs for postoperative pain management after lumbar spine surgery: a meta-analysis of randomized controlled trials. *J Neurosurg Spine.* 2008;9(1):22–31.

24. Dodwell ER, Latorre JG, Parisini E, et al. NSAID exposure and risk of nonunion: a meta-analysis of case-control and cohort studies. *Calcif Tissue Int.* 2010;87(3):193–202.

25. Reuben SS, Ekman EF. The effect of cyclooxygenase-2 inhibition on analgesia and spinal fusion. *J Bone Joint Surg Am.* 2005;87(3):536–542.

26. Rivkin A, Rivkin MA. Perioperative nonopioid agents for pain control in spinal surgery. *Am J Health Syst Pharm.* 2014;71(21):1845–1857.

27. Marret E, Flahault A, Samama CM, Bonnet F. Effects of postoperative, nonsteroidal, antiinflammatory drugs on bleeding risk after tonsillectomy: meta-analysis of randomized, controlled trials. *Anesthesiology.* 2003;98(6):1497–1502.

28. Ofman JJ, MacLean CH, Straus WL, et al. A metaanalysis of severe upper gastrointestinal complications of nonsteroidal antiinflammatory drugs. *J Rheumatol.* 2002;29(4):804–812.

29. Yilmaz MZ, Sarihasan BB, Kelsaka E, et al. Comparison of the analgesic effects of paracetamol and tramadol in lumbar disc surgery. *Turk J Med Sci.* 2015;45(2):438–442.

30. Shahid M, Manjula BP, Sunil BV. A comparative study of intravenous paracetamol and intravenous tramadol for postoperative analgesia in laparotomies. *Anesth Essays Res.* 2015;9(3):314–319.

31. Periáñez-Párraga L, Martínez-López I, Ventayol-Bosch P, et al. Drug dosage recommendations in patients with chronic liver disease. *Rev Esp Enferm Dig.* 2012;104(4):165–184.

32. McNeil Consumer Healthcare. Tylenol (acetaminophen) product information. 2013.

33. Gertler R, Brown HC, Mitchell DH, Silvius EN. Dexmedetomidine: a novel sedative-analgesic agent. *Proc (Bayl Univ Med Cent).* 2001;14(1):13–21.

34. White PF, Eng MR. Intravenous anesthetics. In: Barash PG, Cullen BF, eds. *Clinical Anesthesia.* Philadelphia, PA: Wolters Kluwer Health/Lippincott Williams & Wilkins; 2013:478–500.

35. Bekker A, Sturaitis MK. Dexmedetomidine for neurological surgery. *Neurosurgery.* 2005;57(1 Suppl):1–10; discussion 1–10.

36. Eilers H. Intravenous anesthetics. In Pardo MC, Miller RD, eds. *Basics of Anesthesia.* Philadelphia, PA: Elsevier/Saunders; 2011:99–114.

37. Tanskanen PE, Kyttä JV, Randell TT, Aantaa RE. Dexmedetomidine as an anaesthetic adjuvant in patients undergoing intracranial tumour surgery: a double-blind, randomized and placebo-controlled study. *Br J Anaesth.* 2006;97(5):658–665.

38. Maze M, Scarfini C, Cavaliere F. New agents for sedation in the intensive care unit. *Crit Care Clin.* 2001;17(4):881–897.

39. Kamibayashi T, Maze M. Clinical uses of alpha2-adrenergic agonists. *Anesthesiology.* 2000;93(5):1345–1349.

40. Precedex [product information]. Abbott Park, IL: Abbott Laboratories; 2001.dexmedetomidine.com/Precedex.pdf

41. Hwang W, Lee J, Park J, Joo J. Dexmedetomidine versus remifentanil in postoperative pain control after spinal surgery: a randomized controlled study. *BMC Anesthesiol.* 2015;15:21.

42. Bekker A, Haile M, Kline R, et al. The effect of intraoperative infusion of dexmedetomidine on the quality of recovery after major spinal surgery. *J Neurosurg Anesthesiol.* 2013;25(1):16–24.

43. Kong VK, Irwin MG. Gabapentin: a multimodal perioperative drug? *Br J Anaesth.* 2007;99(6):775–786.

44. Ho KY, Gan TJ, Habib AS. Gabapentin and postoperative pain--a systematic review of randomized controlled trials. *Pain.* 2006;126(1-3):91–101.

45. Yu L, Ran B, Li M, Shi Z. Gabapentin and pregabalin in the management of postoperative pain after lumbar spinal surgery: a systematic review and meta-analysis. *Spine (Phila Pa 1976).* 2013;38(22):1947–1952.

46. Bafna U, Rajarajeshwaran K, Khandelwal M, Verma AP. A comparison of effect of preemptive use of oral gabapentin and pregabalin for acute post-operative pain after surgery under spinal anesthesia. *J Anaesthesiol Clin Pharmacol.* 2014;30(3):373–377.

47. Stasiowska MK, Ng SC, Gubbay AN, Cregg R. Postoperative pain management. *Br J Hosp Med (Lond).* 2015;76(10):570–575.

48. Clivatti J, Sakata RK, Issy AM. Review of the use of gabapentin in the control of postoperative pain. *Rev Bras Anestesiol.* 2009;59(1):87–98.

49. Khan ZH, Rahimi M, Makarem J, Khan RH. Optimal dose of pre-incision/post-incision gabapentin for pain relief following lumbar laminectomy: a randomized study. *Acta Anaesthesiol Scand.* 2011;55(3):306–312.

50. Wuis EW, Dirks MJ, Termond EF, et al. Plasma and urinary excretion kinetics of oral baclofen in healthy subjects. *Eur J Clin Pharmacol.* 1989;37(2):181–184.

51. Mezler M, Muller T, Raming K. Cloning and functional expression of GABA(B) receptors from Drosophila. *Eur J Neurosci.* 2001;13(3):477–486.

52. Cundy KC, Annamalai T, Bu L, et al. XP13512 [(+/-)-1-([(alpha-isobutanoyloxyethoxy) carbonyl] aminomethyl)-1-cyclohexane acetic acid], a novel gabapentin prodrug: II. Improved oral bioavailability, dose proportionality, and colonic absorption compared with gabapentin in rats and monkeys. *J Pharmacol Exp Ther.* 2004;311(1):324–333.

53. Leo RJ, Baer D. Delirium associated with baclofen withdrawal: a review of common presentations and management strategies. *Psychosomatics.* 2005;46(6):503–507.

54. Wiffen P, Collins S, McQuay H, et al. Anticonvulsant drugs for acute and chronic pain. *Cochrane Database Syst Rev.* 2005;(3):CD001133.

55. Mula M, Pini S, Cassano GB. The role of anticonvulsant drugs in anxiety disorders: a critical review of the evidence. *J Clin Psychopharmacol.* 2007;27(3):263–272.

56. Dauri M, Faria S, Gatti A, et al. Gabapentin and pregabalin for the acute post-operative pain management. A systematic-narrative review of the recent clinical evidences. *Curr Drug Targets.* 2009;10(8):716–733.

57. Imamura S, Kushida C. Gabapentin enacarbil (XP13512/GSK1838262) as an alternative treatment to dopaminergic agents for restless legs syndrome. *Expert Opin Pharmacother.* 2010;11(11):1925–1932.

58. Kukkar A, Bali A, Singh N, Jaggi AS. Implications and mechanism of action of gabapentin in neuropathic pain. *Arch Pharm Res.* 2013;36(3):237–251.

59. Pickering AE, McCabe CS. Prolonged ketamine infusion as a therapy for complex regional pain syndrome: synergism with antagonism? *Br J Clin Pharmacol.* 2014;77(2):233–238.

60. Loftus RW, Yeager MP, Clark JA, et al. Intraoperative ketamine reduces perioperative opiate consumption in opiate-dependent patients with chronic back pain undergoing back surgery. *Anesthesiology.* 2010;113(3):639–646.

61. Aveline C, Hetet HL, Vautier P, et al. Peroperative ketamine and morphine for postoperative pain control after lumbar disk surgery. *Eur J Pain.* 2006;10(7):653–658.

62. Subramaniam K, Subramaniam B, Steinbrook RA. Ketamine as adjuvant analgesic to opioids: a quantitative and qualitative systematic review. *Anesth Analg.* 2004;99(2):482–495, table of contents.

63. Himmelseher S, Durieux ME. Ketamine for perioperative pain management. *Anesthesiology.* 2005;102(1):211–220.

64. White PF. The changing role of non-opioid analgesic techniques in the management of postoperative pain. *Anesth Analg.* 2005;101(5 Suppl):S5–22.

65. Choi DM, Kliffer AP, Douglas MJ., Dextromethorphan and intrathecal morphine for analgesia after Caesarean section under spinal anaesthesia. *Br J Anaesth.* 2003;90(5):653–658.

66. Weinbroum AA, Rudick V, Paret G, Ben-Abraham R. The role of dextromethorphan in pain control. *Can J Anaesth.* 2000;47(6):585–596.

67. King MR, Ladha KS, Gelineau AM, Anderson TA. Perioperative dextromethorphan as an adjunct for postoperative pain: a meta-analysis of randomized controlled trials. *Anesthesiology.* 2016;124(3):696–705.

68. Siu A, Drachtman R. Dextromethorphan: a review of N-methyl-d-aspartate receptor antagonist in the management of pain. *CNS Drug Rev.* 2007;13(1):96–106.

69. Ilkjaer S, Bach LF, Nielsen PA, et al. Effect of preoperative oral dextromethorphan on immediate and late postoperative pain and hyperalgesia after total abdominal hysterectomy. *Pain.* 2000;86(1-2):19–24.

70. Kawamata T, Omote K, Kawamata M, Namiki A. Premedication with oral dextromethorphan reduces postoperative pain after tonsillectomy. *Anesth Analg.* 1998;86(3):594–597.

71. Weinbroum AA, Bender B, Bickels J, et al. Preoperative and postoperative dextromethorphan provides sustained reduction in postoperative pain and patient-controlled epidural analgesia requirement: a randomized, placebo-controlled, double-blind study in lower-body bone malignancy-operated patients. *Cancer.* 2003;97(9):2334–2340.

72. Fawcett WJ, Haxby EJ, Male DA. Magnesium: physiology and pharmacology. *Br J Anaesth.* 1999;83(2):302–320.

73. Tramer MR, Schneider J, Marti RA, Rifat K. Role of magnesium sulfate in postoperative analgesia. *Anesthesiology.* 1996;84(2):340–347.

74. Do SH. Magnesium: a versatile drug for anesthesiologists. *Korean J Anesthesiol.* 2013;65(1):4–8.

75. Iseri LT, French JH. Magnesium: nature's physiologic calcium blocker. *Am Heart J.* 1984;108(1):188–193.

76. Mebazaa MS, Ouerghi S, Frikha N, et al. Is magnesium sulfate by the intrathecal route efficient and safe? *Ann Fr Anesth Reanim.* 2011;30(1):47–50.

77. Levaux Ch, Bonhomme V, Dewandre PY, et al. Effect of intra-operative magnesium sulphate on pain relief and patient comfort after major lumbar orthopaedic surgery. *Anaesthesia.* 2003;58(2):131–135.

78. Aglio LS, Stanford GG, Maddi R, et al. Hypomagnesemia is common following cardiac surgery. *J Cardiothorac Vasc Anesth.* 1991;5(3):201–208.

79. Durlach J, Bac P, Bara M, Guiet-Bara A. Physiopathology of symptomatic and latent forms of central nervous hyperexcitability due to magnesium deficiency: a current general scheme. *Magnes Res.* 2000;13(4):293–302.

80. Guo BL, Lin Y, Hu W, et al. Effects of systemic magnesium on post-operative analgesia: is the current evidence strong enough? *Pain Physician.* 2015;18(5):405–418.

81. Jabbour HJ, Naccache NM, Jawish RJ, et al. Ketamine and magnesium association reduces morphine consumption after scoliosis surgery: prospective randomised double-blind study. *Acta Anaesthesiol Scand.* 2014;58(5):572–579.

82. Wacker WE, Parisi AF. *Magnesium metabolism. N Engl J Med.* 1968;278(13):712–717.

83. Vejlsted H, Eliasen P. Postoperative serum level and urinary excretion of magnesium following heart surgery. *Scand J Thorac Cardiovasc Surg.* 1978;12(2):91–94.

84. Gupta K, Vohra V, Sood J. The role of magnesium as an adjuvant during general anaesthesia. *Anaesthesia.* 2006;61(11):1058–1063.

85. Harless M, Depp C, Collins S, Hewer I. Role of Esmolol in perioperative analgesia and anesthesia: a literature review. *AANA J.* 2015;83(3):167–177.

86. Collard V, Mistraletti G, Taqi A, et al. Intraoperative esmolol infusion in the absence of opioids spares postoperative fentanyl in patients undergoing ambulatory laparoscopic cholecystectomy. *Anesth Analg.* 2007;105(5):1255–1262, table of contents.

87. Bhawna, Bajwa SJ, Lalitha K, et al. Influence of esmolol on requirement of inhalational agent using entropy and assessment of its effect on immediate postoperative pain score. *Indian J Anaesth.* 2012;56(6):535–541.

88. Shukla S, Gupta K, Gurha P, Sharma M, Sanjay R, Shukla R, Rana S. Role of beta blockade in anaesthesia and postoperative pain management after major lower abdominal surgery. *The Internet Journal of Anesthesiology.* 2009;25(1).

89. Lee SJ, Lee JN. The effect of perioperative esmolol infusion on the postoperative nausea, vomiting and pain after laparoscopic appendectomy. *Korean J Anesthesiol.* 2010;59(3):179–184.

90. Wilson ES, McKinlay S, Crawford JM, Robb HM. The influence of esmolol on the dose of propofol required for induction of anaesthesia. *Anaesthesia.* 2004;59(2):122–126.

91. Sum CY, Yacobi A, Kartzinel R, et al. Kinetics of esmolol, an ultra-short-acting beta blocker, and of its major metabolite. *Clin Pharmacol Ther.* 1983;34(4):427–434.

92. Fischer LG, Bremer M, Coleman EJ, et al. Local anesthetics attenuate lysophosphatidic acid-induced priming in human neutrophils. *Anesth Analg.* 2001;92(4):1041–1047.

93. Kranke P, Jokinen J, Pace NL, et al. Continuous intravenous perioperative lidocaine infusion for postoperative pain and recovery. *Cochrane Database Syst Rev.* 2015;7:CD009642.

94. Rowland M, Thomson PD, Guichard A, Melmon KL. Disposition kinetics of lidocaine in normal subjects. *Ann N Y Acad Sci.* 1971;179:383–398.

95. Devor M, Wall PD, Catalan N. Systemic lidocaine silences ectopic neuroma and DRG discharge without blocking nerve conduction. *Pain.* 1992;48(2):261–268.

96. Hahnenkamp K, Durieux ME, Hahnenkamp A, et al. Local anaesthetics inhibit signalling of human NMDA receptors recombinantly expressed in Xenopus laevis oocytes: role of protein kinase C. *Br J Anaesth.* 2006;96(1):77–87.

97. Yardeni IZ, Beilin B, Mayburd E, et al. The effect of perioperative intravenous lidocaine on postoperative pain and immune function. *Anesth Analg.* 2009;109(5):1464–1469.

98. Kim KT, Cho DC, Sung JK, et al. Intraoperative systemic infusion of lidocaine reduces postoperative pain after lumbar surgery: a double-blinded, randomized, placebo-controlled clinical trial. *Spine J.* 2014;14(8):1559–1566.

99. Farag E, Ghobrial M, Sessler DI, et al. Effect of perioperative intravenous lidocaine administration on pain, opioid consumption, and quality of life after complex spine surgery. *Anesthesiology*. 2013;119(4):932–940.

100. Goldstein J. Caffeine as an analgesic adjuvant. *Inflammopharmacology*. 2001;9(1,2):51–61.

101. Peroutka SJ, Lyon JA, Swarbrick J, et al. Efficacy of diclofenac sodium softgel 100 mg with or without caffeine 100 mg in migraine without aura: a randomized, double-blind, crossover study. *Headache*. 2004;44(2):136–141.

102. Moore RA, Derry CJ, Derry S, et al. A conservative method of testing whether combination analgesics produce additive or synergistic effects using evidence from acute pain and migraine. *Eur J Pain*. 2012;16(4):585–591.

103. Derry S, Wiffen PJ, Moore RA. Single dose oral ibuprofen plus caffeine for acute postoperative pain in adults. *Cochrane Database Syst Rev*. 2015;7:CD011509.

104. Derry CJ, Derry S, Moore RA. Caffeine as an analgesic adjuvant for acute pain in adults. *Cochrane Database Syst Rev*. 2014;12:CD009281.

105. Sawynok J. Methylxanthines and pain. *Handb Exp Pharmacol*. 2011(200):311–329.

106. Baranidharan G, Das S, Bhaskar A. A review of the high-concentration capsaicin patch and experience in its use in the management of neuropathic pain. *Ther Adv Neurol Disord.*, 2013;6(5):287–297.

107. Derry S, Moore RA. Topical capsaicin (low concentration) for chronic neuropathic pain in adults. *Cochrane Database Syst Rev*. 2012(9):CD010111.

108. Anand P, Bley K. Topical capsaicin for pain management: therapeutic potential and mechanisms of action of the new high-concentration capsaicin 8% patch. *Br J Anaesth*. 2011;107(4):490–502.

109. Martindale W, Reynolds JEF, eds. *Martindale: The Extra Pharmacopoeia*. 32nd ed. London: The Pharmaceutical Press; 1999.

110. Finnerup NB, Attal N, Haroutounian S, et al. Pharmacotherapy for neuropathic pain in adults: a systematic review and meta-analysis. *Lancet Neurol*. 2015;14(2):162–173.

111. Colvin AC, Wang CF, Soens MA, et al. Prolonged cutaneous analgesia with transdermal application of amitriptyline and capsaicin. *Reg Anesth Pain Med*. 2011;36(3):236–240.

112. Savage PEA. Efficacy and safety of a single intraoperative administration of highly purified capsaicin formulation for management of postoperative pain associated with total knee arthroplasty: a randomized phase 3 trial. *J Pain*. 2009;10(4):S53.

113. Hartrick CT, Pestano C, Carlson N, Hartrick S. Capsaicin instillation for postoperative pain following total knee arthroplasty: a preliminary report of a randomized, double-blind, parallel-group, placebo-controlled, multicentre trial. *Clin Drug Investig*. 2011;31(12):877–882.

114. Zittel TT, Meile T, Jehle EC, Becker HD. Intraperitoneal capsaicin treatment reduces postoperative gastric ileus in awake rats. *Langenbecks Arch Surg*. 2001;386(3):204–211.

4

Perioperative Opioid Analgesics of Use in Pain Management for Spine Surgery

Kenneth Fomberstein, Marissa Rubin, Dipan Patel, John-Paul Sara, and Abhishek Gupta

INTRODUCTION

For moderate to severe postoperative pain, parenteral opioids have long been the cornerstone of treatment. They work by stimulating central and peripheral μ and κ receptors, leading to inhibition of voltage-gated calcium channels and increased potassium influx. This results in reduced neuronal excitability, thereby inhibiting the ascending transmission of painful stimuli. Additionally, they activate descending inhibitory pathways [1].

Opioids as a class have been used for many years in both the acute and chronic pain settings, especially in orthopedic surgery. Perioperative pain control can be complicated by preoperative chronic use of opioids, leading to opioid tolerance and opioid hyperalgesia. Opioid-tolerant patients may have a 2- to 5-fold higher postoperative opioid requirement compared to patients who are not chronic opioid users [2]. Mechanisms possibly involved in the development of opioid tolerance include receptor desensitization, internalization, second-messenger switching, receptor dimerization, and more [3]. Dose escalation of opioids in patients with inadequate pain control is often limited by tolerance and drug adverse effects, which differ even with differing routes of administration. Furthermore, there is blunted improvement in therapeutic effect with increasing doses of some opioids despite continued worsening of adverse effects [4–7].

Opioid cross-tolerance can occur when the use of one opioid increases the amount of a second opioid needed to have the same analgesic effect. For example, some studies have shown that remifentanil, an ultra-short-acting opioid used widely as an

Table 4.1 Common opioid receptors

Receptor	Subtypes	Example of Selective Agonist(s)	Example of Selective Antagonist
μ (μ) opioid receptor (MOR)	μ_1	Fentanyl	Cyprodime
	μ_2	Morphine	
kappa (κ) opioid receptor (KOR)	κ_1	U50488[a]	Nor-binaltorphimine
	κ_2		
	κ_3		
delta (δ) opioid receptor (DOR)	δ_1	DADLE[b]	Naltrindole
	δ_2		

[a] (−)-(*trans*)-3,4-dichloro-*N*-methyl-*N*-[2-(1-pyrrolidinyl)cyclohexyl]benzeneacetamide.

[b] [D-Ala2, D-Leu5] enkephalin.

References 10–14.

analgesic in the perioperative period, increases the morphine consumption of patients postoperatively [8]. Opioid receptors are part of the G-protein coupled receptor (GPCR) super family of receptors, and different opioids often act on the same subtype of opioid receptors. An important mechanism involved in generating cross-tolerance is opioid receptor desensitization produced by chronic stimulation of the receptor by a previously used opioid. Desensitization is qualified as a reduction in signal transduction. Molecular mechanisms involved in opioid receptor desensitization include phosphorylation of the receptors by kinases, receptor uncoupling from G-proteins, and opioid receptor trafficking (see Table 4.1) [9].

Side effects of opioids can affect a patient's recovery from surgery. Specifically, constipation, nausea, vomiting, pruritus, oversedation, and respiratory depression can lead to the need for additional pharmacologic intervention and longer hospital stays. Postoperative sedation is particularly a problem when there is need for frequent neurological exams, as is the case in many spine surgeries [10]. Since the enteric nervous system expresses all of the major subtypes of opioid receptors, gut motility and secretory processes are inhibited by opioids. Therefore, one of the most bothersome problems patients on opioids report postoperatively is constipation. Constipation can sometimes be avoided by using nonopioid regimens; however, this is not always possible if pain is severe. Physicians typically prescribe laxatives, administer prokinetic drugs, or sometimes use opioid receptor antagonists to treat constipation postoperatively (see Box 4.1) [11].

Box 4.1 Common Side Effects of Opioids

- Respiratory depression
- Constipation
- Nausea/Vomiting
- Pruritus
- Oversedation

Reference 1.

Opioid conversion refers to the change in administration route of an opioid, while *opioid rotation* is a term used to reflect the change from one opioid to another. Both methods are used (often simultaneously) to alleviate side effects caused by the first opioid, as well to reduce pain [7,12,13]. A change to a second medication may improve pain control due to incomplete cross-tolerance between opioids—thus reducing the opioid load and/or side effects—and individual variations in opioid pharmacodynamics and pharmacokinetics [7].

There is no consensus of opinion on the subjects of both conversion and rotation. Information from manufacturers, reference materials, and online reviews all show high variability among conversion ratios. There have been many attempts at equianalgesic dose conversion tables, but all have been mainly derived from expert opinion or single-dose studies [12–16]. The clinician must consider individual patient situations which affect tolerance, metabolism, and available routes of delivery. Comorbidities including previous opioid exposure, psychiatric history, renal/hepatic/pulmonary disease, potential drug–drug interactions, and genetic factors affecting metabolism must be taken into consideration [7,12–15,17–19]. Errors are best avoided by knowledge of opioid pharmacology, awareness of the limits of equianalgesic tables, application of conversion/rotation guidelines, and tailoring opioid use to individual patient characteristics and response (see Tables 4.2 and 4.3) [7,17].

A two-step guideline widely used since introduction in 2009 involves an online calculator to find the equianalgesic dose, which is then lowered by 25–50% for initial administration. This is followed by frequent reassessment of pain level and deliberate and incremental increases until desired therapeutic effect is achieved [7,17,20]. Many practitioners use similar techniques as a guide to complement their clinical experience and aid clinical judgment, but individual situations remain the primary drivers of clinical decision-making [7,12,19,20]. Route of administration options include oral, transdermal patch, subcutaneous, intramuscular, intravenous, transmucosal, and rectal administration [7]. It is pertinent to consider changes in onset of action as well as bioavailability as these differing pharmacokinetics may be used advantageously to address pain in a multimodal approach. For example, a transdermal patch may be applied for a basal dose, along with additional short-acting medications to be administered on an as-needed basis for breakthrough pain [7,15].

Table 4.2 Example of an opioid equianalgesic dosing table

	Morphine	Hydromorphone (Dilaudid)	Oxycodone	Fentanyl
Morphine 10 mg intravenous equivalent dose	30 mg PO/10 mg intravenous	7.5 mg PO/ 1.3–1.5 mg intravenous	20 mg PO	0.1 mg intravenous
Oral-to-parenteral dosing ratio (PO:IV) (mg: mg)	3:1	5:1	N/A	N/A
Half-life	1.7–3.3 hours	2–3 hours	N/A	1.5–6 hours

References 17, 24–26.

Table 4.3 Intraoperative opioid use

	Morphine	Fentanyl	Hydromorphone	Sufentanil	Remifentanil
Common intraoperative dose (IV)	IM 0.05–0.2 mg/kg IV 0.03–0.15 mg/kg	IV 2–50 µg/kg	IM 0.02–0.04 mg/kg IV 0.01–0.02 mg/kg	IV 0.25–20 µg/kg	IV infusionLoading: 1 µg/kg Maintenance: 0.5–20 µg/kg/min
Time to peak effect (IV)	20 min	6 min	10–15 min	6 min	2 min
Duration of action (IV) (nontolerant patient)	120–240 min	7 min	120–180 min	7 min	5–10 min half-life after stopping infusion
Equipotent dose (IV)	10 mg	0.1 mg (100 µg)	1.5 mg	.01 mg (10 µg)	0.1 mg (100 µg)
Metabolism	Hepatic phase 2 glucuronidation	Hepatic CYP3A4-mediated N-dealkylation	Hepatic phase 2 glucuronidation	Hepatic CYP3A4-mediated N-dealkylation	Plasma esterases

References 12, 27–33.

FENTANYL

Fentanyl is the most commonly used opioid in modern anesthesia practice. Fentanyl was developed to provide enhanced analgesic properties and potency with fewer secondary effects compared with the prototype opioid, morphine [23]. Compared to morphine, fentanyl is 100 times more potent and does not cause the histamine release with resultant hypotension. When used during anesthesia, fentanyl is able to dampen sympathetic response to noxious stimuli associated with intubation, skin incision, and overall surgical stress response [24].

The lipophilic structure of fentanyl allows it to rapidly cross the blood–brain barrier to exert its effects on the brain [24]. Fentanyl has an onset of action of about 2 minutes, time to peak effect of about 4 minutes, and an elimination half-life of about 2–4 hours. The short duration of action of fentanyl after a single dose is secondary to rapid uptake and redistribution into adipose tissue. After large or multiple doses, however, redistribution is less effective in removing fentanyl due to its long elimination half-time [23]. Fentanyl is metabolized by the liver into the inactive metabolite, norfentanyl, which is excreted in bile and urine. Thus, compared to morphine, fentanyl is safe to use in patients with renal failure [24].

The high lipid solubility and rapid redistribution also provides fentanyl with a unique clinical application: the ability to be administered via multiple delivery systems and routes. Fentanyl can be administered via intravenous (bolus injection, infusion, patient-controlled analgesia [PCA]), neuraxial (epidural, intrathecal), intramuscular, transdermal, transmucosal (oral or intranasal), and inhalational routes [23]. Intrathecal administration provides the most potent and complete analgesia. Fentanyl is well suited for intravenous PCA administration due to the latency to peak effect site concentration after bolus injection and the effective, convenient format.

Fentanyl's use during neurosurgery as well as in the perioperative period as a whole has become fairly well established. Regardless of the route of administration, fentanyl exhibits many of the common adverse effects associated with opioid use such as respiratory depression, pruritus, urinary retention, and nausea and vomiting, requiring vigilant monitoring [23].

HYDROMORPHONE

Hydromorphone is a long-acting semisynthetic opioid that is about 5–10 times more potent than morphine. The onset of analgesia occurs slightly faster than morphine due to its greater lipid solubility but more slowly than the highly lipid-soluble fentanyl [25]. The peak effect occurs in 10–20 minutes when administered intravenously, and the elimination half-life is 2.5 hours. Hydromorphone is metabolized into its active metabolites dihydromorphine and dihydroisomorphine and the inactive metabolite hydromorphone-3-glucuronide. This inactive metabolite can accumulate in patients with renal failure, leading to neuroexcitation and cognitive impairment [24]. Hydromorphone is used both in the acute pain setting as well as for chronic cancer pain. It can be administered via intravenous, neuraxial, intramuscular, subcutaneous, and oral routes.

Postoperatively, hydromorphone is very commonly used for pain control with PCA. Differences between the clinical pharmacology of hydromorphone and morphine may potentially make hydromorphone a better choice of drug for PCA. With the standard

8–10 minute PCA dosing interval, the hydromorphone dose will be close to peak effect while a morphine bolus will not [26]. Hydromorphone exhibits the traditional opioid-related adverse effects such as nausea, vomiting, respiratory depression, sedation, cognitive impairment, and pruritus. However, it has been stated that, compared to morphine, these side effects are much less intense with hydromorphone [24].

REMIFENTANIL

Remifentanil was designed to achieve a specific clinical goal: to have an opioid that is rapid-acting and easily titratable to match the dynamic conditions met with during the perioperative period. At the molecular level, remifentanil was designed with specialized structure-metabolism properties in mind [21]. The ester structure of the opioid allows it to be broken down by ester hydrolysis. Once hydrolyzed, the drug loses its μ opioid receptor agonist activity. The ubiquitous nonspecific esterases responsible for hydrolysis are found in red blood cells and tissues. Of note, patients with pseudocholinesterase deficiency do not show a varied response to remifentanil [27].

The unique pharmacokinetic profile of remifentanil can be used to rapidly achieve the desired response. The terminal elimination half-life of remifentanil is less than 10 minutes, and the context-sensitive half-time is only 3 minutes. The biotransformation is rapid, and the duration of an infusion has minimal effect on wake-up time regardless of dose [27]. In contrast to other opioids, remifentanil does not accumulate and does not require dosing based on hepatic function. The main metabolite is renally excreted and does not demonstrate any clinical effects. On the pharmacodynamic level, remifentanil exhibits a short latency to peak effect and is slightly less potent than fentanyl. Due to its preparation, which contains glycine, remifentanil is not approved for epidural or spinal usage [28].

The role of remifentanil in current clinical practice has become fairly well established. Clinical indications for the use of remifentanil include rapid recovery after surgery, fluctuating anesthesia requirements, or difficulty with opioid titration [21]. The agent may also be used for PCA, sedation in the ICU setting, and treatment of obstetric pain [10]. Most commonly, remifentanil is used during total intravenous anesthesia (TIVA) in conjunction with propofol. This method is used very frequently in neurosurgery cases and provides faster emergence than other anesthetics. It is unclear, however, whether remifentanil-propofol (REMI-TIVA) or fentanyl-propofol (FENT-TIVA) is superior in these cases. Studies of emergence and anesthesia times have shown no difference between the two [24].

One important side effect of remifentanil is hyperalgesia, or abnormally heightened sensitivity to pain, resulting in an escalating need for pain control. Opioid-induced hyperalgesia may occur with all opioids, but the incidence is higher when remifentanil is used [29]. The mechanisms are not completely understood, but one study by Wang et al. suggests that remifentanil-induced postoperative hyperalgesia may be related to the activation of the δ opioid receptors (DOR) and the resulting increase in N-methyl-D-aspartate (NMDA).

receptor expression, membrane trafficking, and current in the dorsal horn of the spinal cord. The authors suggest that a DOR antagonist, naltrindole, may be a potential therapeutic strategy to treat hyperalgesia [29].

Sufentanil is the most potent opioid used in clinical practice. It is 10 times more potent than fentanyl and is more intrinsically efficacious at the μ opioid receptor [21,30,31]. It is highly protein-bound, exhibits the typical opioid side-effect profile, and is cleared by hepatic metabolism as most other opioids are; however, it does not cause myocardial depression as morphine, meperidine, and inhalational anesthetics do. On the contrary, it shows good hemodynamic stability as well as recovery from intubation [21,31–33]. This feature, shared with fentanyl, makes sufentanil a good choice of analgesic for a patient with a poor cardiac profile.

Dosed as a bolus, the latency to peak concentration is slightly longer than fentanyl, with rapid decline of effect, making sufentanil a good choice for PCA or to achieve rapid control of breakthrough pain [21,31]. Doses need not be weight-adjusted for individuals with nonextremes of body mass index [34]. When sufentanil or remifentanil were combined with propofol for craniotomy, less analgesic medication was required within the first hour postoperatively when sufentanil was the agent of choice [35].

Due to a large volume of distribution, the time to steady-state concentration of a sufentanil infusion (without bolus) is too long for most procedures, which diminishes its use as an infusion intraoperatively. Nonetheless, the rate of decrease of concentration after discontinuing a continuous infusion at steady-state is faster than fentanyl or alfentanil, owing to a short context-sensitive half-time [21,30,34,36]. This, conversely, may be clinically irrelevant as one study found no difference in time to extubation after spine surgery when compared to fentanyl in TIVA [37]. Of note, there is a marked reduction in extubation times and improved immediate postoperative consciousness associated with the use of remifentanil compared with sufentanil [30]. Nevertheless, sufentanil may be more suitable and easier to administer than remifentanil in the setting of planned postoperative mechanical ventilation and postponed awakening, similar to fentanyl, but with improved response time after terminating a long-term infusion compared to fentanyl.

During intraoperative evoked potential monitoring, sufentanil behaves similarly to other opioids with reduced amplitude and increased latency of auditory evoked potentials, and small but stable to no effect on motor and somatosensory evoked potentials [38–43]. Intrathecal administration of sufentanil upon termination of single-level lumbar discectomy has been shown to improve analgesia and speed recovery [44]. Postoperatively, patients may benefit from as-needed or patient-controlled intravenous dosing, as well as recently available sublingual tablets with an improved safety profile that may aid those patients not yet tolerating oral intake [45–49].

Unlike remifentanil, sufentanil is approved for use in epidural and spinal anesthesia. High satisfaction has been achieved after major spine surgery with patient-controlled epidural analgesia (PCEA) consisting of ropivacaine and sufentanil; additionally, intrathecal sufentanil has been used with success for patients with intractable pain via an implantable drug delivery system; however, there is a concern for the formation of a granuloma as with all intrathecally delivered medications [50,51].

METHADONE

The origin of the synthetic opioid methadone dates back to the 1930s. Methadone has gained popularity for its cost-effective success in managing patients with acute, chronic, neuropathic, and cancer-related pain in neonates, children, and adults [52]. Early studies of perioperative use of methadone date back to the 1980s. However, even with the results of multiple studies showing advantageous use in regards to decreased pain scores, opioid consumption, and time to supplemental analgesics, methadone has not gained popularity in its use perioperatively among anesthesia providers. Methadone still carries a stigma of having previously been used to detoxify heroin users, which has limited acceptance in its use to control pain [53].

The mechanism of methadone is multimodal. Primarily, its benefits are a result of μ receptor agonism in the brain and spinal cord. In the brain, μ agonism in central pain processing centers such as the periaqueductal gray (PAG) allow for its beneficial effects in reducing pain. Methadone's action in spinal cord is located mainly in the substantia gelatinosa, where its inhibition on C fiber afferents results in a reduction of substance P presynaptically and hyperpolarization of second-order neurons postsynaptically, eventually leading to a decrease in afferent pain signals traveling to the brain. Traditionally, opioids have been shown to activate NMDA receptors via second-messenger systems. However, methadone has the unique function of also serving as a noncompetitive NMDA-receptor antagonist. This mechanism of action mirrors that of the commonly implemented anesthetic medication ketamine [52,53]. Experimental studies have shown this additional function to be beneficial, rendering methadone less sensitive to tolerance since its ED50 was not altered after previous exposure to morphine [54].

Intravenous methadone has the advantage of a rapid onset of action (approximately 5–10 minutes), which rivals that of two other highly lipophilic opioids, sufentanil and fentanyl. However, the disadvantage of methadone is the long, unpredictable half-life, which can range based on the individual anywhere from 8–90 hours [55]. Following a single bolus dose of intravenous methadone, the onset to analgesia is approximately 10–20 minutes with a duration of 4–8 hours, which is less than the excretion time. This can put a patient at risk of drug accumulation after repeated doses. When administered orally, it may be detected in the plasma after 30 minutes and takes approximately 2.5–3 hours to reach peak plasma concentration [55]. Methadone is metabolized in the liver via N-demethylation and mainly CYP2B6. It does not have a prodrug or any active metabolites. Caution must be taken in patients with liver failure. In light of the drug's unpredictable metabolism, the influence on adverse effects may be augmented in this patient demographic. Methadone's renal clearance is minimal, therefore it has been utilized in patients with compromised renal function, including hemodialysis-dependent patients, without adverse effect. It is worth mentioning that it is administered in racemic form with the R-form being more potent as a μ agonist and the S-form responsible for the NMDA antagonist properties. The pharmacokinetic profile is similar in pediatrics and healthy adults. Methadone's pharmacokinetics involve extensive binding to plasma proteins, which can contribute to increases in acute phase reactants including plasma proteins such as acid α-glycoprotein, thus contributing to even more pharmacokinetic unpredictability. Another unique characteristic to note is methadone's ability to gradually redistribute from the tissues into the intravascular compartment after withdrawing the drug, thereby maintaining a small plasma concentration. This may explain why this opioid is less prone to induce withdrawal syndrome [56–58].

Perioperative use of methadone gained popularity following multiple peer-reviewed published studies. One study in particular showed that adult patients undergoing multilevel thoracolumbar spine surgery had decreased opioid consumption, less overall pain at 48 hours postoperatively, decreased need for intravenous opioid PCA, and had no increases in opioid-related adverse events when given 0.2 mg/kg of intravenous methadone following intubation [55]. Dose adjustments are frequently implemented in the elderly as metabolism of methadone and risk of respiratory depression are of particular concern in this patient population [59]. The beneficial effects on decreased total opioid consumption in this study were attributed to methadone's unique ability to function as an NMDA antagonist, which also results in decreased incidence of opioid-induced hyperalgesia (OIH) [59–61]. Of note, likely due to the induction of CYP3A4 and P glycoprotein by St. John's wort, of which methadone is a substrate, caution should be used in the combination of these two medications. St. John's wort can precipitate withdrawal in methadone users due to its ability to decrease plasma concentrations by an average of 47% (19–60%) [62].

Methadone demands special attention due to the risk of accumulation and intoxication, especially during the first days of use and during analgesic dose titration. Buildup of this opioid and rapid redistribution may induce respiratory depression with doses as low as 30 mg in nontolerant individuals and with higher doses in tolerant individuals, and it has been shown to result in respiratory depression at 30–45 minutes after a single bolus of up to 30 mg. Methadone-induced respiratory depression peaks after the analgesic peak is achieved and is maintained for a longer period, especially in the beginning of treatment [63,64]. Dose-dependent increases in QT interval may also occur and should be monitored. Most practitioners utilize a baseline electrocardiogram (ECG) to assess the risk–benefit ratio of initiating methadone treatment. Follow up ECGs may be obtained to monitor the effects on QT interval prolongation in high-risk patients. However, after literature review, most authors recommend that patients with risk factors be submitted to ECG before starting treatment and during dose titration [64].

When intravenously administered, it is recommended to record ECG in the following moments: before starting therapy, after 24 hours of use, whenever there is significant dose increase, and whenever there is major clinical alteration (electrolyte abnormality, congestive heart failure, initiation of other QT prolongation medications). Electrolyte monitoring is also recommended for patients at higher risk [65–67]. The risk for torsade de pointes is directly proportional to QT interval duration and is higher when this interval is greater than 500 msec, in addition to methadone doses of greater than 100 mg/day [68]. Approximately 30% of analgesic-related deaths in the United States in 2009 were attributed to methadone, although this drug accounts for just 2% of opioid consumption (see Box 4.2) [69].

PATIENT-CONTROLLED ANALGESIA

An important aspect to consider when providing anesthetic care is the adequate management and treatment of intraoperative and postoperative pain. Untreated pain in the postoperative patient has the potential to lead to significant deleterious effects. Studies have shown an association that links postoperative pain to increased length

Box 4.2 Recommended ECG Monitoring with intravenous Methadone Treatment

- Baseline ECG before treatment initiation
- After 24 hours of use
- With significant dose increases
- When there is major clinical alteration (e.g. electrolyte abnormalities)

References 76–78.

of hospital stay, morbidity, pulmonary complications, and delirium [21]. For cognitively intact adults, PCA is now considered the preferred method for the management and delivery of postoperative pain relief. PCA is a technique of pain management that provides the patient with the ability to administer his own analgesia on demand [10]. The PCA delivery technique is based on the improved understanding of the physiology and mechanisms of pain and helps to reduce the potential for adverse clinical complications.

Traditionally, analgesics have been delivered orally or parenterally when a patient reports discomfort to a healthcare professional. In modern practice, PCAs are more frequently being utilized as they have been deemed more efficacious in providing analgesia. Patients are generally agreeable and even favor PCAs because this technique restores control to the patient when it comes to managing his own pain and recovery. In comparison to traditional methods, PCA has been shown to have a greater safety profile, provide better analgesia, decrease the total amount of drug administered, and hasten the return to physical activity [21]. PCA can be delivered via a number of routes, including oral, parenteral, neuraxial, and peripheral nerve catheter. The five variables associated with all modes of PCA include bolus dose, incremental (demand) dose, lockout interval, background infusion rate, and 1- and 4-hour limits (see Box 4.3) [10].

Once the PCA has been started, the anesthesiologist places limits on the number of doses per unit of time that will be administered to the patient. The lockout interval is set to allow a minimum time interval between subsequent doses. If a continuous background infusion is implemented, the delivery system has the ability to provide the patient the option to administer additional bolus doses [21]. The most commonly used agents are morphine, hydromorphone, and fentanyl. In patients with renal failure, hydromorphone is recommended, but fentanyl may also be used as it does not have active metabolites [10,24,70].

Box 4.3 Important Variables Associated with PCA

- Bolus dose
- Incremental (demand) dose
- Lockout interval
- Background infusion rate
- and 4-hour limits

Reference 12.

PCA generally has a high safety profile, and routine monitoring is not always necessary. Given the risk of respiratory depression with opioid usage, however, pulse oximetry, capnography, and respiratory rate monitoring may be utilized. Capnography is generally reserved for patients with substantial comorbidities who have an increased risk of opioid toxicity. Common side effects of PCA are the typical opioid-related effects, such as nausea and vomiting, pruritus, sedation, and confusion [10].

MORPHINE

Morphine is the prototypical opioid by which all others are compared. Available in many dosing routes including parenteral, oral, rectal, transdermal, neuraxial, subcutaneous, intramuscular, and intraarticular, morphine is the most used and most recognized opioid worldwide [71,72]. Adverse reactions including histamine release, leading to hypotension and anaphylactoid reactions, have caused fentanyl to upend morphine as the intraoperative opioid of choice. However, morphine remains favorable, partially due to its prolonged latency to peak effect, approximately 20 minutes, causing less respiratory depression after intravenous bolus, as well as its prolonged duration of action compared to fentanyl, up to 4 hours compared to up to 1 hour [71].

These characteristics make morphine a common choice for postoperative analgesia via PCA, but premedication can be beneficial as well [73]. In fact, preoperative extended-release oral morphine (30 mg) has been shown to reduce postoperative morphine requirements in patients scheduled for spine surgery without inducing side effects [74].

Morphine, similar to most opioids, undergoes 90% hepatic metabolism, the major active metabolite being morphine-6-glucuronide (M6G), a strong μ receptor agonist with high receptor affinity [22]. M6G has a major contribution to the overall analgesic effect; one study estimated mean contributions as 96.6%, 85.6%, 85.4%, and 91.3% after oral, subcutaneous, intravenous, and rectal administration of morphine, respectively. In patients with renal insufficiency, 97.6% of the analgesic effect is caused by M6G when morphine is given orally [75]. The other major metabolite is morphine-3-glucuronide (M3G), which has shown neuroexcitatory effects in animals but little analgesic effect [22].

Epidural morphine via loading dose or continuous infusion in combination with local anesthetic has been utilized to minimize total postoperative opioid dose but has led to increased respiratory depression with mixed results for GI side effects [76–78]. Liposomal morphine has proved efficacious as a single-shot depot injection (10–20 mg) into the lumbar epidural space immediately after surgery, with significant pain control up to 48 hours [78–80]. However, this technique has been utilized in abdominal, pelvic, lower extremity, breast, and gynecologic surgeries and has been minimally tested in spine surgery [76,78,80].

Morphine can also be delivered intrathecally, directly affecting dorsal horn neurons, with excellent postoperative analgesic efficacy and prolonged duration of action compared to other opioids [81]. The optimal single-shot intrathecal dose appears to be 0.075–0.15 mg; above this dose, an analgesic ceiling effect reveals diminishing increase in analgesia [82]. In chronic pain patients, intrathecal administration is typically achieved using an implantable morphine pump [83]. These patients may present for revision procedures, so knowledge of time and location of implantation, duration of function, and type of medication and dosage is important. These pumps may cause granulation tissue to develop, as well, with subsequent central nervous system inflammatory reaction or increasing intracranial pressure and their expected neurological sequelae [84]. Documented side effects to intrathecal morphine, in addition to pruritus, respiratory depression, hypotension, and nausea, include hypothermia, treatable with lorazepam, and hypopituitarism [85,86].

OXYCODONE

Oxycodone has been used clinically since 1917. In the United States, oral oxycodone combined with acetaminophen has been used primarily to treat moderate pain. Unlike morphine, which acts only on μ receptors, oxycodone is both a μ and κ receptor agonist. Oral controlled-release opioids have several advantages over immediate-release opioids including reduced number of administrations and more uniform analgesia due to steady, less peak-and-trough plasma levels. Controlled-release oxycodone (CRO) is marketed primarily for chronic pain. When compared to controlled-release morphine, CRO is almost twice as potent with three times the oral bioavailability. It has been found to have a reduced incidence of side effects in cancer patients [87].

CROs effects on postoperative pain and analgesic consumption have been studied in the context of several types of surgery. One study investigated the effects of perioperative coadministration of CRO with intravenous morphine compared to intravenous morphine with placebo in patients undergoing lumbar discectomy, a common orthopedic and neurosurgical procedure. The results indicated that 20 mg of CRO perioperatively significantly reduced intravenous morphine consumption postoperatively and also reduced opioid side effects while providing better analgesia. These findings were similar to results in other studies centered on different kinds of surgical procedures [87].

TAPENTADOL

Tapentadol is an oral medication with a unique dual mechanism: it is a μ opioid receptor agonist and norepinephrine reuptake inhibitor [88]. It is considered a short-acting, moderate to weak opioid used for acute, chronic, and neuropathic pain, with potency on the order of 18 times weaker than intravenous morphine [89,90]. It has an improved side-effect profile over other opioid receptor agonists with decreased incidence of gastrointestinal and respiratory depression [91].

Tapentadol is partially metabolized by hepatic enzymes CYP2D6, CYP2C9, and CYP2C19 and should be used in caution in hepatic failure or with medications affecting the rate of function of these enzymes [90]. While it does not affect serotonin levels as does tramadol, another opioid with dual mechanism, possible interactions with medications resulting in increased norepinephrine levels, including monoamine oxidase inhibitors (MAOIs), selective serotonin reuptake inhibitors, Serotonin-norepinephrine reuptake inhibitors, and tricyclic antidepressants, warrants judicious use [90].

REFERENCES

1. Lai LT, Ortiz-Cardona JR, Bendo AA. Perioperative pain management in the neurosurgical patient. *Anesthesiol Clin.* 2012;30(2):347–367.

2. Armaghani SJ, Lee DS, Bible JE, et al. Preoperative opioid use and its association with perioperative opioid demand and postoperative opioid independence in patients undergoing spine surgery. *Spine (Phila Pa 1976)*. 2014;39(25):E1524–E1530.

3. Kiraly K, Caputi FF, Hanuska A, et al. A new potent analgesic agent with reduced liability to produce morphine tolerance. *Brain Res Bull*. 2015;117:32–38.

4. Pereira J, Lawlor P, Vigano A, et al. Equianalgesic dose ratios for opioids: a critical review and proposals for long-term dosing. *J Pain Symptom Manage*. 2001;22(2):672–687.

5. Daitch J, Frey ME, Silver D, et al. Conversion of chronic pain patients from full-opioid agonists to sublingual buprenorphine. *Pain Physician*. 2012;15(3 Suppl):ES59–ES66.

6. Natusch D. Equianalgesic doses of opioids—their use in clinical practice. *Pain.Br J Pain*. 2012;6(1):43–46.

7. Reardon DP, Anger KE, Szumita PM. Pathophysiology, assessment, and management of pain in critically ill adults. *Am J Health Syst Pharm*. 2015;72(18):1531–1543.

8. Smith HS, Peppin JF. Toward a systematic approach to opioid rotation. *J Pain Res*. 2014;7:589–608.

9. Nowoczyn M, Marie N, Coulbault L, et al. Remifentanil produces cross-desensitization and tolerance with morphine on the mu-opioid receptor. *Neuropharmacology*. 2013;73:368–379.

10. Butterworth J, Mackey DC, Wasnick J. *Morgan and Mikhail's Clinical Anesthesiology*. 5th ed. New York: McGraw-Hill Education; 2013.

11. Marie N, Aguila B, Allouche S. Tracking the opioid receptors on the way of desensitization. *Cell Signal*. 2006;18(11):1815–1833.

12. Holzer P. New approaches to the treatment of opioid-induced constipation. *Eur Rev Med Pharmacol Sci*. 2008;12(Suppl 1):119–127.

13. Setnik B, Roland CL, Sommerville KW, et al. A multicenter, primary-care-based, open-label study to assess the success of converting opioid-experienced patients with chronic moderate-to-severe pain to morphine sulfate and naltrexone hydrochloride extended-release capsules using a standardized conversion guide. *J Pain Res*. 2015;8:347–360.

14. Patanwala AE, Duby J, Waters D, Erstad BL. Opioid conversions in acute care. *Ann Pharmacother*. 2007;41(2):255–266.

15. Shaheen PE, Walsh D, Lasheen W, et al. Opioid equianalgesic tables: are they all equally dangerous? *J Pain Symptom Manage*. 2009;38(3):409–417.

16. Vissers KC, Besse K, Hans G, et al. Opioid rotation in the management of chronic pain: where is the evidence? *Pain Pract*. 2010;10(2):85–93.

17. Gordon DB, Stevenson KK, Griffie J, et al. Opioid equianalgesic calculations. *J Palliat Med*. 1999;2(2):209–218.

18. Fine PG, Portenoy RK. Establishing "best practices" for opioid rotation: conclusions of an expert panel. *J Pain Symptom Manage*. 2009;38(3):418–425.

19. Hale ME, Nalamachu SR, Khan A, Kutch M. Effectiveness and gastrointestinal tolerability during conversion and titration with once-daily OROS(R) hydromorphone extended release in opioid-tolerant patients with chronic low back pain. *J Pain Res*. 2013;6:319–329.

20. Brant JM. Opioid equianalgesic conversion: the right dose. *Clin J Oncol Nurs*. 2001;5(4):163–165.

21. Knotkova H, Fine PG, Portenoy RK. Opioid rotation: the science and the limitations of the equianalgesic dose table. *J Pain Symptom Manage*. 2009;38(3):426–439.

22. Smith HS. Opioid metabolism. *Mayo Clin Proc*. 2009;84(7):613–624.

23. Peng PW, Sandler AN. A review of the use of fentanyl analgesia in the management of acute pain in adults. *Anesthesiology*. 1999;90(2):576–599.

24. Barash P, et al. *Clinical Anesthesia*. 7th ed. [ebook without multimedia]. Wolters Kluwer Health; 2013.

25. Murray A, Hagen NA. Hydromorphone. *J Pain Symptom Manage*. 2005;29(5 Suppl):S57–S66.

26. Hong D, Flood P, Diaz G. The side effects of morphine and hydromorphone patient-controlled analgesia. *Anesth Analg*. 2008;107(4):1384–1389.

27. Manullang J, Egan TD. Remifentanil's effect is not prolonged in a patient with pseudo-cholinesterase deficiency. *Anesth Analg*. 1999;89(2):529–530.

28. ULTIVA [package insert]. Rockford, IL: Mylan Institutional LLC; 2011.

29. Thomas B. Remifentanil versus fentanyl in total intravenous anesthesia for lumbar spine surgery: a retrospective cohort study. *J Clin Anesth*. 2015;27(5):391–395.

30. Rosow CE. Sufentanil citrate: a new opioid analgesic for use in anesthesia. *Pharmacotherapy*. 1984;4(1):11–19.

31. Wang C, Li Y, Wang H, et al. Inhibition of DOR prevents remifentanil induced postoperative hyperalgesia through regulating the trafficking and function of spinal NMDA receptors in vivo and in vitro. *Brain Res Bull*. 2015;110:30–39.

32. Viviand X, Garnier F. [Opioid anesthetics (sufentanil and remifentanil) in neuro-anaesthesia]. *Ann Fr Anesth Reanim*. 2004;23(4):383–388.

33. Saari TI, Ihmsen H, Mell J, et al. Influence of intensive care treatment on the protein binding of sufentanil and hydromorphone during pain therapy in postoperative cardiac surgery patients. *Br J Anaesth*. 2014;113(4):677–687.

34. Andrianopoulou A, Triandaphillidis A, Bakatselou V, et al. Evaluation of sufentanil as a supplement to anaesthesia in lengthy spinal surgery. *J Int Med Res*. 1994;22(1):40–46.

35. Gepts E, Shafer SL, Camu F, et al. Linearity of pharmacokinetics and model estimation of sufentanil. *Anesthesiology*. 1995;83(6):1194–1204.

36. Gerlach K, Uhlig T, Hüppe M, et al. Remifentanil-propofol versus sufentanil-propofol anaesthesia for supratentorial craniotomy: a randomized trial. *Eur J Anaesthesiol*. 2003;20(10):813–820.

37. Schraag S, Mohl U, Hirsch M, et al. Recovery from opioid anesthesia: the clinical implication of context-sensitive half-times. *Anesth Analg*. 1998;86(1):184–190.

38. Kalkman CJ, Leyssius AT, Bovill JG. Influence of high-dose opioid anesthesia on posterior tibial nerve somatosensory cortical evoked potentials: effects of fentanyl, sufentanil, and alfentanil. *J Cardiothorac Anesth*. 1988;2(6):758–764.

39. Kimovec MA, Koht A, Sloan TB. Effects of sufentanil on median nerve somatosensory evoked potentials. *Br J Anaesth*. 1990;65(2):169–172.

40. Plourde G, Boylan JF. The long-latency auditory evoked potential as a measure of the level of consciousness during sufentanil anesthesia. *J Cardiothorac Vasc Anesth*. 1991;5(6):577–583.

41. Borrissov B, Langeron O, Lille F, et al. Combination of propofol-sufentanil on somatosensory evoked potentials in surgery of the spine [in French]. *Ann Fr Anesth Reanim*. 1995;14(4):326–330.

42. Schwender D, Weninger E, Daunderer M, et al. Anesthesia with increasing doses of sufentanil and midlatency auditory evoked potentials in humans. *Anesth Analg*. 1995;80(3):499–505.

43. Subramanian A, Wanta BT, Fogelson JL, et al. Time to extubation during propofol anesthesia for spine surgery with sufentanil compared with fentanyl: a retrospective cohort study. *Spine (Phila Pa 1976)*. 2014;39(21):1758–1764.

44. Thees C, Scheufler KM, Nadstawek J, et al. Influence of fentanyl, alfentanil, and sufentanil on motor evoked potentials. *J Neurosurg Anesthesiol*. 1999;11(2):112–118.

45. Abrishamkar S, Karimi M, Safavi M, et al. Effects of intraoperative-intrathecal sufentanil injection on postoperative pain management after single level lumbar discectomy. *Middle East J Anaesthesiol.* 2010;20(6):839–844.

46. Melson TI, Boyer DL, Minkowitz HS, et al. Sufentanil sublingual tablet system vs. intravenous patient-controlled analgesia with morphine for postoperative pain control: a randomized, active-comparator trial. *Pain Pract.* 2014;14(8):679–688.

47. Jove M, Griffin DW, Minkowitz HS, et al. Sufentanil sublingual tablet system for the management of postoperative pain after knee or hip arthroplasty: a randomized, placebo-controlled study. *Anesthesiology.* 2015;123(2):434–443.

48. Minkowitz HS, Candiotti K. The role of sublingual sufentanil nanotabs for pain relief. *Expert Opin Drug Deliv.* 2015;12(5):845–851.

49. Ringold FG, Minkowitz HS, Gan TJ, et al. Sufentanil sublingual tablet system for the management of postoperative pain following open abdominal surgery: a randomized, placebo-controlled study. *Reg Anesth Pain Med.* 2015;40(1):22–30.

50. Schenk MR, Putzier M, Kügler B, et al. Postoperative analgesia after major spine surgery: patient-controlled epidural analgesia versus patient-controlled intravenous analgesia. *Anesth Analg.* 2006;103(5):1311–1317.

51. Gupta A, Martindale T, Christo PJ. Intrathecal catheter granuloma associated with continuous sufentanil infusion. *Pain Med.* 2010;11(6):847–852.

52. Udelsmann A, Maciel FG, Servian DC, et al. Methadone and morphine during anesthesia induction for cardiac surgery. Repercussion in postoperative analgesia and prevalence of nausea and vomiting. *Rev Bras Anestesiol.* 2011;61(6):695–701.

53. Stoelting RK, Hillier SC. *Pharmacology and physiology in anesthetic practice.* Philadelphia, PA: Wolters Kluwer Health; 2005.

54. Gottschalk A, Durieux ME, Nemergut EC. Intraoperative methadone improves postoperative pain control in patients undergoing complex spine surgery. *Anesth Analg.* 2011;112(1):218–223.

55. Angst MS, Clark JD. Opioid-induced hyperalgesia: a qualitative systematic review. *Anesthesiology.* 2006;104(3):570–587.

56. Payne R, Inturrisi CE. CSF distribution of morphine, methadone and sucrose after intrathecal injection. *Life Sci.* 1985;37(12):1137–1144.

57. Garrido MJ, Troconiz IF. Methadone: a review of its pharmacokinetic/pharmacodynamic properties. *J Pharmacol Toxicol Methods.* 1999;42(2):61–66.

58. Sharma A, Tallchief D, Blood J, et al. Perioperative pharmacokinetics of methadone in adolescents. *Anesthesiology.* 2011;115(6):1153–1161.

59. Kharasch ED. Intraoperative methadone: rediscovery, reappraisal, and reinvigoration? *Anesth Analg.* 2011;112(1):13–16.

60. Callahan RJ, Au JD, Paul M, et al. Functional inhibition by methadone of N-methyl-D-aspartate receptors expressed in Xenopus oocytes: stereospecific and subunit effects. *Anesth Analg.* 2004;98(3):653–659, table of contents.

61. Lee M, Silverman SM, Hansen H, et al. A comprehensive review of opioid-induced hyperalgesia. *Pain Physician.* 2011;14(2):145–161.

62. Eich-Höchli D, Oppliger R, Golay KP, et al. Methadone maintenance treatment and St. John's Wort—a case report. *Pharmacopsychiatry.* 2003;36(1):35–37.

63. Sjogren P, Jensen NH, Jensen TS. Disappearance of morphine-induced hyperalgesia after discontinuing or substituting morphine with other opioid agonists. *Pain.* 1994;59(2):313–316.

64. Ehret GB, Desmeules JA, Broers B. Methadone-associated long QT syndrome: improving pharmacotherapy for dependence on illegal opioids and lessons learned for pharmacology. *Expert Opin Drug Saf.* 2007;6(3):289–303.

65. Cruciani RA. Methadone: to ECG or not to ECG. That is still the question. *J Pain Symptom Manage.* 2008;36(5):545–552.

66. Stringer J, Welsh C, Tommasello A. Methadone-associated Q-T interval prolongation and torsades de pointes. *Am J Health Syst Pharm.* 2009;66(9):825–833.

67. Modesto-Lowe V, Brooks D, Petry N. Methadone deaths: risk factors in pain and addicted populations. *J Gen Intern Med.* 2010;25(4):305–309.

68. Walker G, Wilcock A, Carey AM, et al. Prolongation of the QT interval in palliative care patients. *J Pain Symptom Manage.* 2003;26(3):855–859.

69. Wilcock A, Beattie JM. Prolonged QT interval and methadone: implications for palliative care. *Curr Opin Support Palliat Care.* 2009;3(4):252–257.

70. Dean M. Opioids in renal failure and dialysis patients. *J Pain Symptom Manage.* 2004;28(5):497–504.

71. Miller RD, Pardo M. *Basics of Anesthesia.* Philadelphia, PA: Elsevier Health Sciences; 2011.

72. Zou Z, An MM, Xie Q, et al. Single dose intra-articular morphine for pain control after knee arthroscopy. *Cochrane Database Syst Rev.* 2016(5):CD008918.

73. Fitzgibbon DR, Ready LB. Drug choices for intravenous and spinal analgesia. *Eur Surg Res.* 1999;31(2):108–111.

74. Bellissant E, Estèbe JP, Sébille V, Ecoffey C. Effect of preoperative oral sustained-release morphine sulfate on postoperative morphine requirements in elective spine surgery. *Fundam Clin Pharmacol.* 2004;18(6):709–714.

75. Klimas R, Mikus G. Morphine-6-glucuronide is responsible for the analgesic effect after morphine administration: a quantitative review of morphine, morphine-6-glucuronide, and morphine-3-glucuronide. *Br J Anaesth.* 2014;113(6):935–944.

76. Wilartratsami S, Sanansilp V, Ariyawatkul T, et al. The effect of epidural low-dose morphine-soaked microfibrillar collagen sponge in postoperative pain control after laminectomy and instrumented fusion: a randomized double-blind placebo-controlled study. *J Med Assoc Thai.* 2014;97(Suppl 9):S62–S67.

77. Zotou A, Siampalioti A, Tagari P, et al. Does epidural morphine loading in addition to thoracic epidural analgesia benefit the postoperative management of morbidly obese patients undergoing open bariatric surgery? A pilot study. *Obes Surg.* 2014;24(12):2099–2108.

78. Karamese M, Akdağ O, Kara İ, et al. The comparison of intrathecal morphine and IV morphine PCA on pain control, patient satisfaction, morphine consumption, and adverse effects in patients undergoing reduction mammoplasty. *Eplasty.* 2015;15:e15.

79. Viscusi ER, Martin G, Hartrick CT, et al. Forty-eight hours of postoperative pain relief after total hip arthroplasty with a novel, extended-release epidural morphine formulation. *Anesthesiology.* 2005;102(5):1014–1022.

80. Sumida S, Lesley MR, Hanna MN, et al. Meta-analysis of the effect of extended-release epidural morphine versus intravenous patient-controlled analgesia on respiratory depression. *J Opioid Manag.* 2009;5(5):301–305.

81. Lugo, RA, Kern SE. Clinical pharmacokinetics of morphine. *J Pain Palliat Care Pharmacother.* 2002;16(4):5–18.

82. Sultan P, Gutierrez MC, Carvalho B. Neuraxial morphine and respiratory depression: finding the right balance. *Drugs.* 2011;71(14):1807–1819.

83. Wilkes D. Programmable intrathecal pumps for the management of chronic pain: recommendations for improved efficiency. *J Pain Res.* 2014;7:571–577.

84. Deer TR, Prager J, Levy R, et al. Polyanalgesic Consensus Conference--2012: consensus on diagnosis, detection, and treatment of catheter-tip granulomas (inflammatory masses). *Neuromodulation.* 2012;15(5):483–495; discussion 496.

85. Ryan KF, Price JW, Warriner CB, Choi PT. Persistent hypothermia after intrathecal morphine: case report and literature review. *Can J Anaesth*. 2012;59(4):384–388.

86. Xenidis M, Pandya N, Hames E. Effects of intrathecal opioid administration on pituitary function. *Pain Med*. 2013;14(11):1741–1744.

87. Paulozzi LJ, Ryan GW. Opioid analgesics and rates of fatal drug poisoning in the United States. *Am J Prev Med*. 2006;31(6):506–511.

88. Fidman B, Norgid A. Role of tapentadol immediate release (Nucynta) in the management of moderate-to-severe pain. *Pharmacy and Therapeutics*. 2010;35(6):330–357.

89. Singh DR, Nag K, Shetti AN, Krishnaveni N. Tapentadol hydrochloride: a novel analgesic. *Saudi J Anaesth*. 2013;7(3):322–326.

90. Tapentadol [CID 9838022]. PubChem: Open Chemistry Database. https://pubchem. ncbi.nlm.nih.gov/compound/Tapentadol

91. Hale M, Upmalis D, Okamoto A, et al. Tolerability of tapentadol immediate release in patients with lower back pain or osteoarthritis of the hip or knee over 90 days: a randomized, double-blind study. *Curr Med Res Opin*. 2009;25(5):1095–1104.

5 Local Anesthetics

Donna-Ann Thomas, Kay Lee, Hassan Rayaz, Sabrina DaCosta

Local anesthetics, if utilized properly, can be a powerful tool in perioperative pain control. They are good adjuvants to traditional modes of anesthesia and analgesia while offering unique qualities of their own. Understanding the pharmacodynamics and pharmacokinetics of local anesthetics allows for utilization in the perioperative period that significantly improves patient pain control as well as their surgical experience.

MECHANISMS OF ACTION OF LOCAL ANESTHETICS

Anatomy of Nerves

Nerves comprise neurons, connective tissues, and vasculature. It is this anatomical structure that must be taken into consideration when performing nerve blocks (Figure 5.1). Local anesthetics inhibit the function of nerves.

Nerves are made up of single cell units called *neurons*. Each neuron is made up of the cell body (also known as the soma) and two different types of functional cellular extensions called the dendrites and the axon. The cell body contains the nucleus and is the coordinating center of the neuron. The dendrites are cellular extensions from the cell body that receive incoming signals. Each cell has several dendrites while having only one axon. The axon comprises the nerve fiber extending from the cell body that delivers outgoing messages. The nerve fiber can be myelinated or unmyelinated. The myelination or lack of myelination of a nerve plays a major role in local anesthetic function [1].

The connective tissue forms the matrix that holds the nerve fibers together. Individual nerve fibers are surrounded by the endoneurium. Each fascicle or group of nerve fibers is surrounded by the perineurium. Finally, the epineurium surrounds groups of fascicles to fill out the rest of the neural sheath [2]. There is vasculature within the fascicles.

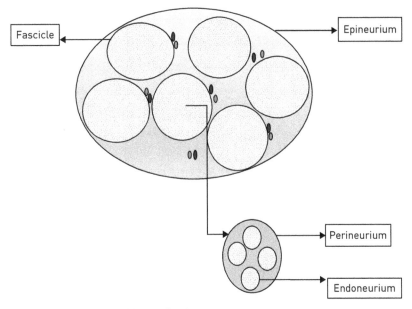

FIGURE 5.1 The anatomy of the peripheral nerve.

Electrophysiology of Neural Conduction and Voltage-Gated Sodium Channels

At the cellular level, the cell membrane creates an environment via active transport in which there are higher levels of extracellular sodium and higher levels of intracellular potassium. The resting membrane potential of these cells is between −60 and −90 mV [3]. When stimulated appropriately with a sufficiently strong enough incoming signal, often via the dendrites, sodium channels open with a net influx of sodium ions into the cell. The net effect of this is that the cell membrane depolarizes (the membrane potential comes closer to zero) and produces an *action potential*, an all-or-nothing response that opens up more sodium channels and increases the number of potassium channels. This influx of sodium ions into the cell and efflux of potassium channels outside of the cell propagate the action potential moving forward through the axon. This is how outgoing messages are transmitted from the neuron [4]. Opening of sodium channels initiates the depolarization needed to ultimately transmit a signal. Blocking these sodium channels is instrumental in blocking signals from neurons that transmit signals of pain.

Molecular Mechanisms of Local Anesthetics

Local anesthetics traverse the cell membrane and bind to sodium channels, rendering them inactive. Local anesthetic molecules cross the lipid bilayer of the cell and bind to an intracellular portion of the sodium channel (i.e., the α subunit). Binding of the α subunit of the sodium channel renders the channel inactive, resulting in no propagation of signal from the neuron. This blockade often occurs at the axon [5].

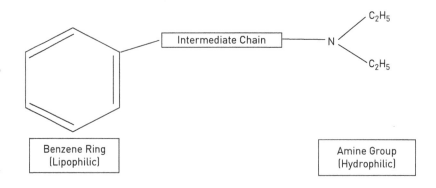

FIGURE 5.2 Local anesthetics have a benzene ring. This benzene ring is lipophilic and linked to an amine group by an intermediate chain. The intermediate chain contains either an amide or an ester which determines the class of the local anesthetic.

Pharmacology and Pharmacodynamics

The chemical properties of local anesthetics have a relationship to their activity and potency. The structure of local anesthetics is comprised of three major portions: the hydrophilic tertiary amine, the lipophilic aromatic moiety (benzene ring), and the linking group that connects them (Figure 5.2). It is this linking group that determines the class of the local anesthetic. The linking group can be an ester or an amide [6].

For the most commonly used local anesthetics, the same principles of pharmacodynamics can be applied to both ester and amide groups. Local anesthetics are weak bases with pKa values greater than 7.4. The pKa value is the pH at which 50% of the medication is ionized and 50% is nonionized and is a major determinant of speed of onset. The closer the pKa value of the local anesthetic is to the pH of the extracellular environment, the faster the onset. The most important determinant of duration of blockade is the lipid solubility. Recall that the local anesthetic molecule must cross the lipid bilayer of the neuron and attach to the intracellular α subunit of the sodium channel in order to inactivate the sodium channel and halt the propagation of signal. The more lipid soluble the local anesthetic molecule is, the easier it is for more molecules to cross the lipid bilayer and gain access to that intracellular α subunit and maintain duration of blockade [7].

Local anesthetics with an ester linking group between the hydrophilic amine and lipophilic aromatic groups make up the *ester* group. Esters as a class can be identified by their generic names, where the generic name of the anesthetic only has one "i" in the word. Tetracaine, for example, is an ester local anesthetic, whereas lidocaine is an amide local anesthetic (two "i's" in the name). Ester local anesthetics are metabolized by plasma cholinesterase in the bloodstream. They are metabolized to alcohol and para-aminobenzoic acid (PABA). It is this PABA derivative that is more likely to cause allergic reactions in patients.

Local anesthetics with an *amide* linking group between the hydrophilic amine and lipophilic aromatic groups make up the amide group. They are metabolized by the liver. As just mentioned, local anesthetic generic names with two "i's" in the word are part of the amide group (e.g., lidocaine) [8]. Tables 5.1–5.3 show the properties and uses of commonly used esters and amides.

Table 5.1 Ester local anesthetics

Drug	pKa	Concentration (%)	Maximum dose (mg/kg)	Location	Onset	Duration (min)
Benzocaine	3.5	<20%	Not Available (max 200 mg total)	Topical	Slow	30–60
Chloroprocaine	9.1	1	12	Infiltration	Fast	30–60
		2	12	PNB	Fast	30–60
		2–3	12 (max 800 mg or 1,000 mg with epi total)	Epidural	Fast	30–60
Cocaine	8.6	4–10	3 (max 150 mg total)	Topical	Fast	30–60
Procaine	8.9	10	12 (max 1,000 mg total)	Spinal	Fast	30–60
Tetracaine	8.4	0.5	3	Topical	FastFast	30–60
			3 (max 20 mg total)	Spinal		120–360

Reference 34.

PNB, peripheral nerve block.

Speed of local anesthetic onset is affected by (1) pKa (lower resulting in faster onset), (2) lipid solubility (higher solubility resulting in slower onset), and (3) higher concentration plus the total dose of local anesthetic (results in a faster onset due to increase solution concentration creating a diffuse gradient). Duration of local anesthetic is affected by (1) protein binding (increased protein binding results in a longer duration), (2) lipid solubility, and (3) plasma esterase deficiency for ester anesthetics.

Additives

Vasoconstrictors can be used to prolong the duration of blockade. Vasoconstriction at the site of the local anesthetic injection can decrease uptake and metabolism of the local anesthetic, thus prolonging duration. *Epinephrine* is the most commonly used vasoconstrictor. Epinephrine concentrations of 1:400,000 to 1:200,000 can be used [9], with the 1:400,000 concentration possibly causing some vasodilation of the neural vasculature instead of vasoconstriction, thereby avoiding compromise of blood flow to the nerves themselves [10].

Less than 3% of the commercially prepared local anesthetic exists as the lipid-soluble neutral form. The neutral form is important for penetration into the neural cytoplasm, whereas the charged form interacts with the local anesthetic receptor within the sodium channel. The alkalinization of the local anesthetics increases the ratio of

Table 5.2 Amide local anesthetics

Drug	pKa	Concentration (%)	Maximum dose (mg/kg)	Location	Onset	Duration (min)
Bupivacaine	8.1	0.25	3 (max 175 mg/225 mg with epi total)	Infiltration	Fast	120–480
		0.5–0.75	3 (max 150 mg total)	Epidural	Moderate	120–300
		0.25–0.5	3 (max 150 mg total)	PNB	Slow	240–720
		0.5–0.75	3 (max 20 mg total)	Spinal	Fast	60–240
Lidocaine	7.8	0.5–1	7 with epi	Infiltration	Fast	60–240
		1.5–2	7 with epi	Epidural	Fast	60–120
		0.25–0.5	7 with epi	IV Regional	Fast	30–60
		1–1.5	7 with epi	PNB	Fast	120–180
		1.5–5	7 with epi	Spinal	Fast	30–60
		4	7 with epi	Topical	Fast	30–60
			4.5 without epi			
			(Max 300 mg without epi. total. Max 500 mg with epi total)			
Mepivacaine	7.6	0.5–1	7 with epi	Infiltration	Fast	60–240
		1.5–2	7 with epi	Epidural	Fast	60–180
		1–1.5	7 with epi	PNB	Fast	120–240
		2–4		Spinal	Fast	60–120
			(Max 400 mg total /500 mg with epi total) (100 mg Max for Spinal total)			

Agent	pKa	Concentration (%)	Max dose (mg/kg)	Route	Onset	Duration (min)
Prilocaine	7.9	0.5–1	8	Infiltration	Fast	60–120
		2–3	8	Epidural	Fast	60–180
		0.25–5	8	IV Regional	Fast	30–60
		1.5–2	8 (Max 600 mg total)	PNB	Fast	90–180
Ropivacaine	8.2	0.2–0.5	3 (Max 200 mg total)	Infiltration	Fast	120–360
			3 (Max 200 mg total)	Epidural	Moderate	120–360
			3 (Max 250 mg total)	PNB	Slow	300–480

Reference 34.

PNB, peripheral nerve block.

Speed of local anesthetic onset is affected by (1) pKa (lower resulting in faster onset), (2) lipid solubility (higher solubility resulting in slower onset), and (3) higher concentration plus the total dose of local anesthetic (results in a faster onset due to increase solution concentration creating a diffuse gradient).

Duration of local anesthetic is affected by (1) protein binding (increased protein binding results in a longer duration), (2) lipid solubility, and (3) liver disease will increase duration of amide anesthetics.

Prilocaine at greater than 600 mg can cause methemoglobinemia.

Table 5.3 Uses for local anesthetics

Chemical class	Local anesthetic	Site	Metabolism
Esters	Cocaine	Topical	Hepatic carboxyl-esterase
	Chloroprocaine (Nesacaine)	Epidural Infiltration PNB	Plasma esterases
	Benzocaine (Americaine)	Topical	
	Procaine (Novocain)	Infiltration	
	Tetracaine (Pontocaine)	Spinal	
Amides	Bupivacaine (Marcaine)	Epidural Infiltration PNB Spinal	Hepatic cytochrome P450-linked enzymes
	Dibucaine (Nupericaine)	Spinal	
	Lidocaine (Xylocaine)	EpiduralInfiltration PNB Spinal	
	Meplvacaine (Carbocaine)	EpiduralInfiltration PNB	
	Prilocaine (Citanest)	EpiduralInfiltration PNB	
	Ropivacaine (Naropin)	EpiduralInfiltration PNB	

Reference 34.

PNB, peripheral nerve block.

local anesthetic existing as the lipid-soluble neutral form and shortens the onset time of the local anesthetic blockade.

Opioids have multiple central and peripheral mechanisms of analgesic action. Addition of opioids to central neuraxial local anesthetics results in synergistic analgesia [11] with exception of chloroprocaine, which proved to decrease the effectiveness of opioids co-administered epidurally [12].

α2-Specific agonists such as clonidine produce analgesia via supraspinal and spinal adrenergic receptors [13]. Clonidine also has direct inhibitory effects on peripheral nerve conduction [14]. Studies show that clonidine improves the duration of analgesia by about 2 hours, both with intermediate and long-acting local anesthetic via either neuraxial or peripheral nerve blocks [15].

Dexamethasone, a steroid, combined with intermediate to long-acting local anesthetics, increases the duration of analgesia by approximately 50% for peripheral nerve blocks [16]. However, its mechanism of action and potential side effects are not fully understood yet.

PHARMACOKINETICS OF LOCAL ANESTHETICS

The administered dose of local anesthetics and the rates of systemic absorption, tissue distribution, and drug elimination determine the plasma concentration of the local anesthetic. Elevated concentrations can have undesirable effects on other electric-sensitive systems, such as the cardiovascular system and the central nervous system (CNS).

Systemic Absorption

The site of injection, the dose, the drug's intrinsic pharmacokinetic properties, and the addition of a vasoactive agent determine the rate of local anesthetic system absorption.

The vascularity of the tissue plays the major role in determining the rate of drug absorption. Local anesthetics deposited in vessel-rich tissues will achieve higher peak plasma levels faster. Thus, the rate of systemic absorption is greatest with *intercostal* nerve blocks, followed by *caudal* and *epidural* injections, *brachial plexus* block, and *femoral* and *sciatic* nerve blocks in decreasing order.

The rate of systemic absorption and the peak plasma level are directly proportional to the dose of local anesthetic at a given site of injection. This relationship is nearly linear and independent of the drug concentration and the speed of injection [17].

The rate of systemic absorption varies with individual local anesthetics. Lipid solubility determines both the potency and the duration of action of local anesthetics by facilitating their transfer through membranes and binding the drug close to the site of action. This transfer decreases the rate of metabolism by plasma esterase and liver enzymes. In general, more potent, lipid-soluble agents are associated with a slower rate of absorption than are less lipid-soluble agents.

At low concentrations, the rate of vascular absorption of more potent agents is lower than less potent agents because they cause more vasoconstriction [18]. At high concentrations, vasodilatory effects predominate for most local anesthetics.

Distribution

Systemically absorbed local anesthetics are rapidly distributed throughout the body. However, different local anesthetic concentrations are seen among organ systems. The distribution pattern is determined by organ perfusion, the partition coefficient between compartments, and plasma protein binding [19]. Well-perfused organs, such as the heart and the brain, have higher drug concentrations and subsequently are more prone to local anesthetic toxicity.

Elimination

The chemical property of local anesthetics determines the metabolic pathway for clearance. Aminoesters are hydrolyzed by plasma cholinesterases. Aminoamides are transformed by hepatic carboxylesterases and cytochrome P450 enzymes. The clearance of aminoamide local anesthetics can be delayed in severe liver disease, and, subsequently, significant drug levels may accumulate [20].

Clinical Pharmacokinetics

By understanding the pharmacokinetics of local anesthetics, one can predict the peak plasma level and subsequently avoid the toxic dose administration.

The correlation of systemic plasma levels between the dose of local anesthetic and weight is often inconsistent [21]. The effect of gender on clinical pharmacokinetics of local anesthetics is not well defined [22], but pregnancy may decrease clearance [23].

Cardiac and hepatic diseases will alter expected pharmacokinetic parameters of local anesthetics; thus, lower doses of local anesthetics should be used. On the other hand, renal disease has little effect on pharmacokinetic parameters.

CLINICAL USE OF LOCAL ANESTHETICS

A eutectic mixture of lidocaine and prilocaine can be applied topically to skin to alleviate the sharp, painful sensation associated with needle insertions. Most commonly, local infiltration of the dermis with lidocaine or bupivacaine can provide quick onset anesthesia appropriate for minor, superficial procedures.

A regional anatomic approach of local anesthetics can provide a wider and greater coverage area. *Bier block*, or intravenous administration of local anesthetics to a limb under pneumatic compression, can accomplish anesthesia and analgesia specific to that limb. Peripheral nerve blocks, or direct application of local anesthetics to a set of nerves or to the plexus, such as brachial or lumbar plexus, can accomplish anesthesia and analgesia in the distribution of those nerves. Local anesthetics also can be deposited centrally near the nerve roots, either intrathecally in the lumbar cistern or epidurally in the cervical, thoracic, lumbar, and caudal regions of the spine.

The duration of anesthesia and analgesia with local anesthetics can be extended with continuous infusion via an indwelling catheter.

TOXICITY OF LOCAL ANESTHETICS

Local anesthetics readily cross the blood–brain barrier and can cause CNS toxicity. At low plasma concentrations, mild sensory disturbances, such as tinnitus, blurred vision, dizziness, tongue paresthesia, or circumoral numbness are observed. At high concentration, CNS excitatory and seizure activities predominate. At very high concentration or with rapid increase, this may progress to generalized CNS depression and coma, followed by respiratory depression and arrest [24].

Cardiovascular toxicity is seen at a higher plasma concentration than that for CNS toxicity. Hypotension; dysrhythmias, such as prolongation of PR interval and QRS complex duration; and myocardial depression are seen initially with all local anesthetics. However, more potent agents such as bupivacaine and ropivacaine have been associated with devastating outcomes such as fatal cardiovascular collapse and complete heart block [25].

Box 5.1 Local Anesthetic Systemic Toxicity (LAST)

The LAST pharmacologic treatment is different from other cardiac arrest scenarios:
- Get Help
- Initial Focus
  - Airway management: ventilate with 100% oxygen
  - Seizure suppression: benzodiazepines are preferred; AVOID propofol in patients having signs of cardiovascular instability
  - Alert the nearest facility having cardiopulmonary bypass capability
- Management of Cardiac Arrhythmias
  - Basic and Advanced Cardiac Life Support (ACLS) will require adjustment of medications and perhaps prolonged effort
  - AVOID vasopressin, calcium channel blockers, β-blockers, or local anesthetic
  - REDUCE epinephrine dose to <1 µg/kg
- Lipid Emulsion (20%) Therapy
  - Bolus 1.5 mL/kg (lean body mass) intravenously over 1 minute
  - Continuous infusion 0.25 mL/kg/min
  - Repeat bolus once or twice for persistent cardiovascular collapse
  - Double the infusion rate to 0.5 mL/kg/min if blood pressure remains low
  - Continue infusion for at least10 minutes after attaining circulatory stability
  - Recommended upper limit: Approximately 10 mL/kg lipid emulsion over the first 30 minutes
- Post LAST events at www.lipidrescue.org and report use of lipid to www.lipidregistry.org

In treating systemic toxicity from local anesthetics, lipid emulsion may act as a plasma "sink" to absorb tissue-bound local anesthetics [26]. The American Society of Regional Anesthesia and Pain Medicine has published a checklist for treatment of Local Anesthetic Systemic Toxicity (LAST). See Box 5.1 [27].

Local anesthetics also can cause histopathologic changes consistent with neuronal injuries on nerve fibers directly. Intrafascicular injections result in more histologic changes than either extrafascicular or extraneural injections [28]. In large concentrations, all local anesthetics can produce dose-dependent damage, but in clinically relevant concentrations, they appear generally safe [29].

Transient neurologic symptoms (TNS), such as pain or sensory abnormalities in lower back, buttocks, or lower extremities, are mainly seen after lidocaine spinal anesthesia with incidences of 4–40%. This phenomena can also be seen with other local anesthetics [30]. However, TNS has not resulted in permanent neurologic injury, and there is no clear dose relation to TNS [31]. Lidocaine, the lithotomy position, and ambulatory anesthesia are associated with increased risk of TNS [32].

Local anesthetics can cause histopathologic changes in skeletal muscles and subsequent muscle pain and dysfunction clinically. However, most myotoxic injuries are subclinical and appear entirely reversible [33] [rue immunologic reactions to local anesthetics are rare. The majority of hypersensitivity reactions are seen with aminoester agents, most likely due to their metabolism to PABA. Also, preservatives, such as methylparaben and metabisulfite, seen in many local anesthetic preparations can trigger allergic reactions.

REFERENCES

1. Lin Y, Liu S. Local anesthetics. In: Barash P, ed. *Clinical Anesthesia*. 7th ed. Philadelphia, PA: Lippincott William and Wilkins; 2013.
2. Hadzic A, Franco C. Essential regional anesthesia anatomy. In: Hadzic A, ed. *Hadzic's Peripheral Nerve Blocks and Anatomy for Ultrasound-Guided Regional Anesthesia*. 2nd ed. New York: McGraw Hill; 2012:3–28.
3. Scholz A. Mechanism of anaesthetics on voltage-gated sodium and other ion channels. *Br J Anaesth*. 2002;89:52–61.
4. Gadsden J. Local anesthetics: clinical pharmacology and rational selection. In: Hadzic A, ed. *Hadzic's Peripheral Nerve Blocks and Anatomy for Ultrasound-Guided Regional Anesthesia*. 2nd ed. New York: McGraw Hill; 2012:29–40.
5. Maheshwari K, Naguib M. Local Anesthetics. In *Stoelting's Pharmacology & Physiology in Anesthetic Practice*. 5th ed. Philadelphia, PA: Wolters Kluwer; 2015:282–313.
6. Horlocker T. Local Anesthetic agents: pharmacology. In: *Faust's Anesthesiology Review*. 4th ed. Canada: Elsevier Saunders; 2015:269–271.
7. Gadsden J. Local anesthetics: clinical pharmacology and rational selection. In: Hadzic A, ed. *Hadzic's Peripheral Nerve Blocks and Anatomy for Ultrasound-Guided Regional Anesthesia*. 2nd ed. New York: McGraw Hill; 2012:29–40.
8. Maheshwari K, Naguib M. Local anesthetics. In: *Stoelting's Pharmacology & Physiology in Anesthetic Practice*. 5th ed. Philadelphia, PA: Wolters Kluwer; 2015:282–313.
9. Maheshwari K, Naguib M. Local anesthetics. In: *Stoelting's Pharmacology & Physiology in Anesthetic Practice*. 5th ed. Philadelphia, PA: Wolters Kluwer; 2015:282–313.
10. Neal JM. Effects of epinephrine in local anesthetics on the central and peripheral nervous systems: neurotoxicity and neural blood flow. *Reg Anesth Pain Med*. 2003;28:124–134.
11. Walker SM, Goudas LC, Cousins MJ, et al. Combination spinal analgesic chemotherapy: a systematic review. *Anesth Analg*. 2002;95:674. [PMID:12198058]
12. Karambelkar DJ, Ramanathan S. 2-chloroprocaine antagonism of epidural morphine analgesia. *Acta Anaesth Scand*. 1997;41:774. [PMID:9241341]
13. Eisenach JC, De Kock M, Klimscha W. Alpha(2)-adrenergic agonists for regional anesthesia: a clinical review of clonidine (1984–1995). *Anesthesiology*. 1996;85:655. [PMID:8853097]
14. Butterworth JF, Strichartz GR. The α2-adrenergic agonists clonidine and guanfacine produce tonic and phasic block of conduction in rat sciatic nerve fibers. *Anesth Analg*. 1993;76:295. [PMID:8093828]
15. Popping DM, Elia N, Marret, et al. Clonidine as an adjuvant to local anesthetics for peripheral nerve and plexus blocks. *Anesthesiology*. 2009;111:406. [PMID:19602964]
16. Parrington SJ, O'Donnell DO, Chan V, et al. Dexamethasone added to mepivacaine prolongs the duration of analgesia after supraclavicular brachial plexus blockade. *Reg Anesth Pain Med*. 2010;35:422. [PMID:20814282]
17. Morrison LM, Emanuelsson BM, McClure JH, et al. Efficacy and kinetics of extradural ropivacaine: comparison with bupivacaine. *Br J Anaesth*. 1994;72:164. [PMID:8110567]
18. Johns RA, Seyde WC, DiFazio CA, et al. Dose-dependent effects of bupivacaine on rat muscle arterioles. *Anesthesiology*. 1986;65:186. [PMID:3740507]
19. Tucker GT, Mather LE. Pharmacology of local anaesthetic agents. Pharmacokinetics of local anaesthetic agents. *Br J Anaesth*. 1975;47(Suppl):213. [PMID:1148097]

20. Thomson PD, Melmon KL, Richardson JA, et al. Lidocaine pharmacokinetics in advanced heart failure, liver disease, and renal failure in humans. *Ann Intern Med.* 1973;78:499. [PMID:4694036]

21. Braid DP, Scott DB. Dosage of lignocaine in epidural block in relation to toxicity. *Br J Anaesth.* 1996;38:596. [PMID:5917224]

22. Adinoff B, Devous Sr MD, Best SE, et al. Gender differences in limbic responsiveness, by SPECT, following pharmacologic challenge in healthy subjects. *Neuroimage.* 2003;18:697. [PMID:12667847]

23. Tucker GT, Mather LE. Properties, absorption, and disposition of local anesthetic agents. In: Cousins MJ, Bridenbaugh PO, eds. *Neural Blockade in Clinical Anesthesia and Management of Pain.* 3rd ed. Philadelphia, PA: Lippincott-Raven Publishers; 1998:55.

24. Groban L. Central nervous system and cardiac effects from long-acting amide local anesthetic toxicity in the intact animal model. *Reg Anesth Pain Med.* 2003;28:3.

25. Butterworth JF. Models and mechanisms of local anesthetic cardiac toxicity. *Reg Anesth Pain Med.* 2010;35:167. [PMID:20301823]

26. Weinberg GL, Ripper R, Murphy P, et al. Lipid infusion accelerates removal of bupivacaine and recovery from bupivacaine toxicity in the isolated rat heart. *Reg Anesth Pain Med.* 2006;31:296. [PMID:16857549]

27. Neal JM, Bernards CM, Butterworth JF, et al. ASRA practice advisory on local anesthetic systemic toxicity. *Reg Anesth Pain Med.* 2010;35:152–161.

28. Whitlock EL, Brenner MJ, Fox IK, et al. Ropivacaine-induced peripheral nerve injection injury in the rodent model. *Anesth Analg.* 2010;111:214. [PMID:20442258]

29. Selander D. Neurotoxicity of local anesthetics: animal data. *Reg Anesth.* 1993;18:461. [PMID:8110648]

30. Zaric D, Christiansen C, Pace NL, et al. Transient neurologic symptoms after spinal anesthesia with lidocaine versus other local anesthetics: a systematic review of randomized, controlled trials. *Anesth Analg.* 2005;100:1811. [PMID:15920219]

31. Pollock JE, Liu SS, Neal JM, et al. Dilution of lidocaine does not decrease the incidence of transient neurologic symptoms. *Anesthesiology.* 1999;90:445. [PMID:9952151]

32. Pollock JE. Transient neurologic symptoms: etiology, risk factors, and management. *Reg Anesth Pain Med.* 2002;27:581. [PMID:12430108]

33. Zink W, Bohl JRE, Hacke N, et al. The long term myotoxic effects of bupivacaine and ropivacaine after continuous peripheral nerve blocks. *Anesth Analg.* 2005;101:548. [PMID:16037174]

34. Lin Y, Liu S. Local anesthetics. In: Barash P, ed. *Clinical Anesthesia.* 7th ed. Philadelphia, PA: Lippincott William and Wilkins; 2013.

6 Susceptibility of Peripheral Nerves in Diabetes to Compression and Implications in Pain Treatment

Natalia Murinova and Daniel Krashin

INTRODUCTION

Diabetes is a major cause of morbidity and mortality in the developed world, affecting 7% of the adult population in the United States in 2012 [1]. The prevalence of diabetes has increased in almost every nation, with a quadrupling overall of diabetes since 1980 (see Figure 6.1) [2]. The director of the World Health Organization has called the explosive growth of obesity and diabetes a "slow motion disaster"[3]. This great impact on world health is due to two factors: the sharply increasing rate of diabetes and the greatly increased direct and indirect burden associated with the diagnosis of diabetes because diabetics require expenditures on average 2.3 times higher than their nondiabetic peers [1]. This problem will only increase if current trends continue, with diabetes rates in the United States as high as one in three adults by 2050 according to one forecast [4]. So far, attempts to slow or reverse these trends through public health policy and individual initiatives have had limited effect.

Among the many detrimental effects of diabetes on the human body, one of the most significant in terms of quality of life is diabetic neuropathy. This neuropathy, which typically takes the form of a peripheral length-related neuropathy that starts in the feet and later affects the legs, hands, and arms, causes many problems, including chronic burning pain which is often worse at night and is often poorly responsive

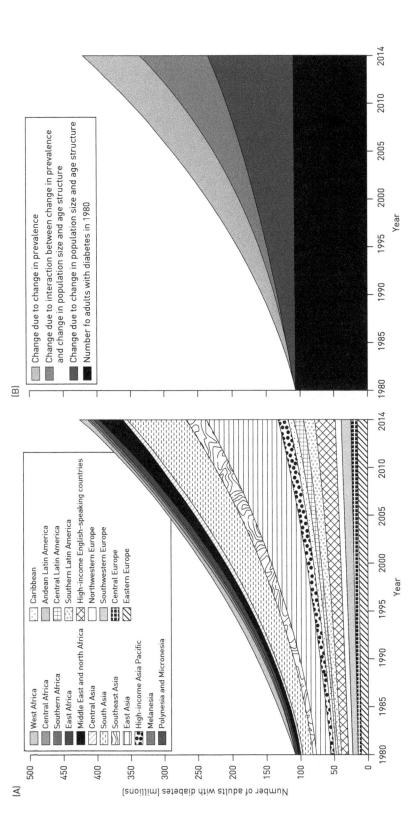

FIGURE 6.1 Trends in the number of adults with diabetes by region (A) and decomposed into the contributions of population growth and aging, rise in prevalence, and interaction between the two (B). NCD Risk Factor Collaboration. Worldwide trends in diabetes since 1980: a pooled analysis of 751 population-based studies with 4.4 million participants. *The Lancet* 2016;387(10027):1513–1530. This image released for free reuse under a Creative Commons License.

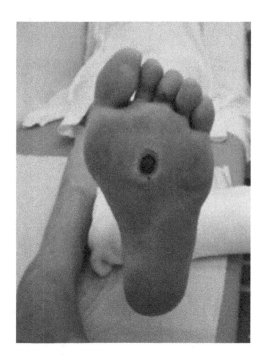

FIGURE 6.2 Foot ulcer associated with diabetic neuropathy. Image courtesy of Wikipedia (https://sr.wikipedia.org/wiki/Hronična_rana#/media/File:Neuropatski_ulkus.JPG) and made freely available under a Creative Commons License.

to neuropathic medications. This neuropathy also contributes to foot injury by worsening motor control and impairing sensation, leading to chronic foot ulcers and infection, and, in later life, frequently to amputation (see Figure 6.2). It is estimated that there is a 25% cumulative risk of lower extremity amputation in patients with diabetic peripheral neuropathy [5]. The decreased sensation also causes functional deficits, which increase fall risks in the elderly and make many everyday tasks of living more difficult.

It has generally been assumed that this progressive neuropathy is primarily due to the underlying metabolic disturbances in diabetes and that little can be done other than to provide tight blood sugar control. However, tight glycemic control has significant risks associated with hypoglycemic episodes and may not be very effective in type 2 diabetes [6]. An alternative hypothesis suggests that at least a portion of the neuropathic symptoms that are so common in diabetes represent increased susceptibility to compressive neuropathy [7]. This hypothesis has received only limited study to date but opens up an exciting new understanding of diabetic neuropathy if confirmed and also raises the possibility of entirely novel treatment approaches being used to treat severe diabetic neuropathy. Decompression of the entrapped nerve would, according to the hypothesis, relieve at least part of the neuropathy, relieving pain and restoring nerve function. This may prevent further complications such as foot ulcers, osteomyelitis, and amputation, as well as decreasing falls and secondary fractures. As this topic is being actively researched and is somewhat controversial, this chapter will seek to present the evidence that supports and contradicts this hypothesis, along with experimental and clinical study information relevant to the topic.

PATHOPHYSIOLOGY OF DIABETIC NEUROPATHY WITH RELEVANCE TO COMPRESSION NEUROPATHY

Diabetes causes a host of metabolic derangements beyond the basic concepts of insulin resistance, pancreatic dysfunction, and elevated blood glucose. However, the chronically elevated blood glucose does play a major role in neurotoxicity, and closer glucose control does appear to improve, though not reverse, diabetic neuropathy, particularly in type 1 diabetes [6]. We will review the most relevant mechanisms here.

The high glucose level leads to increased synthesis of sorbitol via the aldose reductase pathway (the polyol pathway). This has been implicated in the pathogenesis of microvascular disease and neuropathy, and aldose reductase inhibitors may be a promising treatment in diabetic neuropathy as well [8]. Sorbitol is hyperosmotic, causing nerve diameter to increase, which can raise the risk of compression in anatomically narrow areas such the carpal, cubital, or tarsal tunnels [9,10].

Second, axonal transport of nutrients and proteins is affected in diabetes, which impairs neuronal repair efforts during and after nerve compression [11].

The third mechanism is glycation. High serum glucose concentrations result in glucose binding to many components of peripheral nerves, from basement membrane collagen to nerve cell membranes, endovascular linings, and axon cytoskeletons. This results in impaired neural function, microangiopathy, and reduced regenerative capacity. Advanced glycation end-products (AGE) activate the AGE receptor, which further causes oxidative stress to the peripheral nerve. This process of glycation also makes the nerves and support structures more mechanically stiff, increasing their vulnerability to compression and shear forces [12].

ANIMAL MODELS FOR DIABETIC NEUROPATHY AND COMPRESSION

The hypothesis of increased vulnerability to compression neuropathy in diabetes developed from the earlier *double-crush hypothesis*. This hypothesis, which has been largely confirmed experimentally and clinically, states that a nerve suffering proximal injury will be more prone to developing compression injury at a distal point. The classic example of this double-crush phenomenon is the coexistence of either carpal tunnel syndrome or cubital tunnel (ulnar neuropathy at the elbow) with cervical radiculopathy. This was initially proposed by Upton in a paper from 1973 describing that, in 115 subjects with either carpal tunnel or cubital tunnel syndrome, 81 were found to have proximal nerve lesions [13]. Upton suggested that this association was related to "constraints of axoplasmic flow" in the affected neurons.

Nerve compression has been studied in vivo in rats using a Silastic band to squeeze the rat sciatic nerve as a model for chronic nerve compression [14]. Researchers found that a single band that tightly fit, but did not compress, the sciatic nerve did not seem to effect neurophysiology; however, when a second noncompressive band was placed either distally or proximally over the same nerve, nerve conduction diminished rapidly [15]. Using this model, the team proceeded to examine the effects of nerve banding in rats treated with streptozotocin, the standard animal model for diabetic neuropathy [16]. This showed rats with induced diabetes had nerves that were more susceptible to compression than controls.

CLINICAL ASSOCIATION OF DIABETES WITH NERVE COMPRESSION

Electrodiagnostic abnormalities are very common in diabetes. A large study of more than 1,300 diabetic subjects found abnormal peroneal nerve conduction study results in 75%; among asymptomatic subjects, the rate was 66%, with 45% having bilateral abnormalities [17]. In a Canadian study comparing the prevalence of clinical carpal tunnel syndrome and abnormal electrodiagnostic findings in controls and diabetics, the rate of carpal tunnel was 2% in the reference population, 14% in diabetics without peripheral neuropathy, and 30% in those with diabetic neuropathy [18]. However, electrodiagnostic testing alone was not able to distinguish patients with clinical carpal tunnel syndrome from those without.

High-resolution ultrasonography of diabetic patients with neuropathy demonstrated increased nerve cross-section at both compression and noncompression sites. Interestingly, in some cases, posterior tibial nerve swelling was observed consistent with neuropathic symptoms despite normal electrodiagnostic findings [19]. Another study of lower extremity nerve ultrasound in diabetic peripheral neuropathy found that ultrasound findings such as diameter or echogenicity could not distinguish diabetic peripheral neuropathy patients from controls and were not correlated with abnormal electrodiagnostic results [20].

In a recent study of 63 patients with diabetes, 28 had symptomatic carpal tunnel syndrome, but an additional 19 had abnormal findings consistent with carpal tunnel syndrome even though they were asymptomatic [21]. Therefore, the diagnosis of neuropathy remains clinical since neither imaging nor electrodiagnostic testing can provide a gold standard of objective diagnosis.

DIAGNOSTIC APPROACH

The Tinel sign has been suggested as a key indicator of neuropathy as its presence is correlated with axonal compromise, demyelination, and increased irritability [22]. In the specific context of carpal tunnel syndrome, the Tinel sign, along with the Phalen sign, have been found to be highly sensitive, particularly in the setting of paresthesias [23]. A study by Dellon et al. reported that the Tinel sign over the tarsal tunnel was predictive of both pain relief and improved sensation after decompression surgery of the tibial nerve in diabetic patients [24]. The clinical improvement in this study was robust, with mean pain ratings on the visual analog scale (VAS) declining from 8.5 to 2.0. However, in a more recent study, the Tinel sign was not been found to be reliable in the diagnosis of compressive neuropathies according to electrodiagnostic criteria in the lower extremities, with low sensitivity and specificity [25]. This study examined multiple possible compressive sites in each subject without clinically diagnosed neuropathy and used electrodiagnostic criteria as endpoints instead of clinical outcomes; these differences make it very difficult to compare the two studies.

This study found that neuropathy symptom scores were highly correlated with the overall number of Tinel signs evoked out of a possible 18 sites of likely nerve compression [26]. The correlation and number of Tinel signs evoked was much lower in patients not reporting neuropathy symptoms.

ANIMAL MODELS OF DECOMPRESSIVE SURGERY FOR DIABETIC NEUROPATHY

Diabetic neuropathy can be studied in rats using streptozotocin-induced diabetes and observing effects on behavior and gait. Diabetic rats with very high blood glucose were found to have characteristic abnormalities of gait which resolved with normalization of blood sugar; using this as a model, decompressive surgery was performed on a group of rats with induced diabetes, and they were found not to develop the characteristic gait abnormalities [27,28]. Decompression of the sciatic and peroneal nerves in another study using rats bred to develop diabetes likewise found that this procedure prevented the development of sensory and motor changes that would otherwise occur in this breed [29].

A study using a standard method for assessing pain response in rats compared hindfoot withdrawal response to heat in rats with experimentally induced diabetes after sciatic nerve compression with Silastic bands and after the band was removed. The response time to heat increased during the compressive phase of the experiment and decreased after decompression again [30]. An experiment using a very similar paradigm compared nondiabetic rats with sciatic nerve compression and either early or hypersensitivity and thermal hyperalgesia during compression of the nerve, which resolved in both experimental arms after decompression, but more quickly and completely in the group that had the shorter compression period [31].

SURGERY FOR COMPRESSIVE AND DIABETIC NEUROPATHY IN THE LOWER EXTREMITIES

Tarsal tunnel syndrome results from compression of the tibial nerve in the tarsal tunnel formed by the flexor retinaculum on the medial side of the foot. This results in pain behind the medial malleolus radiating to the arch and plantar foot, often associated with numbness and painful paresthesias [32].

Dellon and his surgical group have advocated decompressive surgery that opens not only the tarsal tunnel, but also the distal tunnels (medial, plantar, and the calcaneal), and also stipulate that the patient must ambulate early after surgery to prevent scarring and adhesions of the newly decompressed nerve [33]. He also recommends decompressing the peroneal nerve at two sites: the deep peroneal nerve between the first and second metatarsal heads and the common peroneal nerve below the fibular head. This procedure is sometimes called *Dellon triple surgery.*

ANALYSES OF DECOMPRESSION SURGERY FOR DIABETIC NEUROPATHY

The American Association for Neurology (AAN) issued a practice advisory regarding decompression surgery for diabetic neuropathy in 2006, reporting that this treatment modality should be considered *U* (Unproven) until more high-quality evidence is amassed [34]. The Cochrane Collaboration also published a review of decompressive surgery for symmetrical lower extremity polyneuropathy in diabetes in 2008 by some of the same authors and came to a similar conclusion [34]. The AAN discussion suggests that surgery should be reserved for those cases where focal neuropathy (i.e., chronic nerve compression at a specific site) can be demonstrated with electrodiagnostic studies. However, studies have suggested that nerve compression cannot be reliably diagnosed by electrodiagnostic criteria in the setting of diabetes, as noted in the carpal tunnel study referred to previously [18].

Observational studies have been done showing improved outcomes after decompression in many areas, including low incidence of ulceration, amputation, and hospitalization in treated patients over a prolonged period, compared to other published diabetic cohorts [35]. A more recent analysis of 10 observational studies suggests that decompression surgery appears to improve the symptoms and natural history of compressive neuropathies in diabetic patients [36].

A Chinese observational study of 560 diabetic patients who underwent decompression surgery found healing of existing surface ulcers and no development of new ulcers at 18-month follow-up, no amputations, and improvements in nerve conduction, quantitative sensory testing, and two-point discrimination [37]. Another observational study examined 560 patients with diabetic peripheral neuropathy who underwent Dellon nerve decompression surgery. Postoperative patients showed significant improvements in multiple areas, including nerve conduction, quantitative sensory testing, nerve cross-section on ultrasound, and Toronto clinical scoring system ratings for neuropathy [38].

Multiple randomized controlled trials are currently under way to further assess and define the benefits of decompression surgery. The first randomized controlled trial study to be published, the Lower Extremity Nerve Entrapment Study (LENS), randomized diabetic patients with lower extremity painful neuropathy and Tinel sign at an anatomic compression to four-site nerve decompression in one leg, with the other leg used as control [39]. Visual analogue scale ratings of pain dropped in the treated leg from a mean of 6.5 to 3.5. The pain improvement was maintained at 1 year, although ratings in the monofilament test and two-point discrimination test of sensation were not significantly improved. An additional study performed as part of LENS did not show any benefit of this treatment on postural stability [40]. A third study published as part of LENS examined pain scores and quality of life scores among patients undergoing these treatments. It found that decompression surgery does not improve health-related quality of life but did reduce pain scores by a clinically relevant amount in 42.5% of the diabetic subjects, to 3.5/10, far below the 5.3/10 of the control group [41]. These effects are clearly clinically significant; multiple studies have estimated the minimum clinically significant difference on the VAS to be around 1 point (or 10 mm on a 100-mm scale) [42].

SURGICAL COMPLICATIONS IN DIABETIC PERIPHERAL NEUROPATHY

The systematic review mentioned previously by Baltodano identifies the most common complications of this procedure to be dehiscence (15%) and postoperative wound infection (6%) [36]. The Zhang study only reported two cases of wound dehiscence and one of wound hematoma [37].

However, elective foot surgery in the setting of diabetic neuropathy is always considered risky as postoperative patients with neuropathy can rapidly deteriorate clinically, even to the point of requiring amputation [43]. Patients with diabetic peripheral neuropathy may rapidly develop Charcot foot after revascularization surgery [44] or other surgery [45]. Nonsurgical management should first be exhausted according to the 2000 International Consensus paper on the diabetic foot [46]. Diabetic neuropathy is also an independent risk factor for postoperative wound infection [47].

Studies of orthopedic management in this population are limited, and there are no evidence-based treatment algorithms. Outcomes in ankle fracture repairs are worse in complicated diabetes patients (including those with neuropathy), with higher rates of surgical failure, infection, and need for repeat surgery [48]. Limb-threatening complications include development of Charcot feet and joint deformities [49]. Early detection of these complications is critical; a study of non–surgically induced Charcot joints in diabetics found that outcomes were dramatically worse in those diagnosed later [50]. For all surgeons treating patients in this population, it is necessary to understand the natural history of diabetes as it pertains to orthopedics and to collaborate closely with other diabetic specialists including wound care specialists, endocrinologists, orthotists, infectious disease specialists, and neurologists. In particular, meticulous wound care and improved blood sugar control in the perioperative period has been shown to decrease surgical complications and improve short- and long-term outcomes [51].

CONCLUSION

The medical, social, and economic impact of diabetic peripheral neuropathy is tremendous. The economic impact of foot ulcers and complications such as amputation has been estimated as being a third of the direct costs of diabetes, some $38 billion in 2007 [52]. This problem will only increase if current trends continue, with diabetes rates in the United States as high as one in three adults according to one prediction [4]. So far, attempts to slow or reverse these trends through public health policy and individual initiatives have had limited effect. Even if this changes due to new developments in the field, the cohort of diabetics from the current epidemic will continue to develop severe complications as they age. Management of these patients will urgently require increased availability of specialized foot care including availability of wound care, revascularization surgery, orthopedic surgery, and neurological and endocrine care. The possibility of treating diabetic peripheral neuropathy and preventing some of its most severe and traumatic complications is exciting. Further study and long-term tracking of patients will be needed since these procedures are likely to be cost-effective only over the longer term by avoiding the ever-greater direct and indirect costs of neuropathy, foot ulceration, and amputation [53].

REFERENCES

1. American Diabetes Association. Economic costs of diabetes in the US in 2012. *Diabetes care*. 2013;36(4):1033–1046.
2. NCD Risk Factor Collaboration. Worldwide trends in diabetes since 1980: a pooled analysis of 751 population-based studies with 4.4 million participants. *The Lancet*. 2016;387(10027):1513–1530.

3. Chan M. Obesity and diabetes: the slow-motion disaster: keynote address at the 47th meeting of the National Academy of Medicine. *WHO Director-General's Speeches* 2016; http://www.who.int/dg/speeches/2016/obesity-diabetes-disaster/en/. Accessed December 29, 2016.

4. Boyle JP, Thompson TJ, Gregg EW, Barker LE, Williamson DF. Projection of the year 2050 burden of diabetes in the US adult population: dynamic modeling of incidence, mortality, and prediabetes prevalence. *Popul Health Metr.* 2010;8(1):29.

5. Boulton AJ, Vileikyte L, Ragnarson-Tennvall G, Apelqvist J. The global burden of diabetic foot disease. *Lancet.* 2005;366(9498):1719–1724.

6. Callaghan BC, Little AA, Feldman EL, Hughes RA. Enhanced glucose control for preventing and treating diabetic neuropathy. *Cochrane Database Syst Rev.* 2012 Jun 13;(6):CD007543.

7. Dellon A. A cause for optimism in diabetic neuropathy. *Ann Plast Surg.* 1988;20(2):103.

8. Hotta N, Kawamori R, Fukuda M, Shigeta Y; for Aldose Reductase Inhibitor-Diabetes Complications Trial Study Group. Long-term clinical effects of epalrestat, an aldose reductase inhibitor, on progression of diabetic neuropathy and other microvascular complications: multivariate epidemiological analysis based on patient background factors and severity of diabetic neuropathy. *Diabet Med.* 2012;29(12):1529–1533.

9. Jakobsen J. Peripheral nerves in early experimental diabetes. *Diabetologia.* 1978;14(2):113–119.

10. Burg MB, Kador PF. Sorbitol, osmoregulation, and the complications of diabetes. *J Clin Invest.* 1988;81(3):635.

11. Yagihashi S, Mizukami H, Sugimoto K. Mechanism of diabetic neuropathy: where are we now and where to go? *J Diabetes Investig.* 2011;2(1):18–32.

12. Chen R-J, Lin C-CK, Ju M-S. In situ biomechanical properties of normal and diabetic nerves: an efficient quasi-linear viscoelastic approach. *J Biomech.* 2010;43(6):1118–1124.

13. Upton AM, Mccomas A. The double crush in nerve-entrapment syndromes. *Lancet.* 1973;302(7825):359–362.

14. Mackinnon SE, Dellon AL, Hudson AR, et al. Chronic nerve compression: an experimental model in the rat. *Ann Plast Surg.* 1984;13(2):112–120.

15. Dellon AL, Mackinnon SE. Chronic nerve compression model for the double crush hypothesis. *Ann Plast Surg.* 1991;26(3):259–264.

16. Dellon AL, Mackinnon SE, Seiler WA IV. Susceptibility of the diabetic nerve to chronic compression. *Ann Plast Surg.* 1988;20(2):117–119.

17. Vinik AI, Kong X, Megerian JT, et al. Diabetic nerve conduction abnormalities in the primary care setting. *Diabetes Technol Ther.* 2006;8(6):654–662.

18. Perkins BA, Olaleye D, Bril V. Carpal tunnel syndrome in patients with diabetic polyneuropathy. *Diabetes Care.* 2002;25(3):565–569.

19. Pitarokoili K, Kerasnoudis A, Behrendt V, et al. Facing the diagnostic challenge: nerve ultrasound in diabetic patients with neuropathic symptoms. *Muscle Nerve.* Jun 2016;54(1):18–24.

20. Hobson-Webb LD, Massey JM, Juel VC. Nerve ultrasound in diabetic polyneuropathy: correlation with clinical characteristics and electrodiagnostic testing. *Muscle Nerve.* 2013;47(3):379–384.

21. Han HY, Kim HM, Park SY, et al. Clinical findings of asymptomatic carpal tunnel syndrome in patients with diabetes mellitus. *Ann Rehabil Med.* 2016;40(3):489–495.

22. Burnett MG, Zager EL. Pathophysiology of peripheral nerve injury: a brief review. *Neurosurg Focus.* 2004;16(5):1–7.

23. Ntani G, Palmer KT, Linaker C, et al. Symptoms, signs and nerve conduction velocities in patients with suspected carpal tunnel syndrome. *BMC Musculoskelet Disord.* 2013;14(1):242.

24. Dellon AL, Muse VL, Scott ND. A positive Tinel sign as predictor of pain relief or sensory recovery after decompression of chronic tibial nerve compression in patients with diabetic neuropathy. *J Reconstr Microsurg.* 2012;28(04):235–240.

25. Datema M, Hoitsma E, Roon KI, et al. The Tinel sign has no diagnostic value for nerve entrapment or neuropathy in the legs. *Muscle Nerve.* 2016;54(1):25–30.

26. Shar Hashemi S, Cheikh I, Lee Dellon A. Prevalence of upper and lower extremity Tinel signs in diabetics: cross-sectional study from a United States, urban hospital-based population. *J Diabetes Metab.* 2013;4(245):2.

27. Dellon ES, Dellon AL. Functional assessment of neurologic impairment: track analysis in diabetic and compression neuropathies. *Plast Reconstr Surg.* 1991;88(4):686–694.

28. Dellon AL, Dellon ES, Seiler WA IV. Effect of tarsal tunnel decompression in the streptozotocin-induced diabetic rat. *Microsurgery.* 1994;15(4):265–268.

29. Siemionow M, Sari A, Demir Y. Effect of early nerve release on the progression of neuropathy in diabetic rats. *Ann Plast Surg.* 2007;59(1):102–108.

30. Barac S, Jiga LP, Barac B, et al. Hindpaw withdrawal from a painful thermal stimulus after sciatic nerve compression and decompression in the diabetic rat. *J Reconstr Microsurg.* 2013;29(01):063–066.

31. Pettersson LM, Danielsen N, Dahlin LB. Altered behavioural responses and functional recovery in rats following sciatic nerve compression and early vs late decompression. *J Plast Surg Hand Surg.* 2016;50(6):321–330.

32. Ahmad M, Tsang K, Mackenney P, et al. Tarsal tunnel syndrome: a literature review. *Foot and Ankle Surgery.* 2012;18(3):149–152.

33. Dellon A. The Dellon approach to neurolysis in the neuropathy patient with chronic nerve compression. *Handchir Mikrochir Plast Chir.* 2008;40(06):351–360.

34. Chaudhry V, Russell J, Belzberg A. Decompressive surgery of lower limbs for symmetrical diabetic peripheral neuropathy. *Cochrane Database Syst Rev.* Jul 2008;(3):CD006152.

35. Aszmann O, Tassler PL, Dellon AL. Changing the natural history of diabetic neuropathy: incidence of ulcer/amputation in the contralateral limb of patients with a unilateral nerve decompression procedure. *Ann Plast Surg.* 2004;53(6):517–522.

36. Baltodano PA, Basdag B, Bailey CR, et al. The positive effect of neurolysis on diabetic patients with compressed nerves of the lower extremities: a systematic review and meta-analysis. *Plastic and Reconstructive Surgery–Global Open.* 2013;1(4):e24.

37. Zhang W, Li S, Zheng X. Evaluation of the clinical efficacy of multiple lower extremity nerve decompression in diabetic peripheral neuropathy. *J Neurol Surg A Cent Eur Neurosurg.* 2013;74(02):096–100.

38. Valdivia JMV, Weinand M, Maloney CT Jr, et al. Surgical treatment of superimposed, lower extremity, peripheral nerve entrapments with diabetic and idiopathic neuropathy. *Ann Plast Surg.* 2013;70(6):675–679.

39. van Maurik JFM, van Hal M, van Eijk RP, et al. Value of surgical decompression of compressed nerves in the lower extremity in patients with painful diabetic neuropathy: a randomized controlled trial. *Plast Reconstr Surg.* 2014;134(2):325–332.

40. van Maurik JFM, ter Horst B, van Hal M, et al. Effect of surgical decompression of nerves in the lower extremity in patients with painful diabetic polyneuropathy on stability: a randomized controlled trial. *Clin Rehabil.* 2014;1:8.

41. Macaré van Maurik J, Oomen R, Hal M, et al. The effect of lower extremity nerve decompression on health-related quality of life and perception of pain in patients with painful diabetic polyneuropathy: a prospective randomized trial. *Diabet Med.* 2015;32(6):803–809.

42. Kelly AM. Does the clinically significant difference in visual analog scale pain scores vary with gender, age, or cause of pain? *Acad Emerg Med.* 1998;5(11):1086–1090.

43. Banks D, Gellman R, Davis W. Foot surgery can lead to bone degeneration in diabetic patients. Paper presented at: American Orthopaedic Foot and Ankle Society Annual Winter meeting. Anaheim, CA; 1999.

44. Edelman SV, Kosofsky EM, Paul RA, Kozak GP. Neuro-osteoarthropathy (Charcot's joint) in diabetes mellitus following revascularization surgery: three case reports and a review of the literature. *Arch Intern Med.* 1987;147(8):1504–1508.

45. Fishco WD. Surgically induced Charcot's foot. *J Am Podiatr Assoc.* 2001;91(8):388–393.

46. Apelqvist J, Bakker K, Van Houtum W, et al. International consensus and practical guidelines on the management and the prevention of the diabetic foot. *Diabetes Metab Res Rev.* 2000;16(S1).

47. Wukich DK, Crim BE, Frykberg RG, et al. Neuropathy and poorly controlled diabetes increase the rate of surgical site infection after foot and ankle surgery. *J Bone Joint Surg Am.* 2014;96(10):832–839.

48. Wukich DK, Joseph A, Ryan M, et al. Outcomes of ankle fractures in patients with un-complicated versus complicated diabetes. *Foot Ankle Int.* 2011;32(2):120–130.

49. Connolly JF, Csencsitz TA. Limb threatening neuropathic complications from ankle fractures in patients with diabetes. *Clin Orthop Relat Res.* 1998;348:212–219.

50. Chantelau E. The perils of procrastination: effects of early vs. delayed detection and treatment of incipient Charcot fracture. *Diabet Med.* 2005;22(12):1707–1712.

51. Uhl RL, Rosenbaum AJ, DiPreta JA, et al. Diabetes mellitus: musculoskeletal manifestations and perioperative considerations for the orthopaedic surgeon. *J Am Acad Orthop Surg.* 2014;22(3):183–192.

52. Driver VR, Fabbi M, Lavery LA, et al. The costs of diabetic foot: the economic case for the limb salvage team. *J Vasc Surg.* 2010;52(3):17S–22S.

53. Rankin TM, Miller JD, Gruessner AC, et al. Illustration of cost saving implications of lower extremity nerve decompression to prevent recurrence of diabetic foot ulceration. *J Diabetes Sci Technol.* 2015;9(4):873–880.

7   Cervical Spine

Siddarth Thakur and Salahadin Abdi

INTRODUCTION

Pain emanating from the cervical spine represents a significant diagnostic and therapeutic challenge for clinicians. The problem is due in part to the imprudent use of the term "neck pain" to be synonymous with pain from structures in the cervical spine leading to inappropriate investigations and treatment. The exact prevalence of cervical spine or "neck pain" is difficult to capture due to the variable definitions used in epidemiologic studies, but one systematic review found an average prevalence in the general population to be 23.1% worldwide [1].

Pain from the cervical spine can be best conceptualized by the pattern in which it is expressed; namely, axial or radicular. Most commonly axial or midline pain is believed to originate from degeneration of intervertebral discs (discogenic) or zygapophyseal (facet) joints. Radicular pain manifests as both neck and/or arm pain, frequently occurring when spinal nerve roots are compromised due to compressive forces secondary to disc herniation, degenerative foraminal stenosis, or other causes (e.g., trauma, tumor). Interestingly, large disc herniation has been observed to manifest without symptoms, and severe radicular pain has emerged without evidence of structural abnormality. These observations suggest that additional factors are involved in the etiology of these conditions. One such factor, inflammation, may contribute to nerve root irritation through release of pro-inflammatory mediators (i.e., prostaglandins, leukotrienes, tumor necrosis factors) resulting in the activation of nociceptors. Although it is conceptually accommodating to compartmentalize the etiology of cervical spine pain from a single source, the reality is that multiple structures are often involved, given the complex anatomy of the cervical spine. In this chapter, we will discuss cervical spine anatomy and biomechanics, as well as the etiology, pathophysiology, and management options for axial and radicular neck pain.

The cervical spine is a unique and complex structure because it is highly mobile and requires significant stability due to the weight of the head and constant dynamic mechanical stress occurring with movement. The configuration therefore predisposes the cervical spine to degeneration, which is often painful and increases with age. The cervical spine is made up of 7 vertebrae (C1–C7), 5 intervertebral discs, 12 uncovertebral joints (Luschka), and 14 zygapophyseal (facet) joints. The first two vertebrae, C1 (atlas) and C2 (axis), are structurally unique, and their articulations with the occiput superiorly allows for a significant range of motion between the head and neck. C1 is a ring-shaped vertebra which articulates with the occiput above to form the atlanto-occipital joint (primarily flexion and extension) and with C2 below to form the atlantoaxial joint (primarily axial rotation). The dens of C2 projects superiorly, providing an anchor point for both the occiput and C1, which are secured by the alar and cruciform ligaments. The remaining cervical vertebrae (C3–C7) share a common structure: a vertebral body, intervertebral discs, transverse processes, pedicles, laminae, vertebral arches, and a spinous process. The pedicles have superior and inferior articulations that form the zygapophyseal or facet joints. The five cervical discs connect the interspaces between C2–C7, each with a thick external ring of fibrous cartilage, the annulus fibrosus, which encapsulates an osmotically active colloidal proteoglycan gel, the nucleus pulposus. The nucleus pulposus serves to absorb and evenly distribute compressive forces but with aging it loses its water content, which increases the axial load and shearing forces on posterior spinal elements (including the facet joints). The discs and vertebral bodies are separated by hyaline and fibrocartilaginous end plates. The anterior aspects of the discs and vertebral bodies are covered by the anterior longitudinal ligament, which functions to limit cervical extension. The posterior longitudinal ligament runs along the posterior discs and vertebral bodies, limiting cervical flexion. Additionally, the supraspinous and interspinous ligaments and the ligamentum flavum provide stability with flexion, although they are inconsistently found and often not contiguous in the cervical spine. The muscles supporting movement of the head and neck include flexors, extensors, rotators, and those that assist with lateral flexion. In addition to movement, the muscles also work to protect the spinal cord and spinal nerves when the neck is under mechanical stress, as well as to maintain the cervical spine in a shallow lordosis. The head flexes relative to the neck through the actions of the rectus capitis (anterior, lateral) and longus capitis. The head extends relative to the neck through the action of the rectus capitis (minor and major), obliquus capitis (superior and inferior), and splenius/semispinalis/longissimus capitis, all of which insert on the skull. Neck flexion is achieved by activation of the bilateral sternocleidomastoid (SCM) and scalene muscles. Conversely, neck extension is achieved by action of the splenius/semispinalis/longissimus cervicis. Lateral flexion and rotation are movements supposed by the SCM, semispinalis capitis and cervicis, splenius capitis, and longissimus capitis and cervicis when they are activated ipsilaterally. Other muscles such as the upper trapezius, which originates on the spinous process of C7, occipital protuberance, and superior nuchal line and inserts on the posterior clavicle, are also important to be aware of, as they are often implicated in cervical myofascial pain presenting with axial neck pain.

The neural elements of the cervical spine include the spinal cord and dorsal and ventral roots that join in the vertebral canal to form spinal nerves that give rise to dorsal and ventral rami. The arachnoid and dura matter encase the dorsal and ventral roots, eventually blending into the epineurium of the spinal nerves. The spinal nerves exit at the intervertebral foramen, which is formed by the pedicles of consecutive vertebrae superiorly and inferiorly, facet joints posteriorly, and an uncovertebral joints anteromedially. The vertebral artery lies immediately lateral to the opening of the intervertebral foramen. The C3–C7 nerves exit above their numbered pedicles, respectively, except C8 (as there is no C8 vertebrae), which exits above the first thoracic vertebrae. The spinal nerve occupies the inferior portion of the foramen, with its associated radicular arteries and veins located superiorly. Upon exiting the foramen, the spinal nerves divide into dorsal and ventral rami. The C1–C2 ventral rami innervate the atlanto-occipital and atlantoaxial joints; C1–C4 ventral rami form the cervical plexus innervating the cervical muscle and a portion of the cutaneous innervation of the head and neck; and the C5–T1 ventral rami contribute to the brachial plexus, responsible for most sensory and motor function of the shoulder, arm, and hand. The dorsal rami from the cervical spinal nerves divide further into medial and lateral branches. The medial branches of the C1–C3 are named the suboccipital, greater occipital, and third occipital nerves, respectively. The remaining cervical medial branches innervate their respective facet joints. The majority of the lateral branches of the cervical dorsal rami go on to supply deep paraspinal muscles (i.e., multifidus, semispinalis, longissimus).

A comprehensive understanding of cervical spine anatomy is necessary for interventional management of painful conditions. The orientation of spinal structures and how they vary between cervical, thoracic, and lumbar spine is of particular importance. For example, in the cervical spine, the facets are oriented parallel toward the frontal plane at about 45 degrees to the transverse plane; the structure changes to a more sagittal plane orientation of about 90 degrees to the transverse plane in the lumbar spine. The facet joint is generally innervated by the medial branch of dorsal rami of above and below (e.g., C5–C6 facet is innervated by the C5 and C6 medial branch). However, the actual pattern of innervation is likely more complex than that. The medial branches are located consistently around the dorsolateral aspect of the articular pillar, easily identified on fluoroscopy, and distinctly separate from the vertebral artery and spinal nerve. Furthermore, it is critical to recognize that the unique characteristics of the epidural space, the interspinous ligament, and ligamentum flavum are inconsistently found or are insubstantial above the C7–T1 vertebral space. The C7–T1 space is also the largest epidural space in the cervical spine, making it a safer needle entry site than rostral targets for interventions such as interlaminar epidural steroid injections. Another important landmark is the anterior tubercle of the transverse process of C6, the Chassaignac tubercle, which is present at the level of the cricoid cartilage and easily palpable. Historically it has been used as a target for an initial needle positioning when performing a stellate ganglion block without image guidance. However, the current practice is to use ultrasound or fluoroscopy for this procedure targeting the C6 or C7 vertebral level.

AXIAL NECK PAIN

Etiology and Pathophysiology

Neck pain that is limited to the occipital, cervical, or posterior scapular areas is considered to be axial in nature. Axial pain can result from a variety of causes including degeneration of the intervertebral discs, facet, or uncovertebral joints (cervical spondylosis); whiplash injuries; cervical strain; and myofascial pain. The process of degeneration is thought to occur when intervertebral discs begin to lose height due to dehydration of the nucleus pulposus, creating increased stress on uncovertebral and facet joint biomechanics. The cascade then continues, causing osteophytes, ligamentum flavum hypertrophy, and annular tears with associated pain. In many cases of axial neck pain (e.g., discogenic or facetogenic), the location of pain perceived is highly variable and may even be referred from another site of pathology. Referred pain occurs when pain is perceived in areas that are innervated by different nerves than those of the site of noxious stimulation. It is typically experienced as a poorly localized, deep, diffuse pain and thought to be due to convergence of nociceptive afferents carrying painful information to second-order neurons at the level of the spinal cord that then relay it supraspinally.

Facetogenic Pain

Pain from the facet (zygapophyseal) joints or *facetogenic pain* can occur in the setting of degeneration or be related to flexion-extension type injury secondary to a whiplash event. The prevalence of pain after whiplash is considerable, with estimates of as high as 88% of patients suffering from chronic neck pain [2]. The pain is thought to be due to intraarticular hemorrhage, small fractures, disc contusion, and capsular tears occurring after sigmoid deformation of the cervical spine after collision. However, many of these pathological processes are not easily observed radiographically or reliably detected with physical exam. Therefore, an intraarticular injection or a cervical medial branch block with a small aliquot of local anesthetic may be needed to confirm that pain is in fact originating from a cervical facet. To control for false-positive blocks, different local anesthetics with variable durations of action or a control (saline) injection can be used, as well as multiple blocks (separated in time). Accurate diagnosis is essential; as noted earlier, referred pain is often observed with painful facet joints. Pain from the upper cervical facets (C2–C3) can be experienced in the upper neck and occiput (cervicogenic headache), whereas pain from lower cervical facets (C6–C7) can be experienced around the scapula [3]. In addition to axial neck pain, patients after whiplash often suffer from injuries to soft tissues, spinal nerves, spinal ligaments, and intervertebral discs.

Discogenic Pain

Degenerative disc disease is a common finding that is commonly observed on radiologic examination of older adults; however, the correlation of radiographic findings to clinical symptoms is poor. Therefore, the term "cervical discogenic pain" may be more appropriate. The pain often associated with muscle spasm and tightness, with resultant decreased range of motion. It may be a result of dehydration of the nucleus pulposus with disruption of the annulus and activation of local mechanoreceptors and nociceptors. Two additional factors may play a role; inability to appropriately distribute pressure among the disc, endplates, and facets and an inflammatory component due to local leakage of nuclear material stimulating the annulus, dura mater, posterior longitudinal ligament, dorsal root ganglion, and spinal nerve. Similar to facetogenic pain, the pain patterns from intervertebral discs can be nebulous. Discography has been utilized to elucidate referral patterns; interestingly, the symptoms were often experienced unilaterally, with C5–C6 disc injection causing pain around the shoulder girdle and upper limb, and pain in the periscapular regions occurring with injection of discs from mid to lower cervical segments [4].

Myofascial Pain

Cervical myofascial pain manifests as a regional and referred pain associated with small circumscribed areas of myofascial hyperirritability known as *trigger points*. The identification of trigger points is done through physical examination with palpation of a taut band of skeletal muscle. Trigger points can be both latent, associated with decreased range of motion, or active, with decreased range of motion and associated pain. Direct stimulation by deep palpation of a trigger point can induce characteristic localized and referred pain. The characteristic referral zones of trigger points have been eloquently described by Travell and Simons [5]. In the upper body, the trapezius, levator scapulae, and infraspinatus muscles are commonly involved. Although the precise pathophysiology of trigger points is not well understood, they are likely the result of tension, inflammation, and trauma. In the observed taut bands, it is hypothesized that increased intracellular calcium causes uncontrolled muscle shortening, leading to impaired local circulation with decreased oxygen and nutrient supply to the area.

Other Etiologies

There are numerous other pathological processes that can manifest as axial neck pain. For example, metastatic tumors to the cervical spine may cause vertebral compression fracture with associated mechanical pain. If a tumor in the cervical spine grows, it may cause periosteal stretching with resultant persistent neck pain. Infectious processes such as osteomyelitis, discitis, or epidural abscesses can also manifest with midline pain. Last, even rheumatologic processes such as the numerous seronegative spondyloarthropathies may also present with axial neck pain.

Management

The diverse and complex etiologies of axial neck pain underscore the importance of an individualized treatment plan. Treatment goals should be set early, with emphasis not only on pain relief but also on restoring optimal function. A multimodal approach may be beneficial to achieve these goals.

Pharmacological Management

The pharmacologic interventions for neck pain are not specific, therefore it is reasonable to utilize the World Health Organization (WHO) analgesic ladder to guide clinical management. Although originally designed for the treatment of cancer-related pain, the WHO ladder has been adopted for many painful conditions, including neck pain. Simple analgesics such as acetaminophen and nonsteroidal anti-inflammatory drugs (NSAIDs) are the mainstay of treatment for both acute and chronic neck pain despite limited and inconsistent benefit. In the acute setting, muscle relaxants may be beneficial, but use during the day may be limited due to sedative side effects. If patients with chronic neck pain have coexisting anxiety and depression, tricyclic antidepressants (TCAs) or a serotonin-norepinephrine reuptake inhibitor (SNRI) may be beneficial. The addition of a weak opioid such as tramadol may be necessary for moderate pain not controlled with acetaminophen, NSAIDs, and adjuvant medications. The addition of stronger opioids should be reserved only for the most recalcitrant painful conditions.

Physical Therapy, Complementary and Alternative Medicine

A comprehensive treatment plan should also include physical exercise and posture modification. A formal physical therapy program with a focus on therapeutic exercise, range of motion, neuromuscular reeducation, and establishment of a home exercise program may provide lasting pain relief for patients suffering from chronic axial neck pain. The use of adjunctive modalities such as massage, electromyographic (EMG) biofeedback, transcutaneous electrical stimulation, ultrasound, traction, and acupuncture have shown inconsistent benefit when studied systematically [6]. There has been evidence supporting the use of spinal manipulation when combined with exercise, at least in the short term. For example, one study demonstrated decreased disability scores, greater pain relief, and patient perception of recovery compared to sham ultrasound and usual care [7]. It is also imperative to acknowledge and address any psychosocial problems that patients may have. Cognitive behavioral therapy has been supported in a recent Cochrane review for the treatment of chronic neck pain and related distress when compared to no treatment [8].

Interventional Management

In the cases where conservative management provides inadequate analgesia, several interventional options exist to treat axial neck pain. For facetogenic pain, the diagnosis is supported with localized pain to palpation and a positive response to appropriately performed medial branch blocks or intraarticular facet injections. If the patient outcome is satisfactory with medial branch block or intraarticular facet injections alone, then no further treatment is warranted. However, if the pain relief is short-lived and the patient and clinician feel that ablation of the nerves innervating the facet joint (medial branch radiofrequency neurotomy) would be beneficial, then the procedure should be performed. There is at least fair evidence for the use of percutaneous cervical medial branch radiofrequency neurotomy in providing long-term pain relief in patient's suffering from chronic axial neck pain [9].

The literature evaluating interventions for cervical discogenic pain is much less robust than for lumbar discogenic back pain. Interventions applying heat to the nucleus pulposus to cause denervation or destruction of nociceptors may sound appealing, but this approach is not well studied in cervical discogenic pain and, if performed, must be done so with extreme caution given the proximity of the spinal cord and risk of cord damage with resulting tetraplegia. Other interventions, such as intradiscal platelet-rich plasma, have shown promising results with chronic lumbar discogenic pain but data regarding injection into cervical discs is lacking. Reduction of inflammatory mediators in the disc through intradiscal steroids is conceptually attractive but unfortunately has not consistently shown to be beneficial in lumbar discogenic pain

[10]. The use of cervical epidural steroid injection for chronic cervical discogenic pain is not routine in clinical practice but is a viable option if conservative management fails to provide adequate pain relief. It has been supported in a systematic review, as well as in a clinical trial comparing cervical interlaminar epidural injections of local anesthetic alone versus local anesthetic and steroids with both groups demonstrating pain relief with no detectable difference between the two [11].

The interventional treatment of myofascial pain syndrome includes insertion of a needle with or without the injection of a medication into a hypersensitive trigger point. There has been no consistent support for trigger point injection when studied, although they are frequently used in routine clinical settings. Injection of botulinum toxin has also been performed with inconsistent results, and a Cochrane review performed in 2014 found inconclusive evidence to support its use [12]. Regardless of the intervention therapy undertaken, the treatment is then directed at restoring normal biomechanics and muscle function through an intensive stretching program with the adjuvant use of modalities such as cold and electrical stimulation.

CERVICAL RADICULOPATHY

Etiology and Pathophysiology

Cervical radiculopathy is a neurophysiological dysfunction of a cervical spinal nerve root. It commonly manifests as a unilateral shooting pain and paresthesia in a nerve root distribution with evidence of partial sensory, motor, and/or loss of reflex. It is important to differentiate the radicular pain seen in radiculopathy, which often involves the distal upper extremity, from that of referred pain patterns seen with discogenic, facetogenic, or myofascial pain, as previously described. Furthermore, radiculopathy should be separate from radiculitis, a term used to describe pain and paresthesia in a dermatomal distribution without objective findings of sensory or motor loss and/or loss of reflex. The majority of radiculopathies occur in the setting of nerve root compression with either disc herniation, degenerative spondylosis, or a combination of both. Degenerative of the vertebral disc through disc desiccation, dehydration of the disc with fibrocartilaginous replacement of glycosaminoglycans by fibrocartilage in the nucleus pulposus, causes the so-called degenerative cascade. The degeneration leads to increased stress on the uncovertebral joints, facets, and vertebral end plates leading to ligamentous and osseous hypertrophy. With spondylosis, bone growth, such as osteophytes, can occur around the facet joints and uncovertebral joints resulting in neural foraminal narrowing and nerve root compression. The initial pathophysiology is similar to that hypothesized with axial pain, but the manifestation may be expressed with more radicular than axial pain depending on the relative severity and precise structures involved. Disc herniation occurs when the integrity of fibers in the annulus fibrosus are compromised, leading to the prolapse of material from the nucleus pulposus. The material causes an inflammatory response and impinges on the nerve root, resulting in radiculopathy. The disc herniations can be classified as "soft," often occurring in the acute setting usually in younger patients, or "hard," with more calcified disc material seen with advanced spondylosis and age. Disc herniations can also be classified by location: intraforaminal, posterolateral, and central. Intraforaminal herniations may be seen with acute radiculopathies and affect the exiting nerve root. Posterolateral herniations usually occupy the space between the posterior longitudinal ligament and the uncinate process. Central herniation may result in spinal cord compression and occur when disc material passes through the posterior longitudinal ligament in the setting of advanced spondylosis with osseous hypertrophy that prevents lateral migration of disc material. The specific injury to nerve fiber axons could be related to direct compression or ischemia through interruption in blood flow.

Cervical radiculopathy is diagnosed based primarily on history and physical exam, with supporting evidence from electrodiagnostic and radiological studies. The pattern of symptoms frequently follows the nerve root involved both by dermatome (sensory) and myotome (motor). However, the pain and paresthesia may be nonlocalizing as there is considerable overlap between dermatomes. Muscle testing should be systematic, and neurological weakness must be distinguished from pain-limited weakness. Diminished reflexes should be demonstrated, and multiple reflexes should be checked with particular attention to signs of upper motor neuron involvement (hyperreflexia or presence of Hoffmann's sign) as this may be indicative of cervical spondylotic myelopathy or other central nervous system pathology. Reproduction of symptoms with axial compression and ipsilateral neck extension (Spurling's maneuver) also supports the diagnosis. In radiculopathies, the C7 nerve root is most frequently involved followed by C6, C8, and C5, respectively [13]. The electrodiagnostic examination with nerve conduction studies will show normal sensory nerve action potential (SNAP) latency and amplitude as the lesion is proximal to the dorsal root ganglion (DRG). A test of motor nerve conduction may show abnormality with decreased compound motor action potential (CMAP) amplitude representing axon loss, but this is absent unless symptoms are chronic and severe. Needle electromyography is more sensitive for detecting denervation from a nerve root, and abnormal spontaneous activity with fibrillation and positive sharp waves are demonstrated in proximal muscles (paraspinals) a few days after symptom onset and in distal muscles (intrinsic hand) a few weeks later. Imaging studies such as magnetic resonance imaging (MRI) may be used to support the diagnosis, although providers should recognize that this modality may detect an abnormality not congruent with the patient's symptoms.

Other Etiologies

There is a plethora of conditions that cause symptoms that mimic cervical radiculopathy. A few examples include peripheral entrapment neuropathies (median or ulnar neuropathy), brachial plexopathy, rotator cuff disease, thoracic outlet syndrome, complex regional pain syndrome, herpes zoster, Lyme disease, and neoplasms such as schwannomas, neurofibromas, or Pancoast tumors. The broad differential diagnosis for radicular pain underscores the importance of a comprehensive history, physical, and diagnostic workup.

Management

Given the considerable number of conditions that may present with radicular neck and arm pain, the accurate diagnosis of radiculopathy is necessary to make an optimal treatment plan. The treatment of cervical radiculopathy should focus on pain management, improving neurological symptoms, and preventing recurrent episodes. A conservative multimodal approach consisting of medications, physical therapy, and modalities (e.g., traction) should be implemented prior to more advanced interventions.

Pharmacological Management

Simple analgesics such as acetaminophen or NSAIDs are commonly utilized first-line agents in attempts to control pain in cervical radiculopathy. For those patients who have associated muscle spasms or tightness, muscle relaxants may also be beneficial. Although oral steroids are often utilized, their role in the management of cervical radiculopathy is controversial, and there is a paucity of supporting literature. For instance, a randomized control trial of oral steroid for acute radiculopathy due to a herniated lumbar disc demonstrated no improvement in pain but modest improvement in function at 3 and 52 weeks [14]. Although the study evaluated acute lumbar radiculopathy due to disc herniation, it is reasonable to extrapolate the findings to acute cervical radiculopathy due to disc herniation given the similar pathophysiologic mechanisms. Given that cervical radiculopathy has a considerable component of neuropathic pain, it is reasonable to follow the most recent guidelines for the treatment of neuropathic pain [15]. Specifically, consideration can be given to antidepressants (tricyclics, serotonin-norepinephrine reuptake inhibitors) and opioids such as tramadol, which has a known (weak) serotonin and norepinephrine reuptake inhibition. Additionally, there has been support for the use of membrane stabilizing antiepileptic drugs like gabapentin and pregabalin in radiculopathy, and they are frequently used in clinical practice.

Physical Therapy, Complementary and Alternative Medicine

Physical therapy focusing on decreasing pain and improving function and that includes range of motion, strengthening, biomechanics, and postural education is often employed as a part of the comprehensive treatment of cervical radiculopathy. Although these treatments have limited support in the literature, they have possible benefit and limited harm, making them an appealing option. Furthermore, given the favorable natural course of most cervical radiculopathy, an appreciable difference with treatment using physical therapy compared to that without may be difficult to detect in clinical trials. Cervical traction is another technique wherein a distracting force is applied to relieve pressure on nerve roots; it is thought increase the intervertebral joint spaces. Although theoretically sound, there are limited data supporting the use of traction for the treatment of neck pain. Acupuncture may also be utilized, and its short-term benefit has been demonstrated for neck pain (both axial and radiculopathy).

Interventional Management

Cervical epidural steroid injections can be utilized for patients who do not respond favorably to conservative measures. The use of interlaminar cervical epidural injections have demonstrated moderate evidence in multiple systematic reviews, at least in the short-term (<6 weeks) [16]. The pain relief from epidural steroids may allow patients to avoid surgical intervention. The procedure should be done with fluoroscopic guidance and with extreme caution, using contrast dye to confirm placement and only by clinicians who have been properly trained in the technique. Needle placement should be at the C6–C7 or C7–T1 interspace as the epidural space is widest at these sites and the ligamentum flavum is more discontinuous in the higher cervical spine. Cervical transforaminal epidural steroids injections are purported to deliver medication directly near the site of injury at the nerve root, however, the evidence for the effectiveness is limited. There have not been any randomized, double-blind, controlled trials showing the efficacy or comparative effectiveness when compared to the interlaminar route. Additionally, the complications from cervical transforaminal injections are more common than interlaminar and usually related to neural/vascular trauma or intravascular injection and are potentially fatal. Considering the risk–benefit ratio, it is reasonable to avoid the use of the transforaminal route in favor of the interlaminar route in most cases. In the setting of progressive neurological decline with confirmed nerve root compression on neuroimaging and nonresponse to conservative and interventional management, surgery may be indicated.

CONCLUSION

Neck pain is a common and often challenging condition to manage. The precise etiology of the pain may be difficult to identify because there are many potential pain-generating structures in the cervical spine and surrounding region. It is helpful to delineate the patient's symptoms as axial- or radicular-predominant in order to guide the investigation prior to initiating treatment. The evidence for many commonly used treatment regimens is variable, and therefore an individualized plan is often necessary.

REFERENCES

1. Hoy D, Protani M, De R, et al. The epidemiology of neck pain. *Best Pract Res Clin Rheumatol.* 2010;24:783–792.
2. Barnsley L, Lord S, Bogduk N. Whiplash injury. *Pain.* 1994;58:283–307.
3. Dwyer A, Aprill C, Bogduk N. Cervical zygapophyseal joint pain patterns. I: A study in normal volunteers. *Spine.* 1990;15:453–457.
4. Grubb SA, Kelly CK. Cervical discography: clinical implications from 12 years of experience. *Spine.* 2000;25:1382–1389.
5. Travell J, Simons D. *Myofacial Pain and Dysfunction: The Trigger Point Manual.* Baltimore, MD: Williams & Wilkins; 1992.
6. Harris GR, Susman JL. Managing musculoskeletal complaints with rehabilitation therapy: summary of the Philadelphia panel evidence-based clinical practice guidelines on musculoskeletal rehabilitation interventions. *J Fam Pract.* 2002;51:1042–1048.
7. Walker MJ, Boyles RE, Young BA, et al. The effectiveness of manual physical therapy and exercise for mechanical neck pain: a randomized clinical trial. *Spine.* 2008;33:2371–2378.
8. Monticone M, Ambrosini E, Cedraschi C, et al. Cognitive-behavioral treatment for subacute and chronic neck pain: a Cochrane review. *Spine.* 2015;40:1495–1504.

9. Falco F, Manchikanti L, Datta S, et al. Systematic review of the therapeutic effectiveness of cervical facet joint interventions: an update. *Pain Physician.* 2012;15:E839–868.

10. Zhou Y, Abdi S. Diagnosis and minimally invasive treatment of lumbar discogenic pain—A review of the literature. *Clin J Pain.* 2006;22:468–481.

11. Manchikanti L, Cash KA, Pampati V, et al. Cervical epidural injections in chronic discogenic neck pain without disc herniation or radiculitis: preliminary results of a randomized, double-blind, controlled trial. *Pain Physician.* 2010;13:E265–E278.

12. Soares A, Andriolo RB, Atallah ÁN, et al. Botulinum toxin for myofascial pain syndromes in adults. *Cochrane Database Syst Rev.* Apr 2012;(4):CD007533.

13. Wilbourn AJ, Aminoff MJ. AAEM minimonograph 32: the electrodiagnostic examination in patients with radiculopathies. *Muscle Nerve.* 1998;21:1612–1631.

14. Goldberg H, Firtch W, Tyburski M, et al. Oral steroids for acute radiculopathy due to a herniated lumbar disk: a randomized clinical trial. *JAMA.* 2015;313:1915–1923.

15. Finnerup NB, Attal N, Haroutounian S, et al. Pharmacotherapy for neuropathic pain in adults: a systematic review and meta-analysis. *Lancet Neurol.* 2015;14:162–173.

16. Kaye AD, Manchikanti L, Abdi S, et al. Efficacy of epidural injections in managing chronic spinal pain: a best evidence synthesis. *Pain Physician.* 2015;18:E939–1004.

8 Thoracic Spine Pain

Mark R. Jones, Matthew Novitch,
Graham R. Hadley, Alan D. Kaye,
and Sudhir A. Diwan

BACKGROUND

Spinal pain is a well-recognized pathology that contributes a significant burden to healthcare. Careful measurement estimates that $60–80 billion per year are lost due to reduced work productivity directly attributable to persistent spinal pain [1].

Cervical and lumbar spinal pain benefit from established associations with many pain syndromes, injuries, and degenerative conditions. In contrast, thoracic spinal pain (TSP) receives less attention from clinical, epidemiologic, and genetic research communities owing to a reduced incidence in comparison to pain arising from cervical and lumbar derangement. Approximately 5% of patients referred to outpatient pain clinics endorse thoracic pain, while the annual prevalence of TSP has been estimated to be as high as 34.8% in working adult populations [2–4]. Projections on the lifetime prevalence of TSP vary widely between studies, with estimates ranging anywhere from 1% to 84% [5].

Nevertheless, TSP can be similarly disabling to other forms of spinal pain, imposing significant burdens on the individual and society. Thoracic pain may arise from a multitude of underlying pathologies, including angina pectoris, herpes zoster infection, thoracic disc herniations, pulmonary or pleural tumors, and aneurysms [6]. Furthermore, chronic postoperative pain can occur following surgery, including thoracotomy, sternotomy, coronary artery bypass, or mastectomy [2]. Diaphragmatic, cervical spine, chest, and abdominal visceral disease may also induce referred pain to the thorax from a variety of etiologies such as esophageal carcinoma or motility disorders, pancreatic disease, or pulmonary embolism, for example. TSP may arise from infectious, neoplastic, inflammatory, metabolic, and degenerative conditions that result in pain and disability. For the purposes of this chapter, we will focus on TSP of musculoskeletal origin; however, a thorough history and physical are imperative to avoid overlooking a potentially life-threatening condition. Table 8.1 lists the differential diagnosis for thoracic pain.

Infectious	Herpes zoster/postherpetic neuralgia
	Bornholm disease (pleurodynia or myalgia)
Malignancy	Spinal cord tumor
	Tumor inflicting intercostal neuralgia (e.g., schwannoma, neurofibroma)
	Pleural cavity or chest wall tumor (e.g., metastases, mesothelioma)
Musculoskeletal	Arthropathy (costosternal, costoclavicular, costovertebral, sternoclavicular, facetogenic)
	Discogenic (Intervertebral disc disruption)
	Herniated disc with cord or root compression
	Fracture (vertebral compression fracture, rib fracture)
	Costochondritis
	Myofascial pain syndrome
	Slipping rib syndrome
Iatrogenic	Post-thoracotomy syndrome
	Post-mastectomy syndrome

CLASSIFICATION

TSP is defined as pain experienced between the boundaries of the T1–T12 vertebrae across the posterior aspect of the trunk [5]. Clinically, it is useful to categorize TSP into axial and radicular divisions for purposes of symptom management. Axial TSP is confined to the posterior thoracic region, whereas radicular TSP is characterized by radiating pain in the area innervated by an intercostal nerve.

TSP may be neuropathic, nociceptive, mixed, or idiopathic, and it may originate from intervertebral discs, endplates, vertebrae, facet joints, spinous processes, transverse processes, costochondral junctions, and ligamentous or myofascial structures. Nociceptive pain refers to pain arising from actual or threatened damage to non-neural tissues or as pain secondary activation of the peripheral receptive terminals of primary afferent neurons in response to noxious chemical, mechanical, or thermal stimuli [7]. In contrast, neuropathic pain is secondary to dysfunction or injury to nerves caused by a lesion or disease of the somatosensory nervous system. More commonly, neuropathic pain may arise from peripheral nervous system conditions such as nerve root compression, postherpetic neuralgia, or diabetic neuropathy. Albeit less frequently, central neuropathic pain may also occur, usually via pathologies such as multiple sclerosis, syringomyelia, and spinal cord compressing lesions. Patients often describe neuropathic pain as a burning, tingling, lancinating, or electrical sensation, whereas nociceptive pain is usually characterized as tight, aching, stiff, heavy, and sharp.

ANATOMY

The thoracic spine, much like the cervical and lumbar spine, has vertebral bodies connected by intervertebral discs and longitudinal ligaments, with posterior elements connected by zygapophysial joints [8]. Asymmetry between the heights of the anterior and posterior borders of the thoracic intervertebral discs provides the majority of the kyphotic curvature of thoracic spine. The thoracic spine functions to support axial loading and is distinct from cervical and lumbar regions in that it suspends the rib cage and protects the heart and lungs. The head of each rib typically articulates with the thoracic spine at two places. The head of the rib articulates with the vertebral body, and the tubercle on the neck of the rib articulates with the transverse processes of the vertebra. At T1, T11, and T12, the head of the rib fully articulates with its corresponding numbered vertebra. Range of motion is more limited in the thoracic spine than the cervical and lumbar spines due to the angle of contact between facet joints. In addition, thoracic intervertebral discs are more centrally located, contain smaller volumes, and display a thicker annulus fibrosus composed of a collagen fibers than do lumbar intervertebral discs. Disc shape varies throughout the thoracic spine, with the more elliptical cephalad discs becoming more triangular as they progress caudad before reverting back to elliptical shape at the base of the thoracic spine [9].

The innervation of the thoracic spine is largely homologous to that of the cervical and lumbar levels in regards to the sinuvertebral nerves and courses of the thoracic dorsal rami.

Clinically relevant differences arise in the course of the medial branches of the thoracic dorsal rami. At the cervical and lumbar levels, the medial branches wind around the base of the superior articular process at each segmental level, whereas the thoracic dorsal ramus extends to the end of the transverse process before dividing into medial and lateral branches [10]. Consequently, minimally invasive, diagnostic, and therapeutic procedures targeting the thoracic medial branch must steer toward the transverse process rather than the superior articular process.

AXIAL PAIN

The axial TSP is limited to the posterior thoracic area. Axial TSP is most commonly caused by damage to the thoracic facet joints and intervertebral discs. Several different disease states and conditions may contribute to pathology of these structures. It is important to note that several structures may be affected by pathologies simultaneously, such that both axial and radicular pain are present.

Facetogenic Pain

In populations with localized TSP, the thoracic facet joints are responsible for approximately 42% of symptoms [11]. In comparison, the lumbar facet joints contribute 30% of the total burden for spinal pain. Also known as *zygapophysial joints*, the facet joints of the thoracic region are similar to lumbar and cervical facet joints anatomically as paired diarthrodial articulations between posterior elements of the adjacent vertebrae, although thoracic facet joints project more vertically than their lumbar counterparts [12]. Inflammation of the thoracic facet joints occurs during disease processes such as ankylosing spondylitis and rheumatoid arthritis. Other conditions causing facetogenic pain include thoracolumbar junction syndrome, degeneration, osteoarthritis, and injury. Injury remains the most common source of facet joint pain, as the richly innervated synovium, capsule, and subcostal bone react to insult (e.g., joint stretching, tearing, or capsular fluid distention) with provocation of nociceptors and type-C pain fibers [13].

Thoracic facet joint pain is not a distinct clinical entity. Rather, it remains a diagnosis of exclusion. Patients generally present with continuous pain, which may be unilateral or bilateral in a distinct thoracic area of the back. Neurological findings are notably absent in thoracic facet joint pain. Patients usually present with pain on exam elicited by pressure paravertebral to the symptomatic level. Physical exam cannot definitively pinpoint the facet joint, however, as any maneuver to stress the facet joint will also likely stress several other structures [12].

Many of the rheumatic and inflammatory processes mentioned earlier rely on sensitive genealogic testing for clues, but cannot confirm diagnoses based on the result. For example, the HLA-B27 antigen system is positive in 90–95% of patients with ankylosing spondylitis [14]; a negative result, however, does not rule out the disease. Other, more typical markers of inflammation such as C-reactive protein (CRP) and erythrocyte sedimentation rate (ESR) may provide corroboratory evidence. Imaging studies such as computed tomography (CT) or magnetic resonance imaging (MRI) may be used to rule out the more insidious, life-threatening syndromes as described earlier but are unreliable when used to evaluate thoracic facet joint pain [15]. Strong evidence supports the use of diagnostic medial branch blocks at the appropriate vertebral level for facet joint pain, with sustained diagnosis rates nearing 90% [16]. The associated high false-positive rate mandates at least two consecutive positive blocks for confirmation before more interventions may take place.

Treatment Options

More conservative therapies are typically recommended prior to invasive techniques. Multimodal analgesic therapy is imperative for facetogenic pain. Nonsteroidal anti-inflammatory drugs (NSAIDs) and acetaminophen are considered first-line therapies [15]. Inflammatory arthritis and small joint arthritic pain in particular respond well to NSAIDs, while disease-modifying antirheumatologic drugs and tumor necrosis factor-α (TNF-α) inhibitors are used for the axial spondyloarthropathies. Transcutaneous electrical nerve stimulation (TENS) has demonstrated analgesic benefit for myofascial pain and may be an effective adjunct in concert with pharmacologic and physical therapy for TSP. Last, alternative treatments such as osteopathic manipulation and acupuncture have produced mixed results but may play a role in facet joint pain [17].

Interventional techniques for facet joint pain include the medial branch blocks. In addition to their diagnostic value, these blocks often provide therapeutic analgesia with long-term symptomatic improvement over the course of a year [15]. Radiofrequency ablation of the medial branches may follow diagnostic blocks and has demonstrated effective pain relief of up to a 75% reduction in symptoms 2 months postintervention. Studies examining thoracic facet joint intraarticular injections report limited effectiveness of the technique but a possible role for patients unsuitable for radiofrequency ablation such as those with pacemakers [18]. Regarding more invasive surgical procedures, no convincing evidence currently exists to support surgical intervention for facet joint pain aside from repair of traumatic dislocation [16].

Discogenic Pain

Thoracic intervertebral discs are similar to lumbar and cervical discs in composition; each is constructed of nucleus pulposus, annulus fibrosus, and vertebral endplates

[19]. Earlier in the 20th century, discs were believed to not contain nerve endings, thus rendering them incapable of generating pain [20]. Further research disproved this concept: while normal human discs contain sensory nerve extensions only into the outer third of the annulus, degenerated and herniated discs are more deeply and extensively innervated; nociceptive nerve fibers may indeed penetrate even into the nucleus pulposus [21]. A combination of predisposing genetic factors and chemical and mechanical changes associated with disc degeneration engender a climate hospitable to nerve ingrowth [22,23]. Specifically, disc dehydration promotes delamination and fissuring of the lamellar layers. This altered intervertebral disc matrix biology allows distorted rates and production of angiogenesis, cellular aggrecan (a neurite outgrowth inhibitor), and inflammatory cytokines [24,25]. As degeneration continues, radial tears begin to form in the now highly innervated disc, resulting in the symptoms of discogenic TSP. It is now widely accepted that intervertebral discs can cause chronic upper and mid back pain [26]. Figure 8.1 demonstrates an intervertebral disc with a radial tear in the annulus fibrosus.

Intervertebral disc pain can be difficult to evaluate via routine methodology. Patients often present with a nondescript and unrelenting axial back pain that increases with prolonged sitting or standing. The Valsalva maneuver may incite pain in the afflicted region as well. Imaging modalities such as MRI infrequently correlate with clinical findings, and spinal imaging abnormalities are often present in healthy, asymptomatic individuals [27,28]. There is no benefit in repeat MRI in patients with chronic spine pain [29]. Routine imaging is therefore not recommended as a means of evaluating the pathology behind TSP.

Provocative or analgesic diagnostic discography is currently the only proven diagnostic measure capable of correlating anatomic abnormality with clinical TSP. A prospective study by Jackson et al [30]. reported that CT-guided discography most accurately identified disc pathology in comparison to surgical findings, at a rate of

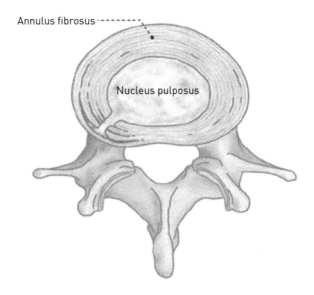

FIGURE 8.1 Illustrated demonstration of an intervertebral disc with a radial tear in the annulus fibrosus [76].

87%. Other studies examining the accuracy and validity of discography have reported false-positive rates ranging from 3% per patient to more than 83% in certain populations [31–33].

Treatment Options

Nonoperative management of discogenic TSP follows a similar protocol to facetogenic TSP. NSAIDs and acetaminophen have shown some efficacy in the management of acute TSP [34]. Opioids are ineffective for chronic TSP but may be considered for acute exacerbations, with clear goals and close monitoring in place [35]. Muscle relaxants have been shown to reduce pain, muscle tension, and immobility in patients with TSP, whereas scant data exist to support the use of neuroleptics [36]. Physical therapy for mobilization and strengthening, in conjunction with multimodal pharmacologic therapy, often provides useful benefits in pain reduction, weight loss, and cardiovascular fitness [37].

After conservative medical management has failed to adequately treat the patient's symptoms, more invasive techniques may be considered. Several minimally invasive intradiscal procedures exist for the treatment of discogenic TSP [38]. Intradiscal electrothermal therapy (IDET) and intradiscal biacuplasty (IDB) provide analgesia by denervating nociceptive tissue within the intervertebral disc through focused, radiofrequency-induced heat ablation. The techniques differ primarily in that IDB uses internally cooled radiofrequency electrodes to achieve more substantial and even heating over the posterior annulus. Percutaneous disc decompression, another intradiscal technique, is employed only for radicular pain and will be discussed later.

Spine surgery does not enjoy a prominent role in the treatment for discogenic TSP. A recent Cochrane database review concluded that surgical decompression or fusion for degenerative disc disease is not supported by any scientific evidence [39]. Several studies have attempted to examine preoperative discography in advance of spinal fusion for discogenic disease; as of yet, the results are conflicting, with no clear benefit based on existing evidence [21].

RADICULAR PAIN

Thoracic segmental pain may originate from many causes and is characterized by radiating pain in the region innervated by the intercostal nerves. Symptoms are typically unilateral and often described as burning, electric, sharp, and lancinating. Pain may be constant or intermittent and may be exacerbated by movement or pressure. The course of the pain is usually helpful in identification of the affected nerve root. Radiculopathy in the thoracic region is the least common spinal radiculopathy because spinal stenosis and foraminal narrowing are modest in most adults [40,41].

Thoracic radiculopathy may present clinically as sensory loss, weakness, reflex loss, and the localization of pain within a certain dermatome. Most often radiculopathy can be diagnosed in a clinical setting without the use of special tests; however, there are several tests that are useful in establishing a definitive diagnosis when a patient presents with radicular TSP. Electromyography (EMG), nerve conduction studies, CT, or MRI with and without contrast are commonly used to aid in diagnosis of radicular pain. It must be noted that each test should only be used to corroborate clinical findings and determine the location best suited for invasive interventions. The self-limiting nature of most TSP radiculopathy, 4–6 weeks on average, begs the question of premature diagnostic testing promoting unnecessary testing and procedures [42]. For example, Lehnert et al. [43] reported that up to 26% of elective outpatient imaging examinations from an academic medical center were inappropriately obtained. Meanwhile, one of the most frequent reasons for ordering an inappropriate CT or MRI was acute or chronic low back pain. Not only can these unnecessary tests needlessly increase healthcare costs for patients, they may not provide any medical benefit, instead leading to actual medical harm [44]. Spinal imaging abnormalities are often present on even healthy, asymptomatic individuals [45].

Needle EMG studies provide evidence for physiological abnormalities that lead to radicular pain [46]. Unfortunately, this study has several limitations (e.g., endorsement of pain and paresthesias alone without the motor involvement needed to produce EMG abnormalities). One major limitation to needle EMG is in patients with polyradiculopathy predominantly affecting the dorsal roots, in whom there may be no abnormalities on needle EMG despite substantial pain because the ventral motor roots would be unaffected. Nerve conduction studies assess a small number of spinal levels and may be used to identify nerve conduction abnormalities in a suspected affected dermatome [46].

MRI is the best study for identifying structural pathology related to radicular pain. Spinal stenosis and other degenerative changes may be seen on MRI, indicating aggravation or compression of the nerve roots which may lead to radicular pain. Figure 8.2 demonstrates radiologic evidence of spinal disease on MRI. Abnormal contrast enhancement of the nerve roots may lead one to a diagnosis of infectious or inflammatory origin [47,48]. Last, lumbar puncture can help rule out leptomeningeal metastases,

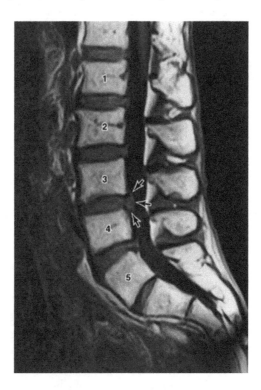

FIGURE 8.2 Radiologic evidence of spinal disease on MRI (arrows) [77].

Lyme meningitis, HIV/AIDS-related polyradiculopathy, and other infectious sources of thoracic spine pathology [49–51].

Musculoskeletal etiologies of thoracic radicular pain include osteoporosis, muscle strain, disc herniation, costovertebral and costotransverse joint dysfunction, and spondylosis. Disc herniation or spondylosis are common etiologies of thoracic radicular pain [2]. Narrowing of the central canal, lateral recess, or the neural foramen due to degenerative changes can lead to nerve root compression, causing radiculopathy in the thoracic region. The intervertebral discs and facet joints may also be damaged due to degenerative causes. Disc herniation is a rupture of the disc material beyond the annulus fibrosus and is due to either protrusion or extrusion. *Protrusion* refers to a complete rupture of disc material in which the base is broader than the dome, and *extrusion* may extend above or below the disc space. With age, the annulus fibrosis itself becomes more fibrotic and less elastic, developing fissures and calcium deposits. As the disc shrinks, the annulus tends to buckle, and a tear or rupture may follow. Other musculoskeletal pathology can cause radicular pain including vertebral metastases, vertebral fracture, vertebral collapse, ankylosing spondylitis, and diffuse idiopathic skeletal hyperostosis [2,52,53].

Infectious processes or neuralgias may also cause radicular pain. Herpes zoster, varicella zoster, cytomegalovirus (CMV), herpes simplex virus, chemical radiculitis, intercostal neuralgia, and other pathological organisms all have been shown to cause thoracic radiculopathy. Nerve roots are completely involved with radiculitis caused by leptomeningeal carcinomatosis, CMV, and herpes zoster and may be compressed, causing compression and ischemia [49]. Herpes zoster, for example, colonizes the dorsal root ganglion, remains latent, and is reactivated, causing an erythematous vesicular maculopapular rash in the dermatome of the affected nerve root.

Other causes radicular pain in the thoracic region include thoracolumbar junction syndrome, slipping rib syndrome, neuropathy secondary to diabetes mellitus, inflammatory conditions such as sarcoidosis, acute inflammatory demyelinating polyradiculoneuropathy, and chemical radiculitis [49–51].

Treatment Options

For pathophysiological conditions such as osteoporosis, muscle strain, disc herniation, costovertebral and costotransverse joint dysfunction, rib fracture, mild ankylosing spondylitis, and spondylosis, conservative therapy should be attempted initially prior to consideration of invasive options. Oral analgesics, oral corticosteroids, avoidance of provocative activities, physical therapy with exercise and increased mobilization, and traction are all acceptable options [54,55]. NSAIDs are the first-line option for the majority of these conditions if patients exhibit adequate renal function. Muscle relaxants are also a common choice to assist in muscle spasm or muscle tightness secondary to nerve dysfunction. Oral glucocorticoids may be used for the inflammatory result of muscle strain and disc herniation. Physical therapy with range of motion exercises, strengthening exercises, and aerobic exercises has been suggested but remains unproved in the literature for radiculopathy [56–59]. The efficacy of epidural steroid injections (ESI) is questioned by conflicting literature; nevertheless, ESI is currently recommended for patients who have undergone 6–8 weeks of conservative therapy with persistent pain without worsening neurological deficit [60,61].

Some musculoskeletal pathology may require more invasive intervention depending on disease progression. Vertebral mass, disc herniation, vertebral collapse, vertebral fracture, severe ankylosing spondylitis, and diffuse idiopathic skeletal hyperostosis may require surgery for definitive treatment. Percutaneous disc decompression, while used more frequently for herniated lumbar intervertebral discs, has demonstrated sustained effectiveness for the treatment of thoracic herniated discs [62]. Vertebroplasty, kyphoplasty, ossification debridement, discectomy, laminectomy, and artificial disc replacement may also be considered for more advanced disease refractory to conservative therapy. Currently, it is only recommended to pursue surgical treatment for radiculopathy if pain symptoms persist longer than 6–12 weeks despite nonsurgical therapy and there is evidence of nerve root compression by MRI or CT [41,63–68]. Some suggest limiting surgical intervention of thoracic radiculopathy to those with progressive myelopathy and neurologic compromise [69].

Infectious processes and inflammatory processes are almost always handled pharmacologically. Herpes zoster or varicella zoster is commonly treated with antiviral therapy and analgesics such as acyclovir and NSAIDs, respectively [70,71]. CMV, herpes simplex virus, chemical radiculitis, intercostal neuralgia, thoracolumbar junction syndrome, slipping rib syndrome, diabetes mellitus, sarcoidosis, and acute inflammatory demyelinating polyradiculoneuropathy are medically managed with respect to their disease process. Symptom management via anti-inflammatory medications, analgesics, and anticonvulsants and antiepileptics such as gabapentin or carbamazepine, in conjunction with resolving medical management of the pathophysiological process, is recommended [2,55,66,69]. In diabetes mellitus, for example, this would mean control of blood sugars via insulin and/or other antidiabetic medications along with antineuropathic medications.

Unique methods exist to directly target thoracic radiculopathy. Spinal manipulation has been suggested to be effective for the treatment of lumbar, cervical, and thoracic radiculopathy. Spinal cord stimulation (SCS) has grown in popularity over recent decades as a treatment for refractory radicular TSP and has proved effective in refractory neuropathic TSP [72,73]. Although a complete overview of the analgesic mechanism behind spinal neuromodulation is beyond the scope of this chapter, it is briefly described as an applied electrical stimulation that inhibits a nociceptive signal from propagating caudally via dorsal pathways. Further research has revealed descending pathways of analgesia that result from SCS in addition to this ascending inhibition [74]. Last, pulsed radiofrequency treatment of the spinal ganglion has been shown to have a short-lasting effect on the reduction of pain [2]. Currently, several reviews evaluating its efficacy have concluded that it is most effective at the lumbar and cervical levels [75].

REFERENCES

1. Gaskin DJ, Richard P. The economic costs of pain in the United States. *J Pain.* 2012;13(8):715–724. doi: 10.1016/j.jpain.2012.03.009. Epub 2012 May 16.
2. van Kleef M, Stolker RJ, Lataster A, et al. Thoracic pain. *Pain Pract.*2010;10(4):327–338.
3. Southerst D, Marchand AA, Côté P, et al. The effectiveness of noninvasive interventions for musculoskeletal thoracic spine and chest wall pain: a systematic review by the Ontario Protocol for Traffic Injury Management (OPTIMa) collaboration. *J Manipulative Physiol Ther.* 2015;38(7):521–531.

4. Fouquet N, et al. Prevalence of thoracic spine pain in a surveillance network. *Occup Med.* 2014;65(2):122–125.

5. Briggs AM, Smith AJ, Straker LM, et al. Thoracic spine pain in the general population: prevalence, incidence and associated factors in children, adolescents and adults. A systematic review. *BMC Musculoskelet Disord.* 2009;10:77.

6. Berger A, Henry L, Goldberg M. Surgical palliation of thoracic malignancies. *Surg Oncol Clin N Am.* 2004;13:429–453, viii.

7. Nijs J, Apeldoorn A, Hallegraeff H, et al. Low back pain: guidelines for the clinical classification of predominant neuropathic, nociceptive, or central sensitization pain. *Pain Physician.* 2015;18(3):E333–E346.

8. Bogduk N. Functional anatomy of the spine. *Handb Clin Neurol.* 2016;136:675–688.

9. Singh V. Thoracic discography. *Pain Physician.* 2004;451–458.

10. Chua WH, Bogduk N. The surgical anatomy of thoracic facet denervation. *Acta Neurochir (Wien).* 1995;136(3-4):140–144.

11. Manchikanti L, Boswell MV, Singh V, et al. Prevalence of facet joint pain in chronic spinal pain of cervical, thoracic, and lumbar regions. *BMC Musculoskelet Disord.* 2004;5:15.

12. Manchikanti L, Boswell MV, Singh V, et al. Comprehensive review of neurophysiologic basis and diagnostic interventions in managing chronic spinal pain. *Pain Physician.* 2009;12(4):E71–E120.

13. Chen C, Lu Y, Kallakuri S, et al. Distribution of A-delta and C-fiber receptors in the cervical facet joint capsule and their response to stretch. *J Bone Joint Surg Am.* 2006;88:1807–1816.

14. Brewerton DA, et al. Ankylosing spondylitis and HL-A 27. *Lancet.* 1973;1(7809):904–907.

15. Brummett CM, Cohen SP. Pathogenesis, diagnosis, and treatment of zygapophyseal (facet) joint pain. In: Benzon HT, Rathmell JP, Wu CL, Turk DC, Argoff CE, Hurley RW, eds. *Practical Management of Pain.* 5th ed. Philadelphia, PA: Elsevier/Saunders; 2014:816–845.

16. Manchikanti L, Kaye AD, Boswell MV, et al. A systematic review and best evidence synthesis of the effectiveness of therapeutic facet joint interventions in managing chronic spinal pain. *Pain Physician.* 2015;18(4):E535–E582.

17. Giles LG, Muller R. Chronic spinal pain: a randomized clinical trial comparing medication, acupuncture, and spinal manipulation. *Spine.* 2003;28:1490–1502.

18. Pope J, Cheng J. Facet (zygapophyseal) intraarticular joint injections: cervical, lumbar and thoracic. In: Huntoon M, Benzon H, Nauroze S, eds. *Spinal Injections and Peripheral Nerve Blocks.* 1st ed., vol. 4. Philadelphia, PA: Elsevier; 2010:129–135.

19. Cohen SP, Larkin TM, Barna SA, et al. Lumbar discography: a comprehensive review of outcome studies, diagnostic accuracy, and principles. *Reg Anesth Pain Med.* 2005;30:163–183.

20. Ikari C. A study of the mechanism of low back pain: the neurohistological examination of the disease. *J Bone Joint Surg Am.* 1954;36:195.

21. Bottros MM, Cohen SP. Lumbar discogenic pain and diskography. In: Benzon HT, Rathmell JP, Wu CL, Turk DC, Argoff CE, Hurley RW, eds. *Practical Management of Pain.* 5th ed. Philadelphia, PA: Elsevier/Saunders; 2014:885–914.

22. Adams MA, McNally DS, Dolan P. "Stress" distributions inside intervertebral discs: the effects of age and degeneration. *J Bone Joint Surg Br.* 1996;78:965–972.

23. Annunen S, Paassilta P, Lohiniva J, et al. An allele of COL9A2 associated with intervertebral disc disease. *Science.* 1999;285:409–412.

24. Podichetty VK. The aging spine: the role of inflammatory mediators in intervertebral disc degeneration. *Cell Mol Biol (Noisy-le-grand).* 2007;53:4–18.

25. Freemont AJ. Watkins A, Le Maitre C, et al. Nerve growth factor expression and innervation of the painful intervertebral disc. *J Pathol.* 2002;197:286–292.

26. Groen GJ, Baljet B, Drukker J. Nerves and nerve plexuses of the human vertebral column. *Am J Anat.* 1990;188:282–296.

27. Jones MR, Kaye AD, Manchikanti L, et al. Pain states, the opioid epidemic, and the critical role for radiologists in clinical practice. *JACR.* In press.

28. Jensen MC, Brant-Zawadzki MN, Obuchowski N, Modic MT, Malkasian D, Ross JS. Magnetic resonance imaging of the lumbar spine in people without back pain. *N Engl J Med.* 331;1994:69–73.

29. Vu T, Al-Grain H, Liu A, et al. The clinical efficacy of repeat magnetic resonance imaging in patients with chronic spine pain. Presented at: the American Pain Society 36th Annual Scientific Meeting; May 17–20, 2017; Pittsburgh, PA.

30. Jackson RP, Becker GJ, Jacobs RR, et al. The neuroradiographic diagnosis of lumbar herniated nucleus pulposus, I: a comparison of computed tomography (CT), CT-myelography, discography, and CT-discography. *Spine.* 1989;14:1356–1361.

31. Wolfer LR, Derby R, Lee JE, et al. Systematic review of lumbar provocation discography in asymptomatic subjects with a meta-analysis of false-positive rates. *Pain Physician.* 2008;11:513–538.

32. Carragee EJ, Tanner CM, Khurana S, et al. The rates of false-positive lumbar discography in select patients without low back symptoms. *Spine.* 2000;25:1373–1380.

33. Yasuma T, Ohno R, Yamauchi Y. False-negative discograms. *J Bone Joint Surg Am.* 1988;70:1279–1290.

34. Van Tulder MW, Scholten RJ, Koes BW, et al. Nonsteroidal anti-inflammatory drugs for low back pain. *Spine.* 2000;25:2501–2513.

35. Benzon H, Raja SN, Spencer SL, Fishman SM, Cohen SP. *Essentials of Pain Medicine.* 3rd ed. Philadelphia, PA: Elsevier/Saunders, 2011.

36. Porter RW, Ralston SH. Pharmacological management of back pain syndromes. *Drugs.* 1994;48:189–198.

37. Van Tulder MW, Malmivaara A, Esmail R, et al. Exercise therapy for low back pain. *Cochrane Database Syst Rev.* 2000;2:CD000335.

38. Kapural L. Intradiscal procedures for the treatment of discogenic lower back and leg pain. In: Benzon HT, Rathmell JP, Wu CL, Turk DC, Argoff CE, Hurley RW, eds. *Practical Management of Pain.* Philadelphia, PA: Elsevier/Saunders; 2014:915–921.

39. Gibson JN, Waddell G, Grant IC. Surgery for degenerative lumbar spondylosis. *Cochrane Database Syst Rev.* 2000;2:CD001352.

40. Kikta DG, Breuer AC, Wilbourn AJ. Thoracic root pain in diabetes: the spectrum of clinical and electromyographic findings. *Ann Neurol.* 1982;11(1):80–85.

41. Sun SF, Streib EW. Diabetic thoracoabdominal neuropathy: clinical and electrodiagnostic features. *Ann Neurol.* 1981;9(1):75–79.

42. Bigos S, Bowyer O, Braen G, et al. *Acute Low Back Problems in Adults. Clinical Practice Guideline No. 14.* Rockville, MD: Agency for Health Care Policy and Research, Public Health Service, U.S. Department of Health and Human Services; 1994. AHCPR Publication No. 95-0642.

43. Lehnert BE, Bree RL. Analysis of appropriateness of outpatient CT and MRI referred from primary care clinics at an academic medical center: how critical is the need for improved decision support? *J Am Coll Radiol.* 2010;7(3):192–197.

44. Hom J, Smith CD, Ahuja N, et al. R-SCAN: imaging for low back pain. *J Am Coll Radiol.* 2016;13(11):1385–1386.

45. Jensen MC, Brant-Zawadzki MN, Obuchowski N, et al. Magnetic resonance imaging of the lumbar spine in people without back pain. *N Engl J Med.* 331;1994:69–73.

46. Fisher MA. Electrophysiology of radiculopathies. *Clin Neurophysiol.* 2002;113(3):317–335. http://www.ncbi.nlm.nih.gov/pubmed/11897532. Accessed August 6, 2017.

47. Koffman B, Junck L, Elias SB, et al. Polyradiculopathy in sarcoidosis. *Muscle Nerve.* 1999;22(5):608–613. http://www.ncbi.nlm.nih.gov/pubmed/10331360. Accessed August 6, 2017.

48. So YT, Olney RK. Acute lumbosacral polyradiculopathy in acquired immunodeficiency syndrome: experience in 23 patients. *Ann Neurol.* 1994;35(1):53–58.

49. Viali S, Hutchinson DO, Hawkins TE, et al. Presentation of intravascular lymphomatosis as lumbosacral polyradiculopathy. *Muscle Nerve.* 2000;23(8):1295–1300. http://www.ncbi.nlm.nih.gov/pubmed/10918273. Accessed August 6, 2017.

50. Grossman SA, Krabak MJ. Leptomeningeal carcinomatosis. *Cancer Treat Rev.* 1999;25(2):103–119.

51. Anders HJ, Goebel FD. Cytomegalovirus polyradiculopathy in patients with AIDS. *Clin Infect Dis.* 1998;27(2):345–352. http://www.ncbi.nlm.nih.gov/pubmed/9709885. Accessed August 6, 2017.

52. Sebastian D. Thoraco lumbar junction syndrome: a case report. *Physiother Theory Pract.* 2006;22(1):53–60. http://www.ncbi.nlm.nih.gov/pubmed/16573246. Accessed August 6, 2017.

53. Udermann BE, Cavanaugh DG, Gibson MH, et al. Slipping rib syndrome in a collegiate swimmer: a case report. *J Athl Train.* 2005;40(2):120–122. http://www.ncbi.nlm.nih.gov/pubmed/15970959. Accessed August 6, 2017.

54. Ellenberg MR, Honet JC, Treanor WJ. Cervical radiculopathy. *Arch Phys Med Rehabil.* 1994;75(3):342–352. http://www.ncbi.nlm.nih.gov/pubmed/8129590. Accessed August 7, 2017.

55. Carette S, Fehlings MG. Clinical practice. Cervical radiculopathy. *N Engl J Med.* 2005;353(4):392–399.

56. Wininger KL, ML, Bester, et al. Spinal cord stimulation to treat postthoracotomy neuralgia: non-small-cell lung cancer: a case report. *Pain Manag Nurs.* 2012;13(1):52–59.

57. van der Heijden GJ, Beurskens AJ, Koes BW, et al. The efficacy of traction for back and neck pain: a systematic, blinded review of randomized clinical trial methods. *Phys Ther.* 1995;75(2):93–104. http://www.ncbi.nlm.nih.gov/pubmed/7846138. Accessed August 7, 2017.

58. Goldie I, Landquist A. Evaluation of the effects of different forms of physiotherapy in cervical pain. *Scand J Rehabil Med.* 1970;2(2):117–121. http://www.ncbi.nlm.nih.gov/pubmed/5523822. Accessed August 7, 2017.

59. Kuijper B, Tans JTJ, Beelen A, et al. Cervical collar or physiotherapy versus wait and see policy for recent onset cervical radiculopathy: randomised trial. *BMJ.* 2009 Oct 7;339:b3883. doi: 10.1136/bmj.b3883

60. Rathmell JP, Benzon HT, Dreyfuss P, et al. Safeguards to prevent neurologic complications after epidural steroid injections. *Anesthesiology.* 2015;122(5):974–984.

61. Benzon HT, Huntoon MA, Rathmell JP. Improving the safety of epidural steroid injections. *JAMA.* 2015;313(17):1713–1714.

62. Graham N, Gross AR, Goldsmith C, Cervical Overview Group the CO. Mechanical traction for mechanical neck disorders: a systematic review. *J Rehabil Med.* 2006;38(3):145–152.

63. Moatz B, Tortolani PJ. Cervical disc arthroplasty: pros and cons. *Surg Neurol Int.* 2012;3(Suppl 3):S216–S224.

64. Gao Y, Liu M, Li T, et al. A meta-analysis comparing the results of cervical disc arthroplasty with anterior cervical discectomy and fusion (ACDF) for the treatment of symptomatic cervical disc disease. *J Bone Joint Surg Am.* 2013;95(6):555–561.

65. Hu Y, Lu G, Ren S, et al. Mid- to long-term outcomes of cervical disc arthroplasty versus anterior cervical discectomy and fusion for treatment of symptomatic cervical disc disease: a systematic review and meta-analysis of eight prospective randomized controlled trials. *PLoS One.* 2016;11(2):e0149312.

66. Bono CM, Ghiselli G, Gilbert TJ, et al. An evidence-based clinical guideline for the diagnosis and treatment of cervical radiculopathy from degenerative disorders. *Spine J.* 2011;11(1):64–72.

67. Storm PB, Chou D, Tamargo RJ. Surgical management of cervical and lumbosacral radiculopathies: indications and outcomes. *Phys Med Rehabil Clin N Am.* 2002;13(3):735–759. http://www.ncbi.nlm.nih.gov/pubmed/12380556. Accessed August 7, 2017.

68. Köse KC, Cebesoy O, Akan B, et al. Functional results of vertebral augmentation techniques in pathological vertebral fractures of myelomatous patients. *J Natl Med Assoc.* 2006;98(10):1654–1658.

69. O'Connor RC, Andary MT, Russo RB, et al. Thoracic radiculopathy. *Phys Med Rehabil Clin N Am.* 2002;13(3):623–644, viii.

70. Tyring SK, Beutner KR, Tucker BA, et al. Antiviral therapy for herpes zoster: randomized, controlled clinical trial of valacyclovir and famciclovir therapy in immunocompetent patients 50 years and older. *Arch Fam Med.* 9(9):863–869. http://www.ncbi.nlm.nih.gov/pubmed/11031393. Accessed August 7, 2017.

71. Shafran SD, Tyring SK, Ashton R, et al. Once, twice, or three times daily famciclovir compared with aciclovir for the oral treatment of herpes zoster in immunocompetent adults: a randomized, multicenter, double-blind clinical trial. *J Clin Virol.* 2004;29(4):248–253.

72. Linderoth B, Meyerson BA. Spinal cord and brain stimulation. In: McMahon SB, Koltzenburg M, Tracey I, Turk D, eds. *Wall & Melzack's Textbook of Pain.* Philadelphia, PA: Elsevier/Saunders; 2013:570–591.

73. Bengt L, Robert DF. Mechanisms of spinal cord stimulation in painful syndromes: role of animal models. *Pain Med.* 2006;7:S14–S26.

74. Zhuang QS, Lun DX, Xu ZW, et al. Surgical treatment for central calcified thoracic disk herniation: a novel l-shaped osteotome. *Orthopedics.* 2015;38(9):e794–e798.

75. van Boxem K, van Eerd M, Brinkhuize T, Patijn et al. Radiofrequency and pulsed radiofrequency treatment of chronic pain syndromes: the available evidence. *Pain Pract.* 2008;8(5):385–393.

76. Kallewaard JW, Terheggen MA, Groen GJ, et al. Discogenic low back pain. *Pain Pract.* 2010;10(6):560–579.

77. Aminoff MJ, Greenberg DA, Simon RP. *Clinical Neurology.* 9th ed. New York: McGraw-Hill; 2015.

9 Lumbosacral Pain

Chang-Yeon Kim, Charles Chang,
Raysa Cabrejo, and James Yue

INTRODUCTION

Spine surgery is one of the most common orthopedic procedures, with more than 500,000 performed annually [1]. Surgery may involve any site in the spine, from cervical to lumbosacral, and ranges from minimally invasive microdiscectomy to major surgeries crossing multiple spinal levels. Such procedures lead to the dissection of soft tissues and muscles, which can cause severe postoperative pain [2]. Many patients also present with preexisting chronic pain conditions or opioid dependencies, may be cognitively impaired, or be very young.

These factors make pain management after spinal surgery a challenging task. Regardless, the effective management of postoperative pain is an essential component of perioperative patient care. Inadequate control of postoperative pain can lead to great anxiety for patients and also contribute to delays in mobilization and discharge, thus increasing the risk for infection, deep venous thrombosis, and poor wound healing [3–5].

The current standard of care for pain management after spinal surgery is opioid administration via intravenous patient-controlled analgesia (PCA), with subsequent conversion to oral opioids and nonsteroidal anti-inflammatory drugs (NSAIDs). Recent developments in pain management have advocated a multimodal approach to analgesia using a combination of simple primary analgesics, opioids, and regional analgesic techniques.

CONVENTIONAL OPEN SURGERY IN THE LUMBAR SPINE

Anterior Approach

Anterior lumbar interbody fusion (ALIF), a common anterior approach to the lumbar spine, avoids extensive damage to the paraspinal muscles and chronic pain associated with posterior lumbar approaches. The surgeon makes an incision at the abdomen and retracts the ureters, common iliac vessels, and the lumbar plexus, which forms within the psoas major muscle. During the retraction of the psoas muscle, injury can occur to the nerve roots and peripheral branches. The sympathetic trunk is also at risk of being severed during the retraction, leading to postsympathectomy dysfunction and manifesting as increased skin temperature, reduced perspiration, dysesthesias, discoloration, and swelling [6,7]. The majority of these symptoms tend to resolve within the year.

Posterior Approach

In posterior lumbar interbody fusion, surgery is performed in the prone position. An incorrect or unmonitored prone position can induce undue pressures and cause nerve palsies, including blindness, brachial pleuropathy, meralgia paresthetica, and flat back syndrome. Posterior surgical entry can also cause direct trauma to the erector spinae muscles, resulting in chronic pain. Prolonged retraction can lead to fibrous tissue replacement of the lumbar paraspinal muscles, known as "fusion disease."8 A major concern when removing the disk and performing the fusion is accidental durotomy, which is more frequent in patients with spinal stenosis. Excessive retraction of the dural sac can risk "battered root syndrome," causing symptoms of nerve root irritation. Either approach to lumbar surgery can result in "failed back surgery syndrome," in which the patient is not physically comfortable without regular medication or treatment and which tends to be described as neuropathic pain.

ENDOSCOPIC SPINAL SURGERY

Endoscopic surgery is performed to minimize blood loss, reduce damage to paravertebral muscles, and preserve ligaments, thus decreasing postoperative pain. These procedures are technically demanding and require a great degree of planning due to limited field of vision and control. The most common endoscopic procedure is the percutaneous endoscopic lumbar diskectomy (PELD). The most damaging complication is missing a fragment during surgery, leading to partial or no relief of preoperative pain. Immediately after surgery, about 30% of patients experience neck pain due to an increase in cervical epidural pressure from the irrigation used during the procedure [9]. Piriformis syndrome presents with low back pain with or without lower leg pain, peaking at about 1 month after surgery in about 13% of patients [10]. Postoperative dysesthesia caused by excessive manipulation of nerve roots or injury to the furcal nerve occurs in 8% of patients. It is localized pain to a dermatome therefore adding to the pain sensation of the patient.

FAST-TRACK POSTSURGICAL PROGRAM

Fast-track programs continue to be implemented because they improve recovery and reduce morbidity of patients. The overall goal is to enact changes in perioperative and postoperative care to reduce "surgical stress." The main components of the approach are early mobilization, oral nutrition, and minimal use of tubes, drains, and catheters [11,12]. For orthopedic patients, the focus has been to first adequately inform the patient, followed by pain relief through oxycodone and paracetamol, with concomitant use of Zofran for the control of nausea. This has been quite effective in reducing length of stay and improving quality of life in patients [13]. However, fast-tracking postsurgical recovery can be traumatic as patients are mobilized for hours and started on oral nutrition as early as the first postoperative day. These tasks are especially difficult to implement in postoperative management for spinal surgery.

APPROACH TO POSTOPERATIVE PAIN MANAGEMENT

For some sequelae of spinal surgery, such as failed back syndrome after lumbar surgery, special techniques involving spinal cord stimulation have shown some promise over conventional medical management [14]. However, for the majority of pain after spinal surgery, a multimodal analgesic regime that combines different classes of analgesics and delivery mechanisms has been the most effective.

Oral Analgesia

In general, oral analgesics offers a safe, simple, and cost-effective method of pain relief. It should always be considered in cases of moderate discomfort with possibility of oral diet [15]. Common classes of oral analgesics include NSAIDs, opioids, gabapentinoids, and acetaminophen.

NSAIDs

Oral NSAIDs have been shown to reduce mild to moderate pain, inflammation, and fever and to improve postoperative ambulation following spinal surgeries [16–18]. They are advantageous for treating patients who have developed opioid tolerance or who are at risk for opioid side effects. However, exclusive use of NSAIDs for analgesia is not recommended after spinal surgery [19], and they are typically used simultaneously with regional blockade or opioids as part of a multimodal analgesic regimen [15,18,20–22].

The major concern with the use of NSAIDs is that they impair bone growth and repair [15], which is problematic after spinal fusion. Cyclooxygenase (COX-2) inhibitors (parecoxib, celecoxib), whose selective action preserves platelet function and minimizes gastric bleeding, are also limited from widespread use because COX-2–dependent production of prostaglandin (PGE2) is important for adequate skeletal regeneration [18]. However, recent evidence has suggested that impaired bone healing results from higher doses and longer duration of treatment with parenteral forms of NSAIDs, and selective usage may reduce opioid consumption without affecting rates of nonunion [18].

The well-known side effects of NSAIDs are platelet dysfunction, risk of hemorrhage, gastric ulceration, and renal toxicity [18]. Absolute contraindications against NSAIDs are concomitant use with anticoagulants, coagulopathy, and active peptic ulcers. Relative contraindications include history of coronary and cerebrovascular disease and liver impairment.

Dosing of oral NSAIDs after spinal surgery has not been standardized as there are many conflicting reports of dosage and effectiveness (Table 9.1). A single preoperative

Table 9.1 Dosing for oral analgesic regimen

Analgesic	Dose
Rofecoxib	Single preoperative dose of 50 mg
Celecoxib	Single preoperative dose of 200 mg
Morphine	20 to 30 mg
Codeine	15 to 60 mg every 6 hours
Tramadol	50 to 100 mg every 4 to 6 hours
Oxycodone	5 to 30 mg every 4 to 6 hours
Hydromorphone	2 to 4 mg every 4 to 6 hours
Gabapentinoids	Single preoperative dose of 300 to 600 mg
Acetaminophen	325 to 650 mg every 4 to 6 hours, not to exceed 4g daily

dose of celecoxib 200 mg or rofecoxib 50 mg has been shown to reduce morphine PCA consumption after 4–8 hours after spinal fusion. While celecoxib did not reduce pain beyond this period, rofecoxib continued to reduce morphine requirements and lower pain scores for 24 hours [23].

Opioids

Oral opioids provide effective relief for moderate to severe pain. The well-known side effects of opioids include nausea, vomiting, pruritus, sedation, and respiratory depression, which are worsened after alteration in GI function due to surgery and can delay patient recovery [15]. Patients may also present with significant opioid dependencies. Providers should ensure that dosing regimens are modified for patients who have developed tolerance, maintaining their baseline narcotic requirements to avoid doses inadequate for severe postoperative pain.

Both immediate and sustained-release forms of oral opioids are employed. Oral morphine and meperidine undergo substantial enterohepatic metabolism, delaying onset and requiring doses that are two to three times higher than parenteral requirements (Table 9.1). Oxycodone is less likely to undergo enterohepatic metabolism and requires smaller doses. Short-acting formulations require repeated dosing every 4–7 hours. Sustained-release opioid preparations require fewer administration intervals, offer longer duration of pain relief (8–12 hours), and necessitate lower doses. Controlled-release oxycodone requires doses at about equal ratio to intravenous PCA morphine [15].

Opioids should be used as a short-term therapy because of the risk of hyperalgesia and addiction. When they are stopped, they should be tapered. Tapering opioids after successful surgery involves replacing short-acting opioids with extended-release products, such as OxyContin, or one with a long half-life, such as methadone. A taper using the original short-acting opioid is also frequently employed, with adjunct therapy such as ondansetron to control opioid-related side affects.

The recommended time scale is a decrease of 10% of the original dose every 5–7 days, until 30% is reached [24]. This reduces the amount and severity of withdrawal symptoms, thus increasing adherence. Drugs that are commonly used to taper are buprenorphine-naloxone and methadone, with no evidence demonstrating that one is superior to the other. To manage withdrawal symptoms, an α_2 adrenergic agonist should be used. At the beginning of the taper, there is a risk for hyperalgesia, which can be treated with nonopioid regimens.

Gabapentin

Gabapentin, an antineuropathic, has been shown to reduce postoperative pain and opioid use. A single dose of 300–600 mg of preoperative oral gabapentin decreases pain scores in the early postoperative period and reduces postoperative morphine consumption in spinal surgery patients. It is generally well tolerated, with the most common side effects including sedation, dizziness, headache, visual disturbance and peripheral edema [25,26].

Acetaminophen

Acetaminophen reversibly inhibits COX and is used as an analgesic for postoperative pain. It is most commonly used as an adjuvant and in combinations with other therapies. Oral acetaminophen in combination with intravenous methocarbamol decreases opioid consumption and increases the effectiveness of physical therapy on postoperative patients [27]. In a study specific to spine surgery, it was shown that oral multimodal analgesia including acetaminophen was better than intravenous PCA, leading to less opioid consumption, nausea, drowsiness, and difficulty with mobilization [26].

Parenteral Therapy

Opioids

The use of parenteral opioids has been the mainstay of analgesia for patients undergoing spinal surgery. Their use, via the intravenous route in particular, is associated with dose-dependent side effects such as respiratory depression, nausea and vomiting, sedation, and gastrointestinal ileus [15,28]. Adequate use of PCA can lessen these side effects, but the incidence rate can still be as high as 71%, with mild to moderate symptoms [28].

Commonly used parenteral opioids include morphine, meperidine, hydromorphone, oxycodone, and fentanyl (Table 9.2). Morphine effectively blocks pain after severe musculoskeletal injury and is commonly used in patients recovering from orthopedic surgery. Analgesia begins 5 and 15 minutes after intravenous and intramuscular administration, respectively. Pain control lasts from 2 to 4 hours, depending on dose and

Table 9.2 Dosing for parenteral analgesic regimen

Analgesic	Dosing
Ketorolac	15 to 30 mg every 6 hours
Propacetamol	1g over 24 hours
Morphine	1 to 3 mg every 5 minutes
Hydromorphone	0.2 to 1 mg every two to three hours
Fentanyl	25 to 50 μg every 5 minutes

site of administration. Administration of morphine may release histamine and has been associated with hypotension and biliary colic [15].

For patients who cannot tolerate the adverse effects of morphine, meperidine and hydromorphone are useful alternatives. However, the parenteral potency of meperidine is one-tenth that of morphine, and its duration of analgesia is two-thirds as long. Normeperidine, a metabolite of meperidine, can accumulate to cause seizures at doses greater than 1 g/day. In contrast, hydromorphone is approximately five times as potent as morphine, has more rapid onset of analgesia, and causes fewer adverse effects. Fentanyl is reserved for patients with hemodynamic instability or high opioid tolerance. It is a potent analgesic, and bolus doses (50–200 μg) or intravenous infusions (50–200 μg/h) are particularly useful in intubated patients [15].

Ketorolac

Ketorolac, the only injectable NSAID formulation available in the United States, has been shown to enhance the effect of narcotics and decrease the narcotics requirement [29]. It has been shown to be as effective as morphine in managing posttraumatic musculoskeletal pain [18,22,29].

Similar to other NSAIDs, there is concern that ketorolac is associated with increased rates of nonunion after spinal fusion [30]. However, there is no definitive consensus regarding ketorolac's effect on nonunion [29], with ketorolac having no significant effects on fusion rates if limited to 48 hours after surgery. Other reports have found that short (<14 days) exposure to normal-dose NSAIDs (ketorolac, diclofenac sodium, celecoxib, or rofecoxib) are safe after spinal fusion. However, short (<14 days) exposure to high-dose ketorolac increased the risk of nonunion, which meant that the effect of perioperative NSAIDs on spinal fusion might be dose-dependent [31].

Propacetamol

Unlike NSAIDs, which inhibit COX enzymes peripherally and may interfere with bone healing, acetaminophen is a centrally acting analgesic and does not have the adverse effects of NSAIDs [32]. Therefore, intravenous propacetamol, a prodrug form of acetaminophen, has found use as an adjunct to opioids after spinal surgery. Propacetamol has been used in Europe for 20 years and was recently approved in the United States under the name Ofirmev in 2010.

Intravenous propacetamol is advantageous in that it avoids the significant side-effect profiles of opioids and NSAIDs. It does not increase nausea, vomiting, and respiratory depression nor does it induce gastrointestinal, hematologic, and renal sequelae [33]. However, there are some disadvantages of using propacetamol as it can be associated with pain at the intravenous injection site and, as in all forms of acetaminophen, is contraindicated in patients with hepatic impairment [34]. Additionally, propacetamol is significantly more expensive ($50/day) than oral or rectal forms of acetaminophen.

Despite some of the reported disadvantages of propacetamol use, it offers significant pain relief while reducing opioid consumption after spinal surgery. A 1 g dose of intravenous acetaminophen, administered over a 24-hour period, can provide rapid and effective analgesia, while inducing only local, minor side effects [35].

intravenous acetaminophen, administered over a 24-hour period, can provide rapid and effective analgesia, while inducing only local, minor side effects [35].

Ketamine

Ketamine, an N-methyl-D-aspartate (NMDA) receptor antagonist, can be used as a standalone drug or as an adjunct to others to reduce pain. Dosing of parenteral ketamine varies, but 1 µg/kg/min perioperative and postoperative ketamine reduced morphine requirements and incidence of nausea and vomiting after microdiscectomy. In another study, it was demonstrated that a 2 µg/kg/min (total bolus: 0.5 mg/kg) infusion of ketamine can reduce the use of fentanyl postoperatively [36].

Patient Controlled Analgesia

Intravenous PCA has been accepted as a superior method to deliver opioid analgesics compared to intermittent divided dosing [2]. Although intravenous PCA is a well-established perioperative pain management tool (dosing in Table 9.3),[37] it is not without disadvantages. Limitations can involve mobility restrictions for patients and long preparation times for staff. Potential safety concerns also exist in the event that intravenous catheters become clotted or infiltrate into subcutaneous tissue. Pump failures and programming errors have also been reported, which can be associated with oversedation and even death [2].

The Ionsys system (fentanyl iontophoretic transdermal system) is a new innovation in PCA administration that overcomes some of the problems in intravenous PCA. The Ionsys system is transdermal and needle-free, self-contained, and preprogrammed. Because the system does not require a pump and related equipment (catheters, tubing, and intravenous poles), it leads to a lower incidence of technology failures or system-related events (SREs). The lower number of SREs decreases the analgesic gaps when transitioning from fentanyl ITS to oral opiates in comparison to intravenous PCA [38–40]. The fentanyl ITS is preprogrammed to release a 40 µg dose over a 10-minute period on activation with a dosing button. The system can deliver up to 6 doses per hour, with a maximum dose of 80 doses in 24 hours, after which the system deactivates [2].

Spinal Analgesia

Spinal blocks involve the clustered injection of analgesics to remove sensation/pain. However, success of the block is highly dependent on adequate training of the administrator. Other factors important to successful administration include quality of

Table 9.3 Intravenous patient-controlled analgesia (PCA) dosing

Opioid	Concentration	Loading dose	Incremental bolus dose	Lockout interval	Maximum in 4 hours
Morphine	1 mg/mL	5–15 mg	0.5–1.5 mg	5–10 min	30 mg
Hydromorphone	0.2 mg/mL	0.5–3 mg	0.1–0.3 mg	6–8 min	6 mg
Fentanyl	20 µg/mL	30–100 µg	10–20 µg	5–6 min	300 µg

113 Lumbosacral Pain

the anatomical landmarks, patient age, and body mass index (BMI) [41]. The location of the injection must also be considered as the risk of error increases as one moves up the spine; therefore, the procedure should not be attempted above L3 [42]. About 7.3% will experience postdural puncture headache due to leakage of cerebrospinal fluid [43], which manifests as a severe and searing headache, drowsiness, dry mouth, fatigue, nausea, dizziness, and itchiness. Although the incidence is low (about 1:150,000), spinal hematoma has also been reported, with a higher risk in patients taking antithrombolytic agents [44]. In addition, patients with underlying spinal canal stenosis or pathology are more prone to neurologic complications after the block [45].

MULTIMODAL PAIN MANAGEMENT

Opioids remain the agents of choice for severe pain after spinal surgery. However, due to their dose-dependent adverse effects, concomitant use of nonopioid analgesic has been advocated to provide a multimodal analgesic regimen. The goal of such a regimen is to decrease opioid dose requirements, thus reducing associated adverse events while still achieve postsurgical pain management goals [15]. A variety of nonopioid analgesic compounds have been studied for multimodal analgesia, including ketorolac, gabapentinoids, acetaminophen, and local anesthetics such as bupivacaine [15,42]. Techniques combining different analgesic delivery methods, such as intrathecal infusion in conjunction with intravenous PCA, have been studied as well. These techniques have shown improved pain scores and reduced opioid consumption, and they remain the ideal strategies for pain control after spinal surgery.

CONCLUSION

The management of pain after spinal procedures remains a challenging task. Surgeons should consider prior use of opioids, pain syndromes related to specific approaches, and individual patient responses to treatment. One mode of analgesia is frequently insufficient to control the pain, and the use of multimodal analgesic regimens combining opioid and nonopioid methods will ensure a more effective recovery.

REFERENCES

1. Rajaee S, Bae H, Kanim L, Delamarter R. Spinal fusion in the united states: analysis of trends from 1998 to 2008. *Spine (Phila Pa 1976)*. 2012;37(1):67–76.
2. Lindley E, Milligan K, Farmer R, et al. Patient-controlled transdermal fentanyl versus intravenous morphine pump after spine surgery. *Orthopedics*. 2015;38(9):e819–e824.
3. Breivik H, Stubhaug A. Management of acute postoperative pain: still a long way to go! *Pain*. 2008;137(2):233–234.
4. Breivik H. Postoperative pain management: why is it difficult to show that it improves outcome? *Eur J Anaesthesiol*. 1998;15(6):748–751.
5. Kehlet H, Jensen T, Woolf C. Persistent postsurgical pain: risk factors and prevention. *Lancet*. 2006;367(9522):1618–1625.
6. Hrabalek L, Sternbersky J, Adamus M. Risk of sympathectomy after anterior and lateral lumbar interbody fusion procedures. *Biomed Pap Med Fac Univ Palacký Olomouc Czechoslov*. 2015;159:318–326.

7. Brau S. Mini-open approach to the spine for anterior lumbar interbody fusion: description of the procedure, results and complications. *Spine J.* 2002;2(3):216–223.

8. Singla N, Rock A, Pavliv L. A multi-center, randomized, double-blind placebo-controlled trial of intravenous-ibuprofen (IV-ibuprofen) for treatment of pain in postoperative orthopedic adult patients. *Pain Med.* 2010;11(8):1284–1293.

9. Joh J, Choi G, Kong B, et al. Comparative study of neck pain in relation to increase of cervical epidural pressure during percutaneous endoscopic lumbar discectomy. *Spine.* 2009;34(19):2033–2038.

10. Kim J, Kim K. Piriformis syndrome after percutaneous endoscopic lumbar discectomy via the posterolateral approach. *Eur Spine J.* 2011;20(10):1663–1668.

11. Wilmore DW, Kehlet H. Management of patients in fast track surgery. *BMJ.* 2001;322(7284):473–476. Accessed November 23, 2015.

12. Kehlet H, Wilmore DW. Evidence-based surgical care and the evolution of fast-track surgery. *Ann Surg.* 2008;248(2):189–198. Accessed November 23, 2015. doi: 10.1097/SLA.0b013e31817f2c1a.

13. Larsen K, Sorensen OG, Hansen TB, et al. Accelerated perioperative care and rehabilitation intervention for hip and knee replacement is effective: a randomized clinical trial involving 87 patients with 3 months of follow-up. *Acta Orthop.* 2008;79(2):149–159. Accessed November 23, 2015. doi: 10.1080/17453670710014923.

14. Kumar K, Taylor R, Jacques L, et al. Spinal cord stimulation versus conventional medical management for neuropathic pain: a multicentre randomised controlled trial in patients with failed back surgery syndrome. *Pain.* 2007;132(1–2):179–188.

15. Sinatra R, Torres J, Bustos A. Pain management after major orthopaedic surgery: current strategies and new concepts. *J Am Acad Orthop Surg.* 2002;10(2):117–129.

16. Nissen I, Jensen K, Ohrström J. Indomethacin in the management of postoperative pain. *Br J Anaesth.* 1992;69:304–306.

17. Turner P, Hagelin C. Motorcycle helmet use and trends before and after Florida's helmet law change. *Journal of the Transportation Research Board.* 2006;1922:183–187.

18. Bajwa S, Haldar R. Pain management following spinal surgeries: an appraisal of the available options. *J Craniovertebr Junction Spine.* 2015;6(3):105–110.

19. Sharma S, Balireddy R, Vorenkamp K, Durieux M. Beyond opioid patient-controlled analgesia: a systematic review of analgesia after major spine surgery. *Reg Anesth Pain Med.* 2012;27(1):79–98.

20. Jirarattanaphochai K, Jung S. Nonsteroidal antiinflammatory drugs for postoperative pain management after lumbar spine surgery: a meta-analysis of randomized controlled trials. *J Neurosurg Spine.* 2008;9:22–31.

21. Sevarino F, Sinatra R, Paige D, et al. The efficacy of intramuscular ketorolac in combination with intravenous PCA morphine for postoperative pain relief. *J Clin Anesth.* 1992;4:285–288.

22. Le Roux P, Samudrala S. Postoperative pain after lumbar disc surgery: a comparison between parenteral ketorolac and narcotics. *Acta Neurochir (Wien).* 1991;141:261–267.

23. Reuben S, Connelly N. Postoperative analgesic effects of celecoxib or rofecoxib after spinal fusion surgery. *Anesth Analg.* 2000;91(5):1221–1225.

24. Burna C, Kulich RJ, Rathmell JP. Tapering long-term opioid therapy in chronic noncancer pain: evidence and recommendations for everyday practice. PubMed-NCBI. http://www.ncbi.nlm.nih.gov/pubmed/?term=Tapering+Long-term+Opioid+Therapy+in+Chronic+Noncancer+Pain+:+Evidence+and+Recommendations+for+Everyday+Practice. Accessed November 23, 2015.

25. Turan A, Karamanlioğlu B, Memiş D, et al. Analgesic effects of gabapentin after spinal surgery. *Anesthesiology.* 2004;100(4):935–938.

26. Rajpal S, Gordon D, Pellino T, et al. Comparison of perioperative oral multimodal analgesia versus IV PCA for spine surgery. *J Spinal Disord Tech.* 2010;23(2):139–145.

27. Looke TD, Kluth CT. Effect of preoperative intravenous methocarbamol and intravenous acetaminophen on opioid use after primary total hip and knee replacement. *Orthopedics.* 2013;36(2 Suppl):25–32. Accessed November 23, 2015. doi: 10.3928/01477447-20130122-54

28. Raw D, Beattie J, Hunter J. Anaesthesia for spinal surgery in adults. *Br J Anaesth.* 2003;91(6):886–904.

29. Pradhan B, Tatsumi R, Gallina J, et al. Ketorolac and spinal fusion: does the perioperative use of ketorolac really inhibit spinal fusion? *Spine (Phila Pa 1976).* 2008;33(19):2079–2082.

30. Glassman S, Rose S, Dimar J, et al. The effect of postoperative nonsteroidal anti-inflammatory drug administration on spinal fusion. *Spine (Phila Pa 1976).* 2008;33(19):2079–2082.

31. Li Q, Zhang Z, Cai Z. High-dose ketorolac affects adult spinal fusion: a meta-analysis of the effect of perioperative nonsteroidal anti-inflammatory drugs on spinal fusion. *Spine (Phila Pa 1976).* 2011;36(7):E471–E468.

32. Hiller A, Helenius I, Nurmi E, et al. Acetaminophen improves analgesia but does not reduce opioid requirement after major spine surgery in children and adolescents. *Spine (Phila Pa 1976).* 2012;37(20):E1225–E1231.

33. Hernández-Palazón J, Tortosa J, Martínez-Lage J, et al. Intravenous administration of propacetamol reduces morphine consumption after spinal fusion surgery. *Anesth Analg.* 2001;92(6):1473–1476.

34. Smith A, Hoefling V. A retrospective analysis of intravenous acetaminophen use in spinal surgery patients. *Pharm Pract (Granada).* 2014;12(3):417.

35. Sinatra R, Jahr J, Reynolds L, et al. Efficacy and safety of single and repeated administration of 1 gram intravenous acetaminophen injection (paracetamol) for pain management after major orthopedic surgery. *Anesthesiology.* 2005;102(4):822–831.

36. Radvansky BM, Shah K, Parikh A, et al. Role of ketamine in acute postoperative pain management: a narrative review. *Biomed Res Int.* 2015;2015:749837. doi: 10.1155/2015/749837

37. Sinatra R, Larach S, Ramamoorthy S. Postsurgical pain-management strategies in abdominal surgery. In: *Surgeon's Guide to Postsurgical Pain Management: Colorectal and Abdominal Surgery.* West Islip, NY: Professional Communications; 2012:245–255.

38. Panchal SJ, Damaraju CV, Nelson WW, et al. System-related events and analgesic gaps during postoperative pain management with the fentanyl iontophoretic transdermal system and morphine intravenous patient-controlled analgesia. *Anesth Analg.* 2007;105(5):1437–1441. Accessed November 23, 2015. doi: 105/5/1437 [pii].

39. Sinatra RS, Jahr JS, Watkins-Pitchford JM. *The Essence of Analgesia and Analgesics.* Cambridge University Press; 2010.

40. Allan L, Hays H, Jensen NH, et al. Randomised crossover trial of transdermal fentanyl and sustained release oral morphine for treating chronic non-cancer pain. *BMJ.* 2001;322(7295):1154–1158. Accessed November 23, 2015.

41. de Filho G, Gomes H, da Fonseca M, et al. Predictors of successful neuraxial block: a prospective study. *Eur J Anaesthesiol.* 2002;19(6):447–451.

42. Reynolds F. Damage to the conus medullaris following spinal anaesthesia. *Anaesthesia.* 2001;56(3):238–247.

43. Lybecker H, Møller J, May O, et al. Incidence and prediction of postdural puncture headache. A prospective study of 1021 spinal anesthesias. *Anesth Analg.* 1990;70(4):389–394.

44. Moen V, Dahlgren N, Irestedt L. Severe neurological complications after central neuraxial blockades in Sweden 1990–1999. *Anesthesiology.* 2004;101(4):950–959.

45. Hebl J, Horlocker T, Kopp S, Schroeder D. Neuraxial blockade in patients with pre-existing spinal stenosis, lumbar disk disease, or prior spine surgery: efficacy and neurologic complications. *Anesth Analg.* 2010;111(6):1511–1519.

10 Lumbar Neurogenic Claudication
Causes and Pain Management Options

Raj J. Gala and James Yue

INTRODUCTION

Lumbar neurogenic claudication refers to the clinical presentation of radiating pain into one or both legs with walking. An element of back pain may also be present. In early to mid-stages of the disease, patients often have no symptoms at rest, but, with ambulation, they often mention discomfort in the thighs, calves, and feet that gradually increases.[1] In advanced stages, the radiating leg pain can be present at rest for long periods of time. The pain often is described as a heaviness or weakness in the legs. Typically, there is improvement with leaning forward or resting. The hallmark pathology of lumbar neurogenic claudication is spinal stenosis, but a narrow canal alone is not usually enough to produce symptoms of claudication. Spinal stenosis is present in other diseases that do not manifest as claudication. In addition, canal narrowing can exist for many years prior to the development of lumbar neurogenic claudication symptoms [1].

CLASSIFICATION

Spinal stenosis arises from a variety of causes, both congenital and acquired. Congenital narrowing of the vertebral canal is a normal variant but is also present in growth disorders, for example. In these conditions, the pedicles may be shorter and closer, so minor degenerative changes may result in symptoms. There are a wide range of conditions that result in acquired stenosis, including trauma, degenerative, iatrogenic, infectious, and neoplastic.

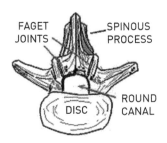
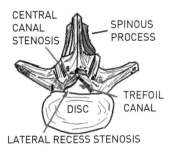

FAGET JOINTS
SPINOUS PROCESS
ROUND CANAL
DISC

CENTRAL CANAL STENOSIS
SPINOUS PROCESS
TREFOIL CANAL
DISC
LATERAL RECESS STENOSIS

FIGURE 10.1 Spinal canals are usually one of three shapes—round, trefoil, and ovoid (not pictured). Patients with trefoil-shaped canals are predisposed to spinal stenosis symptoms as these canals have the smallest cross-sectional area.

ANATOMY

An understanding of normal lumbar anatomy helps to explain how stenosis can result in claudication symptoms. The spinal canal has an anterior border, lateral border, and posterior border. The anterior boundary of the spinal canal comprises the vertebral bodies, intervertebral discs, and the posterior longitudinal ligament (PLL). The pedicles, neural foramen, and the lateral ligamentum flavum make the lateral border of the canal. Last, the spinal canal posterior border is bounded by the lamina, ligamentum flavum, and facet joints. The shape of the spinal canal varies in the normal population (Figure 10.1).

The degenerative pathway of lumbar spinal stenosis, outlined by Kirkaldy-Willis [2], is based on degeneration in the "three-joint complex" of the two posterior facet joints and the intervertebral disc. Impingement and stenosis result from bony alterations such as osteophytes and facet enlargement and also from soft tissue pathology such as hypertrophic ligamentum flavum and disc protrusions (Figure 10.2). Claudication symptoms typically worsen with extension as the hypertrophic ligamentum flavum buckles into the canal. Any added instability, such as degenerative spondylolisthesis, can further narrow the canal and compound the problem. This is most often seen as degenerative anterolisthesis of L4 on L5 (Figure 10.3). This area is predisposed to instability for several reasons [3]: the iliolumbar ligaments attach at the L5 transverse processes, resulting in relatively more motion at L4–L5, and the facet joints at L4–L5 have a more sagittal orientation.

PATHOPHYSIOLOGY

As mentioned earlier, the pathophysiology of neurogenic claudication involves more than simply the presence of spinal stenosis. Various human cadaver and animal studies have been performed to investigate the cause of symptoms. In a cadaver study, it was shown that below a critical size of cauda equina constriction corresponding to a cross-sectional diameter of 60–80 mm^2, nerve root pressures increased [4]. In a canine model, it was shown that 25% constriction of the cauda equina at a single level did not result in neurologic deficit [5]. Other studies have looked at various pressure measurements. While direct electrical and physical changes occur in nerve roots at pressures of 50 mm Hg, there is vascular congestion and decreased solute transport

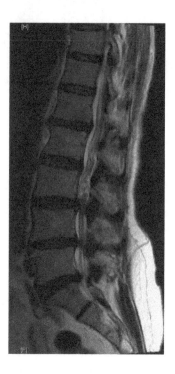

FIGURE 10.2 Example of spinal stenosis on sagittal view of T2 magnetic resonance image (MRI). Note the disc protrusions and hypertrophic ligamentum flavum.

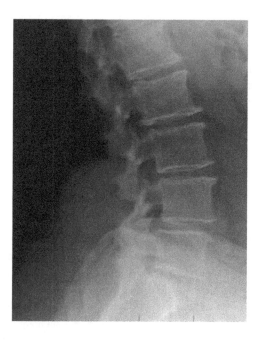

FIGURE 10.3 Example of mild anterolisthesis of L4 on L5 in the setting of degenerative diskovertebral and facet joints.

at pressures as low as 5–10 mm Hg [6]. Constriction and mechanical deformation of nerve roots may result in pain impulses. One study showed that the impulses were of short duration but became prolonged if the nerve tissue had been exposed to suture constriction for 2–4 weeks [7]. This may help explain how long-term stenosis leads to pain. In addition, constriction of nerve tissue in the presence of inflammation is more likely to be painful as compared to having either condition alone [8].

In studies measuring epidural pressure and position, standing with extension produced the highest epidural pressure. Epidural pressure decreased with flexion of the spine and with lying and sitting postures [9]. During walking, epidural pressures waxed and waned, possibly relating to a mechanism for intermittent cauda equina compression.

Patients with lumbar neurogenic claudication often have multiple levels of stenosis. There are many clinical scenarios in which a single level of stenosis does not result in claudication symptoms, such as a slow-growing spinal tumor or a large central disc protrusion. These conditions may just produce back pain, similar to a single level of stenosis from degenerative changes. This has also been corroborated with experimental studies. Using balloons to induce nerve compression at disc levels, a study showed that two adjacent levels of compression at 10 mm Hg each produced far greater reduction of nerve impulse amplitude when compared to a single level of compression at 50 mm Hg [10]. The mechanism for nerve injury from multiple levels of compression includes both diminished arterial blood flow and increased venous congestion. With walking, the capacity for arterial vasodilation is limited. In addition, there will be increased venous return from the lower extremities, potentially leading to enlargement of dural venous spaces, further decreasing the space in the cauda equina [1].

CLINICAL PRESENTATION

Lumbar stenosis is common in the older population. The typical patient with neurogenic claudication is a male over the age of 50. Symptoms usually start in the back and radiate down one or both legs past the knees during walking and are exacerbated with extension. Unlike radicular pain, the symptoms of lumbar neurogenic claudication do not follow a specific dermatomal pattern. Classically, patients describe leaning forward on a grocery cart in order to tolerate going to the store. Uphill walking is usually tolerated better than downhill walking, as uphill walking involves spine flexion and downhill walking involves extension. Patients often tolerate stationary bicycling as compared to treadmill walking for the same reasons. Physical exam in the office may be relatively normal, apart from mild tenderness in the low back. The patient may adopt a position of relative lumbar extension while standing, which may involve slight hip and knee flexion. Neurological examination is often usually normal since the patient is at rest. It may be possible to elicit some deficits after exercise [1].

It is important to check the peripheral circulation as it may be difficult to differentiate vascular claudication from neurogenic claudication. Because the patient population is generally older, it is not infrequent that peripheral arterial disease will be present as well. This may need to be investigated with Doppler studies or arteriography. In contrast to neurogenic claudication, the symptoms of vascular insufficiency usually progress from distal to proximal. Those patients may have rest pain or a baseline level of pain unrelated to the position of the spine. For this reason, bicycling is poorly tolerated, unlike in patients with neurogenic claudication. Pain at night that is relieved with hanging the symptomatic limb over the side of the bed usually is indicative of a vascular cause of claudication. Physical exam may reveal painless extension of the spine as well as shiny legs with no hair. Other differential diagnoses include joint arthritis, sciatic claudication, lumbar spondylosis, peripheral neuropathy, and lumbosacral lesions.

DIAGNOSTIC STUDIES

The diagnostic imaging of patients with neurogenic claudication usually starts with plain X-rays of the lumbar spine. Because most patients are generally older, there is usually some degree of spondylosis on the radiographs (Figure 10.4). The alignment should be checked, and full-length scoliosis films can be obtained if there is concern. It is important to inspect for spondylolisthesis, which may also necessitate flexion-extension films to look for dynamic instability. X-rays can show ossification of soft tissue structures as well as ankylosis of the spine.

Advanced imaging modalities include computed tomography (CT) and magnetic resonance imaging (MRI). While CT scan illustrates bony structures well, it does a poor job of visualizing soft tissue pathology in the spine. This can be improved by injecting contrast dye into the cerebrospinal fluid (CSF) during the CT scan and performing a concomitant myelogram [11]. While this is an invasive procedure, it provides an alternative for patients who cannot undergo an MRI. In addition, it can be helpful when a patient has spinal hardware that limits visibility in MRI.

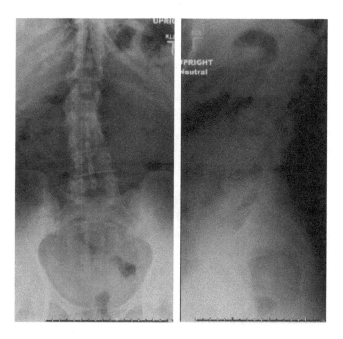

FIGURE 10.4 Anteroposterior (AP) and lateral radiograph of thoracolumbar spine showing spondylosis, as evidenced by narrowed disc spaces, osteophytes, and arthrosis of the facet joints. The AP radiograph shows degenerative scoliosis in the lumbar spine.

As MRI continues to become more feasible and available, it is the study of choice for detecting spinal stenosis. In addition to being noninvasive and nonradiating, MRI provides detailed imaging in all three planes of both bony and soft tissue anatomy. The degree of stenosis can be evaluated, as well as its location, such as central, lateral recess, or neuroforaminal stenosis. MRI can show pathology such as facet cysts, ligamentum hypertrophy, facet hypertrophy, disc herniations, and osteophyte complexes, all of which can contribute to stenosis and symptoms.

Electrodiagnostic studies include electromyography (EMG), nerve conduction studies (NCS), and somatosensory evoked potentials (SSEPs). These studies are not routinely obtained as they have high rates of false-positive and false-negative results [12]. For example, EMG does not evaluate sensory disturbances, which are the most common complaints in neurogenic claudication.

MANAGEMENT

The natural history of symptomatic lumbar spinal stenosis varies. The majority of patients do not deteriorate neurologically with time. It is rare to have rapid neurological decline. Nonoperative treatment works well for a significant number of patients. In a small series of 32 patients followed for 4 years, 70% had no change in their pain, 15% had worse pain, and 15% had improved pain [13]. Initial management involves counseling and educating the patient. Simple changes, such as alteration of lifestyle and physical therapy "Back School," may be enough to improve a patient's quality of life.

There are several other nonsurgical interventions and medical treatments that may help patients, though it is unclear if the interventions improve outcomes as compared to no treatment. No direct comparison studies have been performed, according to a recent literature review, comparing active treatment to no treatment [14]. For this reason, choice of medical treatment is largely based on prior training and experience of the clinician.

PHARMACOLOGIC TREATMENT

Often the first prescribed medications for patients with symptomatic lumbar stenosis are simple analgesics and nonsteroidal anti-inflammatory drugs (NSAIDs). Of note, these drugs have not been studied in patients with lumbar stenosis, so there are no trials comparing their efficacy [14]. For this reason, several medical committees have recommended acetaminophen as initial therapy to avoid the toxicity associated with NSAID use. Because the patient population with this spinal stenosis is generally older, they are more likely to have comorbidities that do not tolerate NSAIDs. Acetaminophen can be dosed up to 4 g/day in most cases and can provide pain relief similar to NSAIDs. Opioid analgesics can also be used, but they carry a risk for altered mental status and sedation in the older population. While they may be beneficial in the short term, narcotics have not been shown to increase walking or standing tolerance in patients in spinal stenosis.

Gabapentin is an antiepileptic drug commonly used to treat neuropathy, such as in diabetic patients. A pilot study performed in 2007 randomized 55 patients with lumbar neurogenic claudication into two groups [15]. Both groups received standard nonoperative treatment such as physical therapy, lumbar bracing, and NSAIDs. The experimental group also received gabapentin. Patients in the gabapentin group had increased walking distance, improved pain scores, and better recovery of sensory disturbances. This study points to the need for larger clinical trials to investigate the potential benefits of gabapentin. The side effects of gabapentin include sedation and drowsiness, which are of concern in an older patient population.

There is not convincing evidence for the use of calcitonin in patients with lumbar stenosis. Calcitonin has been reported to have analgesic and anti-inflammatory effects. It is a polypeptide hormone and produced in the thyroid. Calcitonin receptors are present in osteoclasts, kidneys, and regions of the brain. Calcitonin is often used in the treatment of Paget's disease and may be beneficial in patients with spinal stenosis from Paget's disease. Older studies reported that short courses of calcitonin also seemed to help a few patients without Paget's disease increase their walking distance, but the findings were purely observational [16]. A more recent trial showed no benefit with using intranasal calcitonin as compared with placebo [17]. Other routes of administration include intramuscular or subcutaneous, so further research with larger scale trials may be helpful in determining the efficacy of calcitonin.

PHYSICAL THERAPY

A recent literature review showed inconclusive evidence about the effectiveness of physical therapy as an isolated treatment for spinal stenosis [14]. Even so, given the low risks of physical therapy, it is widely used in the treatment of spinal stenosis and often incorporated into regimens. The goals of physical therapy revolve around strengthening core musculature while limiting extension of the lumbar spine and decreasing lumbar lordosis. For example, hip flexion contractures should be identified and treated as they can be a source of increased lumbar lordosis. Physical therapy can also help with general deconditioning that is usually present in patients with neurogenic claudication as they are less likely to exercise on their own. Stationary bicycling is a low-impact exercise that most patients can tolerate since the posture is relative flexion. Other modalities include elliptical and aquatic training. Physical therapy can also promote social interaction for the patient, help with mood and depression, and assist with weight loss. There are limited studies looking at passive modalities in the treatment of spinal stenosis. These include manipulation, bracing, acupuncture, and transcutaneous electrical nerve stimulation (TENS).

EPIDURAL STEROID INJECTIONS

The injection of steroid into areas of inflammation is common practice in orthopedics. The basis behind epidural steroid injection (ESI) is to target inflammation at stenotic levels in the spine. While the injections can be performed without fluoroscopy, there are high rates of missing the epidural space when fluoroscopy is not used [18]. The injection techniques include caudal, interlaminar, or transforaminal (Figure 10.5). One study showed no difference in pain or walking distance after a single ESI [19], but several case series have demonstrated benefits with multiple steroid injections. In 2002, a prospective series was published of 34 patients treated with a multiple-injection protocol [20]. At 12-month follow-up, 75% of patients had a significant improvement in pain, and 64% of patients reported increase in walking distance. In a retrospective series of 140 patients, 32% of patients reported greater than

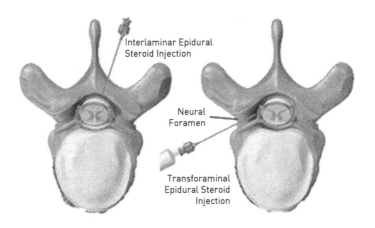

FIGURE 10.5 Diagram of interlaminar versus transforaminal epidural steroid injection. Courtesy S. B. Leavitt, January, 2012.

2 months of pain relief [21]. More than half of the patients reported improvement in their functional abilities, and 74% of patients were at least somewhat satisfied with the ESI treatment. Even patients with severe claudication symptoms can show improvement with a multiple injection protocol. A 1987 study demonstrated that 32% of patients reported good to excellent improvement at an average of 23 months [22]. The caveat with ESI is that it often necessitates stopping anticoagulation and antiplatelets for around 1 week. This poses a challenge for patients who have absolute contraindications to stopping these medications. In addition, it is not uncommon for patients to have transient headaches after ESI. Severe adverse events such as infection or epidural hematoma are rare.

TREATMENT ALGORITHM

Since the natural history is generally favorable in patients with lumbar spinal stenosis, conservative treatment should be the initial management. It is logical to start with the least invasive options, such as physical therapy and gabapentin. Patients who are too sick or fragile to participate in therapy may benefit from bracing or the use of a rolling walker. The next step is the selective use of analgesics, followed by trials of ESI. Aggressiveness of treatment should be based on patient symptoms and not based on spinal canal diameter as measured on imaging. Failure of conservative treatment warrants referral to a spine surgeon, as do signs or findings of cauda equina syndrome.

There are a variety of surgical options for cases that are unresponsive to nonsurgical techniques. The mainstay of surgical treatment includes posterior laminectomy/laminoforaminotomy with or without fusion. Laminectomy techniques involve directly decompressing the compressive source(s) of pain including hypertrophic facets, ligamentum flavum, and herniated disc materials. Indirect decompressive methods have also been described and are often less invasive. These indirect procedures may be effective in early to mid-stage disease and include interlaminar device placements with (Coflex [Paradigm Spine], Figure 10.6) or without (X-Stop [Medtronic], HeliFix [Alphatec], Aperius PercLID [Medtronic], and others) direct forms of decompression [23]. Endoscopic techniques are also being developed [24].

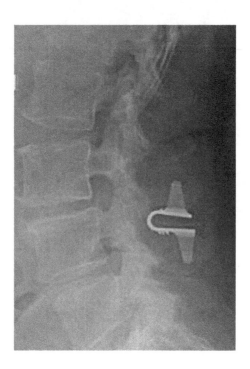

FIGURE 10.6 Radiograph demonstrating the Coflex (Paradigm Spine) interlaminar implant.

CONCLUSION

Lumbar spinal stenosis associated with neurogenic claudication can be a debilitating disease process for many middle- to advanced-age patients. Conservative treatment including aerobic exercise, medication, activity modification, and/or injection therapy is usually sufficient to relieve neurogenic and back pain symptomatology. In recalcitrant cases and in cases associated with spinal instability, direct or indirect surgical techniques with or without spinal stabilization are often beneficial. In those severe cases associated with both stenosis and spinal deformity, both indirect and direct surgical techniques may be required.

REFERENCES

1. Porter RW. Spinal stenosis and neurogenic claudication. *Spine (Phila Pa 1976)*. 1996;21(17):2046–2052.
2. Kirkaldy-Willis WH, Wedge JH, Yong-Hing K, et al. Pathology and pathogenesis of lumbar spondylosis and stenosis. *Spine (Phila Pa 1976)*. 1978;3(4):319–328.
3. Rosenberg NJ. Degenerative spondylolisthesis. Predisposing factors. *J Bone Joint Surg Am*. 1975;57(4):467–474.
4. Schonstrom N, Bolender NF, Spengler DM, et al. Pressure changes within the cauda equina following constriction of the dural sac. An in vitro experimental study. *Spine (Phila Pa 1976)*. 1984;9(6):604–607.
5. Delamarter RB, Bohlman HH, Dodge LD, et al. Experimental lumbar spinal stenosis. Analysis of the cortical evoked potentials, microvasculature, and histopathology. *J Bone Joint Surg Am*. 1990;72(1):110–120.

6. Rydevik B, Brown MD, Lundborg G. Pathoanatomy and pathophysiology of nerve root compression. *Spine (Phila Pa 1976)*. 1984;9(1):7–15.

7. Howe JF, Loeser JD, Calvin WH. Mechanosensitivity of dorsal root ganglia and chronically injured axons: a physiological basis for the radicular pain of nerve root compression. *Pain*. 1977;3(1):25–41.

8. Olmarker K, Nutu M, Storkson R. Changes in spontaneous behavior in rats exposed to experimental disc herniation are blocked by selective TNF-alpha inhibition. *Spine (Phila Pa 1976)*. 2003;28(15):1635–1641; discussion 1642.

9. Takahashi K, Miyazaki T, Takino T, et al. Epidural pressure measurements. Relationship between epidural pressure and posture in patients with lumbar spinal stenosis. *Spine (Phila Pa 1976)*. 1995;20(6):650–653.

10. Olmarker K, Rydevik B. Single- versus double-level nerve root compression. An experimental study on the porcine cauda equina with analyses of nerve impulse conduction properties. *Clin Orthop Relat Res*. 1992(279):35–39.

11. Herno A, Airaksinen O, Saari T, Miettinen H. The predictive value of preoperative myelography in lumbar spinal stenosis. *Spine (Phila Pa 1976)*. 1994;19(12):1335–1338.

12. Plastaras CT. Electrodiagnostic challenges in the evaluation of lumbar spinal stenosis. *Phys Med Rehabil Clin N Am*. 2003;14(1):57–69.

13. Johnsson KE, Rosen I, Uden A. The natural course of lumbar spinal stenosis. *Clin Orthop Relat Res*. 1992(279):82–86.

14. Watters WC, 3rd, Baisden J, Gilbert TJ, et al. Degenerative lumbar spinal stenosis: an evidence-based clinical guideline for the diagnosis and treatment of degenerative lumbar spinal stenosis. *Spine J*. 2008;8(2):305–310.

15. Yaksi A, Ozgonenel L, Ozgonenel B. The efficiency of gabapentin therapy in patients with lumbar spinal stenosis. *Spine (Phila Pa 1976)*. 2007;32(9):939–942.

16. Eskola A, Alaranta H, Pohjolainen T, et al. Calcitonin treatment in lumbar spinal stenosis: clinical observations. *Calcif Tissue Int*. 1989;45(6):372–374.

17. Tafazal SI, Ng L, Sell P. Randomised placebo-controlled trial on the effectiveness of nasal salmon calcitonin in the treatment of lumbar spinal stenosis. *Eur Spine J*. 2007;16(2):207–212.

18. Renfrew DL, Moore TE, Kathol MH, et al. Correct placement of epidural steroid injections: fluoroscopic guidance and contrast administration. *AJNR Am J Neuroradiol*. 1991;12(5):1003–1007.

19. Ng L, Chaudhary N, Sell P. The efficacy of corticosteroids in periradicular infiltration for chronic radicular pain: a randomized, double-blind, controlled trial. *Spine (Phila Pa 1976)*. 2005;30(8):857–862.

20. Botwin KP, Gruber RD, Bouchlas CG, et al. Fluoroscopically guided lumbar transformational epidural steroid injections in degenerative lumbar stenosis: an outcome study. *Am J Phys Med Rehabil*. 2002;81(12):898–905.

21. Delport EG, Cucuzzella AR, Marley JK, et al. Treatment of lumbar spinal stenosis with epidural steroid injections: a retrospective outcome study. *Arch Phys Med Rehabil*. 2004;85(3):479–484.

22. Hoogmartens M, Morelle P. Epidural injection in the treatment of spinal stenosis. *Acta Orthop Belg*. 1987;53(3):409–411.

23. Musacchio MJ, Lauryssen C, Davis RJ, et al. Evaluation of decompression and interlaminar stabilization compared with decompression and fusion for the treatment of lumbar spinal stenosis: 5-year follow-up of a prospective, randomized, controlled trial. *Int J Spine Surg*. 2016;10:6.

24. Hwa Eum J, Hwa Heo D, Son SK, et al. Percutaneous biportal endoscopic decompression for lumbar spinal stenosis: a technical note and preliminary clinical results. *J Neurosurg Spine*. 2016;24(4):602–607.

11 Needle Placement

Kenneth D. Candido and Teresa M. Kusper

INTRODUCTION

Interventional pain management techniques are invaluable tools in the treatment of pain from various etiologies. Knowledge of the relevant anatomy is crucial for the proper placement of the interventional equipment and needles and for appreciating optimal access to the structures of interest. Equally important is familiarity with possible complications and different preventative measures limiting these known complications. The strict adherence to aseptic technique to maintain sterility is a universal practice designed to avoid infectious complications during each and every interventional pain management technique. Equally important is the prevention of vascular complications, often gleaned by inquiring about the history of coagulopathy and use of blood thinning agents. Adequate time intervals for suspending specific anticoagulant or antiplatelet medications must be ascertained prior to any injection technique. An immediate neurological assessment following any interventional procedure is an imperative and mandatory component of every procedure to screen for the new onset of any sensory or motor changes and to demonstrate the intactness of motor and sensory function. The focus of this chapter is to provide a brief description of various interventional pain management injection techniques. A short summary of the relevant anatomy, landmarks used for needle placement, and important safety considerations is provided along with a selection of digital and radiographic photographs depicting the ideal needle placement and contrast flow at or in the immediate proximity of the targeted structures.

EPIDURAL STEROID INJECTION

Indications for epidural steroid injection (ESI) include radicular pain and radiculopathic symptoms in the extremity due to irritation of spinal nerve root(s).

Relevant Anatomy

The epidural space resides between the ligamentum flavum posteriorly and dura mater anteriorly, and extends from the foramen magnum down to the sacrococcygeal ligament. The approximate width of the epidural space is between 3 and 5 mm depending on anatomical site, with lumbar spaces being wider than cervical. This potential space contains spinal nerve roots and the dorsal root ganglion (DRG), small arteries, venous plexuses, and lymphatics along with connective and fatty tissues. The epidural space is bordered by the vertebral body anteriorly, laminae posteriorly, and pedicles laterally. The spinous process of C7 (the vertebrae prominens) is used to identify the C6–C7 interspace, which is most commonly accessed during cervical ESI owing to the largest diameter of the interlaminar space and widest epidural space compared to the other cervical levels. The inferior angles of the scapulae correspond with the T7 spinous process, whereas the tips of the iliac crests demarcate the L4–L5 interspace, which is most frequently accessed during lumbar ESI. The sacral hiatus, used as the entry point for caudal ESI, can be palpated between two sacral cornua at the level of S5.

Needle Placement

In the *interlaminar approach*, an 18- or 20-gauge Tuohy needle tip is placed in the midline of the spine between two consecutive laminae and spinal processes. For bilateral pain, the needle is placed in the midline position, whereas in the presence of unilateral symptoms it is directed toward the affected site using an interlaminar parasagittal approach. Proper needle positioning is confirmed with the anteroposterior (AP) fluoroscopic view. The needle is advanced ventrally through the supraspinous ligament, interspinal ligament, and ligamentum flavum using the lateral fluoroscopic view to assess the depth of the needle advancement. Entry into the epidural space through the ligamentum flavum is confirmed using a loss-of-resistance technique to saline or air and injection of water-soluble, iodine-based contrast dye (Figure 11.1A–E).

The *transforaminal (selective nerve root) approach* is used to place analgesic medication directly around a specific nerve root corresponding with the symptoms manifested by the patient. A blunt-tipped spinal needle is directed toward the inferior aspect of the intervertebral foramen, known as the Kambin's triangle (Figure 11.1F–K).

Safety Precautions

Correct needle trajectory should be verified with periodic or continual fluoroscopic imaging to confirm an adequate distance from vital neural and vascular structures. Ventral depth of the needle is assessed with fluoroscopy and the use of the loss-of-resistance technique to prevent unintentional puncture of the dura and emergence of postdural puncture headache.

SPINAL JOINT INJECTIONS

Atlantoaxial (AA) Intraarticular Injection

Indications

Indications for AA intraarticular injections are cervical pain and cervicogenic headache pain emanating from the AA joint secondary to traumatic event or atlantoaxial arthropathy.

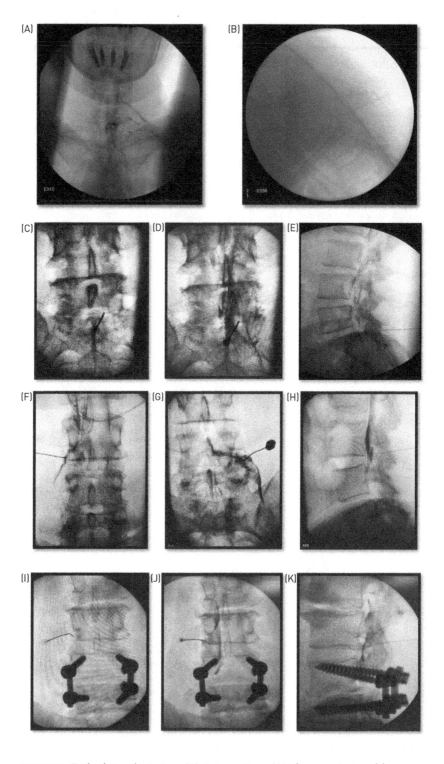

FIGURE 11.1 Epidural steroid injections. (A) Anteroposterior (AP) fluoroscopic view of the midline interlaminar (MIL) Cervical epidural steroid injection (CESI) showing needle seated in the C7–T1 interlaminar space slightly angled toward the right side. (B) Lateral radiograph of the midline interlaminar CESI with needle entering the interlaminar space. (C) AP view of the parasagittal interlaminar (PIL) Lumbar ESI (LESI) with needle accessing the L4–L5 interlaminar

Relevant Anatomy

The AA joint is located between the superior and inferior articulating processes of the axis and atlas, respectively. The vertebral artery runs lateral to the AA joint, whereas the C2 dorsal root ganglion and C2 spinal nerve emerge medial to the AA joint.

Needle Placement

In the posterior approach, the blunt-tipped needle is advanced until the tip is seated in the lateral one-third of the joint space. Optimal needle positioning is confirmed with AP and lateral fluoroscopic views and visualization of contrast dye within the joint capsule (Figure 11.2A,B).

Safety Precautions

Care should be taken not to direct the needle too laterally or medially from the joint space to prevent puncturing the vertebral artery and C2 neural structures, respectively.

Zygapophysial (Facet) Intraarticular Joint Injection, Medial Branch Block, and Radiofrequency Ablation

Facet joint–related pain syndromes (e.g., facet arthropathy) are characterized by well-localized axial spinal pain potentially referred to specific areas that have a dermal representation and mapping. Pain in the cervical area may be referred to the occiput, neck, trapezius muscle, parascapular region, shoulder, and upper arm. Lumbar facet-related pain is referred to the buttocks, groin, and posterior thigh; rarely below the level of the knee.

Relevant Anatomy

The zygapophysial or facet joint is formed by the articulation between the superior articular process of one vertebra and the inferior articular process of the vertebra immediately above it, between the lamina and pedicle. Each facet joint derives its sensory innervation from the medial branches of the dorsal primary ramus at the same vertebral level and from the level above (dual innervation).

FIGURE 11.1 Continued

space. (D) AP view of the PIL LESI demonstrating contrast spread in the lateral epidural space and around the exiting lumbar nerve roots. (E) Lateral view of the PIL LESI with needle placed in the L4–L5 interlaminar space. (F) AP view of the lumbar transformational ESI (LTESI) showing needle tip situated inferior to the pedicle within the left L3–L4 intervertebral foramen with contrast dye outlining left L3 nerve root. (G) AP view of the LTESI with needle tip within the right L4–L5 intervertebral foramen and contrast dye outlining right L4 nerve root. (H) Lateral view of the LTESI with needle at L4–L5 position and contrast flow within the epidural space. (I) AP view of the LTESI in patient with failed back surgery syndrome with needle tip approaching the left L3–L4 intervertebral foramen; surgical screws evident below the needle within the L4 and L5 vertebral bodies. (J) AP view of the LTESI with needle in the final position and contrast spread along the lateral epidural space. (K) Lateral view of the LTESI with needle tip within the L3–L4 intervertebral foramen after injection of the contrast into the epidural space.
Images courtesy of Kenneth D. Candido, MD.

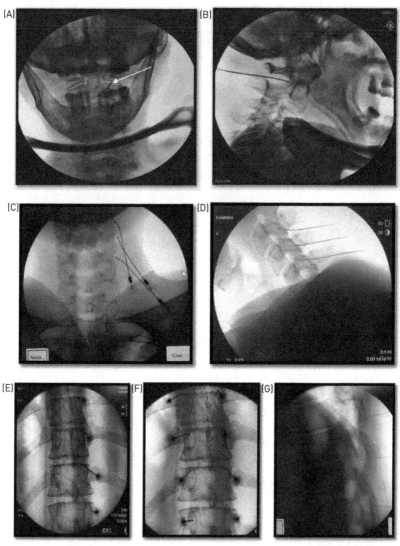

FIGURE 11.2 Spinal joint injections. (A) Anteroposterior (AP) fluoroscopic view of the AA intraarticular joint injection. (B) Lateral view of the atlantoaxial (AA) joint injection with needle placed in the posterolateral aspect of the joint space. (C) AP view of the right cervical medial branch block (MBB) with needles placed at the C3, C4, and C5 articular pillars. (D) Lateral view of MBB of two consecutive cervical facet joints. (E) AP view of right sided thoracic MBB (F) AP view of bilateral thoracic MBB (G) Lateral view of thoracic MBB (H) Digital image of the radiofrequency electrode placement for the left sided cervical RFA of the medial branch nerves (I) AP view of the radiofrequency electrodes in the final positions for RFA of the cervical medial branch nerves (J) Lateral view of the electrodes placed at the cervical articular pillars (K) Digital image demonstrating the placement of radiofrequency electrodes for left sided lumbar MBB. (L) AP view of electrode placement for RFA of lumbar medial branch nerves on the left. (M) Lateral view of electrodes positioned for RFA of the lumbar medial branch nerves. (N) AP view of the intraarticular sacroiliac joint (SIJ) injection showing needle entering the inferior aspect of the joint. (O) AP view of the SIJ injection with the needle in the final position and the contrast outlining the SIJ joint space. (P) Lateral view of needle in the SIJ joint and contrast spread throughout the joint space demonstrating the characteristic inverted letter L configuration. Images courtesy of Kenneth D. Candido, MD.

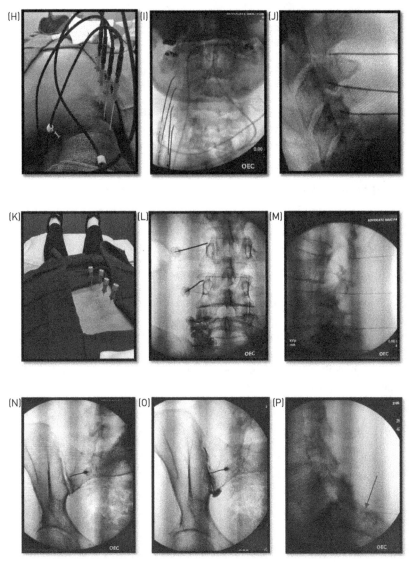

FIGURE 11.2 Continued

Needle Placement

For *intraarticular injection*, the needle is placed into the tissues and is advanced toward the joint space between the superior and inferior articular processes. Needle position is verified with fluoroscopy, and medication is deposited without prior contrast injection due to the limited capacity of the joint.

In *medial branch blocks*, the needle is advanced toward the middle or the waistline of the articular pillar between the pedicle and transverse process of the vertebra near the medial branch nerve (Figure 11.2C-G).

In *radiofrequency ablation*, the final target destination is identical to the medial branch block, but radiofrequency electrodes are used in place of the needles (Figure 11.2H-M).

Safety Precautions

The spinal nerve might be injured if the needle diverges above the joint.

Sacroiliac (SI) Intraarticular Joint Injection

Indication for SI injection is pain in the lower back and/or upper buttock, which may be referred to the groin, greater trochanter, or upper posterolateral thigh areas due to degenerative joint disease or inflammatory conditions, such as ankylosing spondylitis.

Relevant Anatomy

The sacroiliac joint (SIJ) is a diarthrodial joint situated between the sacrum and ilium and is innervated by the contributions from the lumbar plexus and sacral nerve roots.

Needle Placement

The blunt-tipped spinal needle is introduced into the medial aspect of the posterior SIJ joint and is then advanced in the cephalad and ventral direction until it pierces the posterior joint capsule and enters the inferior aspect of the SIJ. The proper needle position is confirmed with fluoroscopic imaging or ultrasound and contrast dye (for fluoroscopy) outlining the joint margins prior to the placement of local anesthetic and steroid solution (Figure 11.2N–P).

Safety Precautions

Complications related to the injection are infrequent; however, there is a rare possibility of injuring visceral organs should the needle be advanced too anteriorly.

SYMPATHETIC BLOCK INJECTIONS

Stellate Ganglion Block

The stellate ganglion (SGB) injection is most commonly employed for the treatment of sympathetically maintained pain syndromes, such as complex regional pain syndrome, postherpetic neuralgia, and vasculopathic syndromes, although the list of clinical indications continues to expand and includes such disparate conditions as posttraumatic stress disorder (PTSD) or breast cancer-related lymphedema.

Relevant Anatomy

The stellate ganglion is formed by the fusion of the inferior cervical ganglion and superior thoracic ganglion in about 80% of individuals. It is located anterior to the longus colli muscle, medial to the vertebral artery, anterior to the neck of the first rib and the transverse process of the seventh cervical vertebra and the uncinate process of the T1 vertebra, and posterior to the subclavian artery and cupola of the lung. The anterior tubercle of the C6 vertebra, known as the Chassaignac tubercle, the cricoid cartilage, and the carotid artery serve as some important landmarks for the injection. The C6 tubercle can be discerned by palpating between the trachea and the sternocleidomastoid muscle at the level of the cricoid cartilage. Retracting the carotid and jugular vessels laterally is used in attempt to minimize vascular injection.

Needle Placement

The location of the ganglion is most commonly accessed via the anterior paratracheal approach. Typically, a blunt-tipped needle is placed at the C6 level rather than at the C7 level, thus decreasing the likelihood of vertebral artery puncture since the artery is enclosed within the foramen transversarium at the C6 level rather than being exposed anterior to the transverse process of C7. Having stated this, there are several authorities who advocate that a C7 approach is anatomically more "correct" as the target for performing SGB, regardless of vertebral artery location. Additionally, there is a lower risk of pneumothorax at the C6 level compared to the C7 level. Once the C6 transverse process is localized, the carotid and jugular vasculature may be retracted laterally before placing the needle. The use of ultrasound guidance and an in-plane approach of needle placement provides some safety in terms of depicting the two-dimensional location of these respective blood vessels. The optimal target location for the needle is at the base of the transverse process inferior to the uncinate process of the C6 vertebra. Needle position is confirmed continuously; aspiration is performed prior to and during contrast injection to rule out intravascular administration of the dye. With ultrasound, it may be possible to witness vascular penetration and injection in real-time without a requirement to refer to ionizing radiation and use of contrast agents. After the correct needle placement is assured, contrast spread can be visualized along the anterolateral margin of the vertebral bodies, reaching the ganglion's proximity at the C7–C1 interspace (Figure 11.3A–C). Successful SGB is characterized by almost immediate development of a Horner's syndrome and increase in the temperature of the ipsilateral arm (Guttman's sign) (Table 11.1).

Safety Precautions

Bilateral SGBs should not be performed due to the risk of blocking bilateral recurrent laryngeal nerves and provoking stridor. Special care must be exercised while maneuvering the SGB needle into its final position to avoid contacting several vital anatomical structures. Avoid intravascular injection by frequent aspiration and use a test dose of a mere 0.25 mL of the intended local anesthetic, which may be sufficient nevertheless to induce a grand mal seizure if even this volume is injected into the nearby vertebral artery.

Lumbar Sympathetic Ganglion (LSNB) Block

Lower extremity pain due to complex regional pain syndrome, peripheral neuropathy, arterial occlusive disease, or postherpetic neuralgia are among the most common

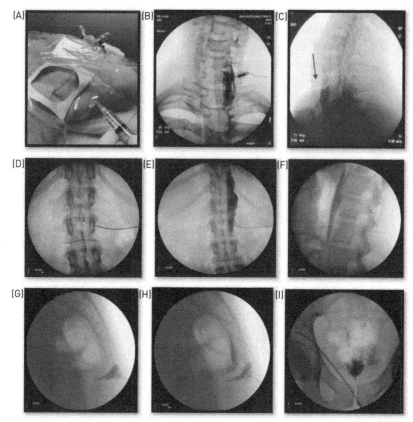

FIGURE 11.3 Sympathetic nerve blocks. (A) Digital image demonstrating proper needle placement between the tracheal and sternocleidomastoid (SCM) muscle for the stellate ganglion block, and contrast injected with frequent aspiration to rule out intravascular placement; head slightly tilted backwards and towards the contralateral side. (B) Anteroposterior (AP) view of the stellate ganglion (SGB); needle seated at the C6 transverse process, contrast spread inferiorly along the anterolateral margin of the vertebral bodies to a T1 level. (C) Lateral fluoroscopic view of the needle at the C6 transverse process and contrast spread during SGB. (D) AP view of the right-sided lumbar sympathetic ganglion block showing needle placement anterolateral to the L2 vertebral body at the level of pedicle. (E) AP view of contrast spread along the right margin of the vertebral bodies during lumbar sympathetic nerve block (LSNB). (F) Lateral view of the LSNB and contrast spread along the anterior margin of lumbar vertebral bodies. (G) Lateral view of the ganglion impar block showing needle placement at the sacrococcygeal junction and injected contrast dye outside the sacro-coccygeal () junction. (H) Lateral view of the ganglion impar nerve block (GINB) with needle advanced through the SC junction and contrast spread along the ventral aspect of the sacrum. (I) AP view of the contrast spread during the GINB. Images courtesy of Kenneth D. Candido, MD.

indications for LSNB. LSNB might also be used to relieve malignancy-related rectal or low back pain.

Relevant Anatomy

Four paired lumbar sympathetic ganglia are located at the level of the second and third lumbar vertebral bodies; occasionally the fourth lumbar and first lumbar as well may have ganglia located at their respective anterior surfaces.

Table 11.1 Features of the successful stellate ganglion block manifested as Horner's syndrome

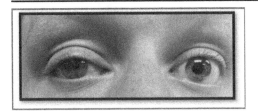

	Iatrogenic Horner's Syndrome
	Drooping of the upper eyelid (ptosis)
	Pupil constriction (miosis)
	Reduced sweating on the ipsilateral side of the face (anhidrosis)
	Sinking of the affected eyeball into the socket (enophthalmos)
	Unilateral conjunctival redness
	Nasal stuffiness

Image courtesy of Kenneth D. Candido, MD.

Needle Placement

The blunt-tipped spinal (typically 22-gauge, 3.5 inches with a curved distal tip) needle is inserted approximately 8–10 cm from the midline at about a 45-degree angle approximately 2 cm below the twelfth rib inferior margin and is directed toward the lower second or upper third lumbar vertebra until it is in contact with the anterolateral middle portion of the pedicle (Figure 11.3D–F).

Safety Precautions

It is imperative to avoid ventral and medial needle displacement to prevent injury to the great vessels (inferior vena cava [IVC] and abdominal aorta [AA]) and the spinal roots, respectively.

Ganglion Impar Block

Indications for the ganglion impar block include perineal, pelvic, and rectal pain.

Relevant Anatomy

The ganglion impar (the ganglion of Walther) is the endpoint of the paired sympathetic chains located in the retroperitoneal cavity at the level of the sacrococcygeal junction.

Needle Placement

The blunt-tipped block needle can be introduced either through the anococcygeal ligament and advanced toward the sacrococcygeal junction or directly through the sacrococcygeal ligament and advanced until the tip is located posterior to the rectum. Proper placement is confirmed by visualizing a comma-shaped contrast spread (Figure 11.3G–I).

Safety Precautions

Use fluoroscopic or ultrasound guidance to minimize the chances of perforation of the rectum or entry into the peritoneal cavity.

PIRIFORMIS MUSCLE INJECTION

This intramuscular injection is used to address pain emanating from the buttock or lower extremity caused by muscle inflammation or spasm or impingement of the sciatic nerve by the piriformis muscle, resulting in "pseudo-sciatica."

Relevant Anatomy

The piriformis muscle spans from the S2 to S4 sacral vertebrae to the medial aspect of the greater trochanter of the femur across the greater sciatic foramen. The sciatic nerve might emerge above, below, or through the piriformis muscle, although it is most commonly ventral to the muscle in more than 85% of individuals. The greater sciatic foramen, lower border of the sacroiliac joint, lateral aspect of the sacrum, and the greater trochanter of the femur serve as landmarks for the identification of the piriformis muscle.

Needle Placement

Injection can be done under the fluoroscopic guidance with contrast dye used to outline the muscle in question and verify the needle placement (Figure 11.4A–C).

Safety Precautions

Verify correct needle placement to prevent injection into the sciatic nerve using either fluoroscopy or ultrasound guidance.

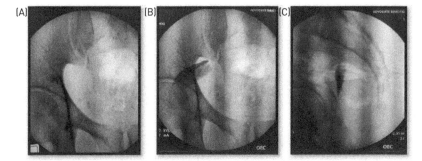

FIGURE 11.4 Piriformis muscle injection. (A) Anteroposterior (AP) view showing needle tip in contact with the border of the greater trochanter. (B) AP view of contrast dye throughout the body of the piriformis muscle. (C) Lateral view of the contrast outlining the piriformis muscle. Images courtesy of Kenneth D. Candido, MD.

Percutaneous Disc Decompression

Percutaneous disc decompression removes the inner nuclear material of a contained intervertebral disc protrusion to alleviate the axial and/or radicular pain caused by disk herniation and irritation of the nearby nerve roots.

Relevant Anatomy

The intervertebral disc is composed of a gel-like internal substance, the nucleus pulposus (NP), and surrounding multiple overlapping concentric rings of the cartilaginous annular fibrosis (AF). It is sandwiched between two contiguous vertebral bodies located anterior to the spinal canal. The DRG and spinal nerve roots emerge bilaterally from the intervertebral foramina posterior to the intervertebral disc.

Needle Placement

After confirmation of a contained disc protrusion on imaging studies and determining candidacy for the procedure, a needle introducer is inserted through the skin, at angles oblique and lateral to the dorsal midline. If fluoroscopy is used, an oblique, 20-degree tilt with flattened end-plates is extremely useful to line up the intended target. The introducer is then advanced down toward the junction of the transverse process and the superior articulating process into the center of the intervertebral disc. Needle placement is verified using AP and lateral fluoroscopy. Once the needle is situated in the central portion of the nucleus pulposus, the stylet is withdrawn and the decompressor unit (using either a coblation technique or one based on Archimedes' rule), is inserted through the introducer and secured in place. Using the nuclear extraction technique, the device is activated and advanced gently and slowly up until reaching the ventral one-third of the vertebral body while confirming the pathway using lateral fluoroscopy. A vacuum is created and the spongy nucleus pulposus is sucked into the decompressor unit and extracted from within the disc, after which the device is carefully retracted through the introducer (Figure 11.5A–F).

Safety Precautions

It is essential to advance the probe slowly and with care not to breach the anterior one-third of the intervertebral disc to prevent intervertebral disc rupture anteriorly, where major vascular structures are found as well. The correct probe path should be monitored continuously with intermittent live fluoroscopy to avoid injury to the adjacent dorsal root ganglia, spinal nerve roots, arterial vessels, and other neighboring structures.

Dorsal Root Ganglion Spinal Stimulation

Dorsal root ganglion stimulation is used in the treatment of persistent extremity pain from causalgia or with radicular features, due possibly to peripheral neuropathic pain syndromes, complex regional pain syndrome, phantom limb pain, or peripheral vascular disease after failure of conservative measures. It provides enhanced paresthesia-free stimulation compared to the traditional spinal cord stimulators.

Relevant Anatomy

Dorsal root ganglia are bundles of cell bodies containing afferent sensory neurons. DRG lie within the intervertebral foramina in the lateral recess of the epidural space.

Needle Placement

An epidural needle is inserted and advanced into the epidural space using the loss-of-resistance to saline technique. Once the epidural space is engaged, the first DRG lead is advanced through the needle near the DRG in the lateral recess of the epidural space. A second needle is introduced at the next level (if indicated based on anatomical mapping) using the loss-of-resistance to saline technique, and this second lead is threaded into the proper location. Strain relief loops are used to minimize migration of these leads, which are finer than conventional spinal cord stimulation leads. Position of the leads is confirmed using AP and lateral fluoroscopy, and stimulation pattern and impedance levels are assessed prior to the placement of the implantable pulse generator at a subsequent date, pending a successful trial period. The needles are withdrawn under continuous live fluoroscopy to make sure the leads do not get displaced, after which the leads are secured with anchors in their final position. A tunnel is created from the dorsal midline to the external pocket where the leads are transferred and secured in their final position (Figure 11.5G–I).

Safety Precautions

Monitor needle advancement and final placement with continual live fluoroscopy to avoid injury to the adjacent DRG, spinal nerve roots, arterial vessels, and other neighboring structures.

Spinal Cord Stimulation

Spinal cord stimulation is used in the treatment of intractable radicular-type pain, failed back surgery syndrome, peripheral neuropathic pain syndromes, complex regional pain syndrome, phantom limb pain, and peripheral vascular disease not responding to conservative treatment measures.

Relevant Anatomy

The epidural space resides between the ligamentum flavum posteriorly and dura mater anteriorly and extends from the foramen magnum down to the sacrococcygeal ligament.

Needle Placement

An epidural needle is inserted and advanced into the epidural space using the loss-of-resistance to saline technique. Once the epidural space is engaged, the first spinal cord stimulator lead is advanced through the needle in a distal to proximal direction and is then situated at a given vertebral level slightly lateral to the dorsal midline. A second needle is introduced adjacent to the first one using the same technique described, and a second 8- or 16-contact lead is threaded from distal to proximal until it is situated parallel to the previous lead. Position of the leads is confirmed with fluoroscopy with common targets being the T7, T8, or T9 intervertebral levels for low back pain, and C2–C3 or C3–C4 for upper extremity pain. The stimulation pattern and impedance levels are assessed prior to the placement of the implantable pulse generator pending the results of a successful trial period. The needles are withdrawn under continuous live fluoroscopy to make sure the leads do not get displaced, after which the leads are secured with anchors in their final position. A tunnel is created from the dorsal midline to the external pocket where the leads are transferred. (Figure 11.5J–L).

Safety Precautions

Absence of cerebrospinal fluid, blood, or paresthesias should be noted during needle advancement; needles should be withdrawn and repositioned if any of these are present.

Vertebroaugmentation (Vertebroplasty and Kyphoplasty)

Vertebroaugmentation techniques are used to restore vertebral height and stability and to reduce pain induced by vertebral compression fractures due to osteoporosis or vertebral neoplasms.

Relevant Anatomy

The middle pedicle of the vertebra is the entry point for the trocar, and the center of the vertebral body is the optimal location for the cement deposition.

Needle Placement

The needle is inserted through the skin and is guided under continuous live fluoroscopy inside of the fractured vertebral body. A drill is inserted and a pathway created toward the anterior third of the vertebra. For kyphoplasty, a balloon catheter is placed inside of the pathway and the balloon is inflated, pushing the bone trabeculae away and creating a cavity within the vertebra. The cavity is filled with polymethylmethacrylate (PMMA) material after the balloon is deflated and retracted. The injected material hardens, thus stabilizing the disrupted vertebral body. (Figure 11.5M–R).

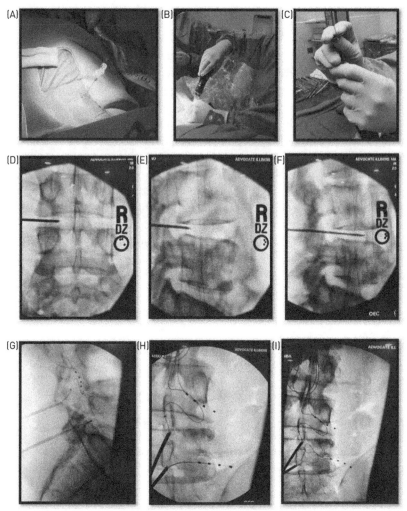

FIGURE 11.5 Advanced spinal techniques. (A) Percutaneous disc decompression (PDD) in patient with contained L4–L5 disc protrusion; introducer needle placed to the left of the dorsal midline. (B) PDD; disc decompressor is inserted through the introducer and guided inside the intervertebral disc. (C) Extracted grayish L4–L5 nucleus pulposus material (1.5 mL) visible along the shaft of the needle. (D) Anteroposterior (AP) fluoroscopic view of the disc decompressor being advanced into the intervertebral disc. (E) Lateral view of the decompressor probe entering the disc space. (F) Lateral view of the decompressor probe approaching the anterior one-third of the IV disc. (G) Lateral view of the DRG stimulator implant showing needle and lead situated at the L4–L5 interspace, and another needle being placed in the L5–S1 interspace. (H) Lateral view of dorsal root ganglia (DRG) stimulator placement showing one lead situated at the L4–L5 level and another one being advanced into the L5–S1 location. (I) Lateral view of DRG stimulator leads in their final positions near two consecutive dorsal root ganglia at L4–L5 and L5–S1 levels. (J) AP view demonstrating the placement of two epidural needles and threading of the spinal cord stimulation (SCS) leads into the epidural space. (K) AP view of two parallel SCS leads within the epidural space. (L) Lateral view showing SCS leads placed inside the epidural cavity. (M) AP view of vertebral augmentation; the trocar positioned at pedicle of T12. (N) AP view of vertebral augmentation demonstrating the unipedicular approach at T12 toward midline. (O) Lateral view showing kyphoplasty balloon deflated emerging from the trocar tip. (P) AP view showing barium-infused methylmethacrylate (MMA) spreading from pedicle to pedicle. (Q) AP view of the vertebral body with MMA after the removal of trocar. (R) Expanded AP view demonstrating MMA placed in T12 vertebral body. Images courtesy of Kenneth D. Candido, MD.

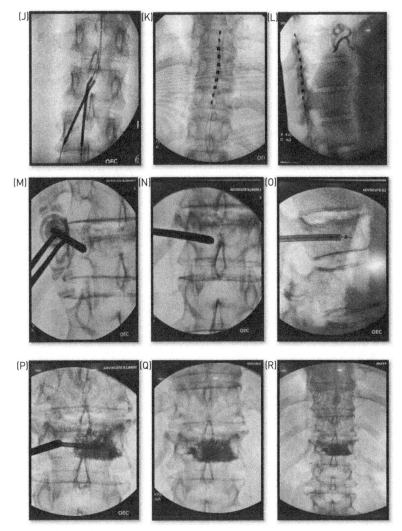

FIGURE 11.5 Continued

Safety Precautions

Visualize trocar advancement to prevent extending beyond the ventral borders of the vertebral body into the spinal cord, dural sac, or nerve roots. PMMA spread should be continuously verified to prevent extravasation posteriorly and damage to the nearby neurovascular structures.

CONCLUSION

Routine and advanced interventional pain management needle placement is essential not only to guarantee success with intended pain-relieving procedures, but also to minimize known complications from these same procedures. It is imperative that interventional pain management physicians comprehend relevant two-dimensional as well as three-dimensional anatomy; appreciate the nuances of identifying that anatomy using ultrasound technology or fluoroscopy; respect anatomical variations that may be commonly found in a general population; and utilize the most appropriate equipment and approaches to successfully perform interventional pain management procedures. This chapter should serve as a primer for some of the more routine as well as advanced therapies, but it should not substitute for hands-on learning and instruction and for ongoing study and learning, which is mandatory for assuring safety, which, for each of these elective procedures, should always be paramount in the mind of the pain management physician.

12 Sacroiliac Pain
Causes and Pain Management Options

Rene Przkora, Richard Cleveland Sims, and Andrea Trescot

INTRODUCTION

There are multiple causes of acute and chronic low back pain (LBP), including discs, nerve roots, and compression fractures. These etiologies are all well visualized on magnetic resonance imaging (MRI) and computed tomography (CT) scans, and they are relatively easy to diagnose. However, the sacroiliac joint (SIJ) is often overlooked as a cause of pain, partially because it is not well visualized on standard imaging and partially because other structures (such as posterior facet joints and L5 nerve roots) can refer to the same area. Recently, renewed interest in the SIJ has spawned a wide range of possible treatment options involving the joint and its surrounding tissues.

HISTORY

In 1938, Haldeman and Soto-Hall [1] were the first to inject the SIJ with procaine, followed by the first fluoroscopically guided procedure by Norman and May in 1956 [2]. Miskew et al. in 1979 successfully aspirated an infected joint under fluoroscopic observation [3], and Hendrix et al. [4] utilized fluoroscopy to inject SIJs for therapeutic purposes in 1982.

ANATOMY OF THE SACROILIAC JOINT

The SIJ lies at the junction of the sacrum and the iliac bones of the pelvis. In the human body, there are two SIJs, one right and one left, with the sacrum between them. The SIJ's function is to transfer the weight of the upper body and spine from the sacrum to the ilium and the lower extremities, thus acting as a shock absorber.

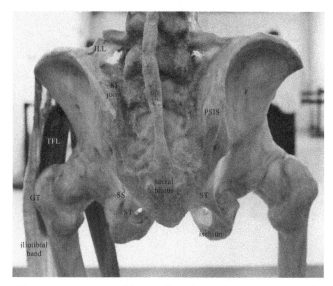

FIGURE 12.1   Ligamentous structures of the sacroiliac joint. PSIS, posterior superior iliac spine; ST, sacrotuberous ligament; SS, sacrospinous ligament; ILL, iliolumbar ligament; GT, greater trochanter; TFL, tensor fascia lata.
Image courtesy of Andrea Trescot, MD.

It is a classified as a diarthrodial synovial joint [5] and has great variability in size, shape, and contour, even within the same individual [6,7]. The SIJ is characterized as a large, auricular-shaped, diarthrodial synovial joint [5] and is in fact the largest axial joint in the body. Despite the synovial classification, only the anterior third of the interface between the sacrum and ilium is a true synovial joint; the rest of the junction comprises an intricate set of ligamentous connections [5]. These ligaments include the *posterior sacroiliac ligament (long sacral ligament), interosseous sacroiliac ligaments, iliolumbar ligament, sacrotuberous ligament*, and the *sacrospinous ligament* (Figure 12.1). This set of ligaments serves to limit movement in all directions. Several muscles surround the joint, including the *gluteus maximus, piriformis*, and *biceps femoris* muscles that also support this joint's stability. The SIJ is innervated by the lumbosacral plexus Figure 12.2), by branches from the superior gluteal (Figure 12.3) and obturator nerves, and by the lateral branches of the posterior sacral nerve roots (Figure 12.4).

SIJ DYSFUNCTION

SIJ pain is becoming widely recognized as a cause of low back pain, accounting for 15–30% of all cases of back pain [8–12]. Degenerative arthrosis of the joint commences at an early age, affecting the iliac cartilage to a greater extent than its sacral counterpart [13], which is thought to be due to the "unphysiological" bending and shearing forces encountered during locomotion [14].

The clinical history of a patient presenting with SIJ dysfunction can be quite diverse but most commonly involves pain in the low back and buttock region. Referred pain patterns into the groin and down the leg can also occur. In one study of 50 patients

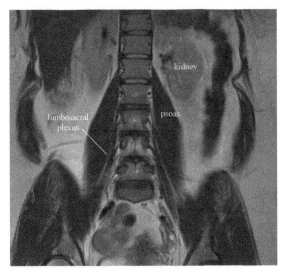

FIGURE 12.2 Coronal magnetic resonance image (MRI) showing the lumbar plexus. Image courtesy of Andrea Trescot, MD.

with injection-confirmed SIJ pain, half of all patients had lower extremity pain associated with SIJ dysfunction. Fifty percent of those patients reported pain distal to the knee and 12% as distal as the foot (Figure 12.5) [15]. This pain can be unilateral or bilateral and may be associated with an inciting event, including a single traumatic injury (44%) or a repetitive injury (21%), or it may be idiopathic (35%) [15].

There are several groups of people who may be predisposed to developing SIJ dysfunction. Pregnant women are at increased risk for SIJ dysfunction, with one study concluding that the 9-month prevalence of back pain was 49% and that 50% of those

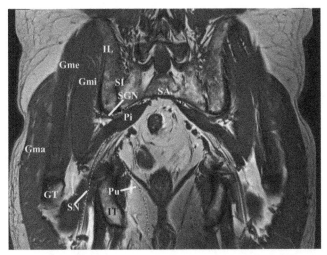

FIGURE 12.3 MRI coronal image. SA, sacrum; SI, sacroiliac joint; IL, ilium; IT, ischial tuberosity; GT, greater tuberosity; Gmi, gluteus minimus; Gme, gluteus medius; Gma, gluteus maximus; PI, piriformis; SGN, superior gluteal nerve; SN, sciatic nerve; PU, pudendal nerve. Image courtesy of Andrea Trescot, MD.

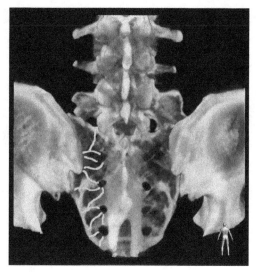

FIGURE 12.4 Posterior lateral branches of the sacral nerves, innervating the sacroiliac joint. Image courtesy of Andrea Trescot, MD.

patients had pain localized in the SIJs [16]. Patients with any type of spinal deformity or leg length discrepancy are predisposed to SIJ dysfunction. In addition, patients with seronegative spondyloarthropathies are also at increased risk for SIJ dysfunction. These include ankylosing spondylitis, enteropathic arthritis, reactive arthritis, psoriatic arthritis, and idiopathic/undifferentiated spondyloarthropathy. Pain in these patients is characterized by morning stiffness and discomfort with gradual improvement throughout the day. This is in stark contrast to that of degenerative SIJ pain, which worsens with normal activities throughout the day and is usually improved with rest. Finally, patients with a history of lumbar or lumbosacral fusion have a propensity

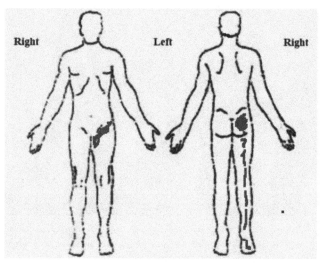

FIGURE 12.5 Pattern of pain seen with sacroiliac joint pathology. Image courtesy of Andrea Trescot, MD.

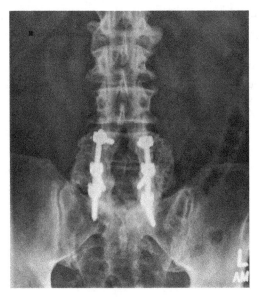

FIGURE 12.6 Lumbar fusion to the sacrum, causing stress at the sacroiliac joint. Image courtesy of Andrea Trescot, MD.

to develop SIJ dysfunction (Figure 12.6). It is well-demonstrated within the literature that the spinal segments adjacent to fusions are at increased risk of degenerative changes.

Diagnosis

As with any diagnosis, a thorough history is an important starting point. There are several physical exam observations (such as pelvic obliquity; see Figure 12.7), as well as maneuvers that have been designed to apply stress to the SIJ and elicit pain. These

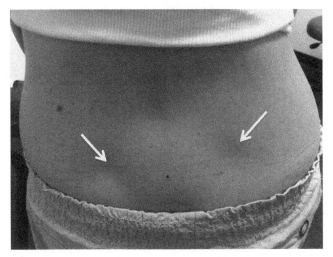

FIGURE 12.7 Pelvic obliquity. Note the asymmetric sacral "dimples" (*arrows*). Image courtesy of Andrea Trescot, MD.

include the *FABER test, Gaenslen test, extension test, Gillet's test, sacroiliac shear test, thigh thrust test, compression test,* and *distraction test.*

- *FABER test:* While the patient is in the supine position, the affected leg near the ankle is placed on the unaffected leg just proximal to the knee. The physician places one hand on the unaffected iliac crest, while the other hand is placed on the medial aspect of the knee on the affected side. A downward force is gently applied to the knee on the affected side. This maneuver will *f*lex, *ab*duct, and *e*xternally *r*otate (FABER) the femur on the affected side. A positive test will elucidate pain over the SIJ and buttock region. A limitation to this test would include patients with preexisting hip and/or knee pain (Figure 12.8).
- *Gaenslen's test:* In the supine position, the affected side thigh and lower leg are hung over the examination table. The unaffected leg is then flexed at the hip and knee while pressing downward over the thigh on the affected side. If pain is felt in the SIJ region on the affected side, then the test is positive. If the patient has any pathology affecting the hip and/or femoral nerve, this physical exam maneuver should be omitted (Figure 12.9).
- *Extension test (Yeoman's test):* With the patient in the prone position, the examiner places one hand over the anterior aspect of the knee with slight elevation while the other hand is applying a downward force over the iliac crest. A positive test is when pain is felt over the posterior SIJ (Figure 12.10).
- *Gillet's test:* With patient standing, the examiner's thumb is placed on the second sacral spinous process while the other thumb is placed on the posterior superior iliac spine (PSIS). Upon maximal flexion of the hip, the PSIS should move inferior to the S2 spinous process. If this occurs, the SIJ is normal. The PSIS will remain at the level of the S2 spinous process or even move superior in a fixed or dysfunctional SIJ.

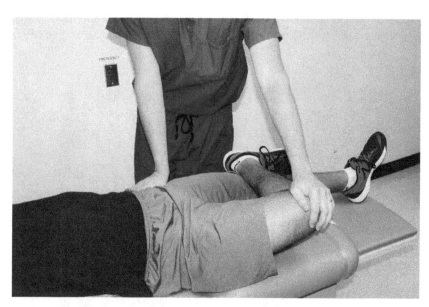

FIGURE 12.8 FABER test. Image courtesy of Rene Przkora, MD.

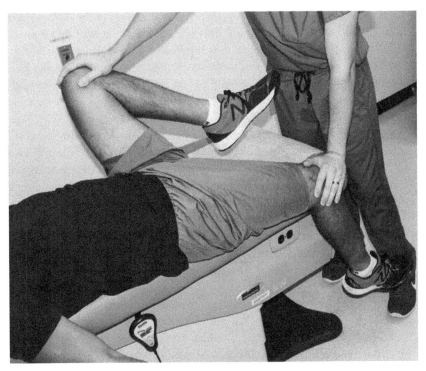

FIGURE 12.9 Gaenslen's test. Image courtesy of Rene Przkora, MD.

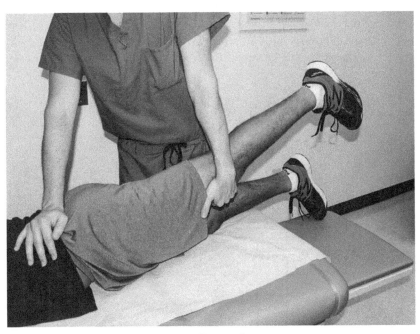

FIGURE 12.10 Extension test. Image courtesy of Rene Przkora, MD.

- *Sacroiliac shear test*: While the patient is prone, the examiner's palm is placed over the posterior iliac wing with shear thrust directed inferiorly, producing a shearing force across the SIJ. If pain is elicited on the affected side, this is a positive test.
- *Thigh thrust test*: In the supine position, the patient flexes both the hip and knee joints to approximately 90 degrees on the affected side. While stabilizing the unaffected hemipelvis, the examiner applies downward force in the axis of the femur on the affected side. A positive test will produce pain in the SIJ.
- *Compression test*: In the lateral decubitus position with the affected side up, the hips are flexed at approximately 45 degrees while the knees are flexed at approximately 90 degrees. A pillow is placed between the knees, and a downward force is applied over the anterior portion of the iliac crest on the affected side. This test is positive if pain is reproduced in the SIJ.
- *Distraction test*: With the patient in the supine position with a pillow under the knees and one arm placed under the lumbar spine, the examiner applies vertical-oriented pressure to the bilateral anterior superior iliac spines in a cross-arm technique. A positive test will produce pain in the SIJ.

Isolating pain from the SIJ complex can prove difficult secondary to other pain triggers when performing these maneuvers. Physical exams specific to the SIJ can produce a painful response in other joints, confounding the diagnosis. For example, the FABER test can stress the hip and/or knee joint, eliciting pain. Gaenslen's test can stress the hip and femoral nerve. Gillet's test can be difficult to perform. Therefore, a single positive test will yield low sensitivity and specificity for SIJ dysfunction; however, a combination of three or more positive tests in the same patient is highly sensitive (85%) and specific (79%) as well as having high positive (77%) and negative predictive values (87%) in a patient with injection-confirmed SIJ pain [17]. Tenderness to palpation over the PSIS can also assist in making the diagnosis (Figure 12.11). This is described by Fortin as the "Fortin finger test" [18] and can be confirmed by X-ray; the test shows tenderness over the PSIS (Figure 12.12). As with any diagnosis, a

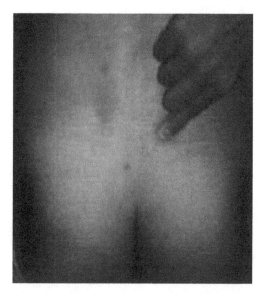

FIGURE 12.11 The "Fortin finger test." Image courtesy of Joseph Fortin, MD.

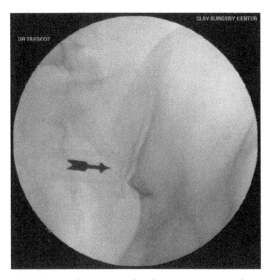

FIGURE 12.12 Fluoroscopic image showing site of tenderness consistent with sacroiliac pathology. Image courtesy of Andrea Trescot, MD.

combination of history, patient symptoms, and physical exam findings will yield the most likely etiology of the patient's pain.

Imaging evaluation of the SIJ, including fluoroscopy (Figure 12.13), CT (Figure 12.14), and MRI (Figure 12.15), have yielded little benefit in making the diagnosis of SIJ dysfunction. Rather, fluoroscopy and MRI may be beneficial in ruling out other causes of SIJ dysfunction (i.e., malignancy, ankylosing spondylitis, and/or fractures). Bone scintigraphy (nuclear medicine bone scan; Figure 12.16) has excellent specificity but poor sensitivity for identifying SIJ dysfunction [19].

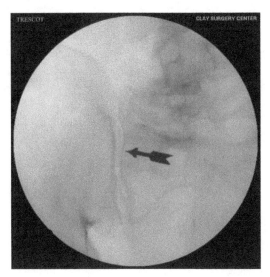

FIGURE 12.13 Fluoroscopic image showing tenderness consistent with diathesis (disruption) of the sacroiliac joint rather than the L5 spondylosis. Image courtesy of Andrea Trescot, MD.

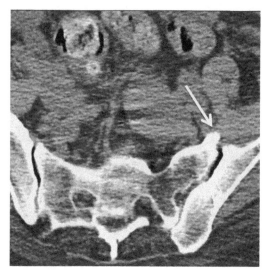

FIGURE 12.14 Axial computed tomography (CT) scan showing sacroiliac disruption (*arrow*). Image courtesy of Andrea Trescot, MD.

The current gold standard for diagnosis of SIJ dysfunction is SIJ injection under fluoroscopy (Figure 12.17) or CT guidance (Figure 12.18) using a local anesthetic solution [20]. Some consider confirmatory diagnosis only after significant pain relief (>75%) in two separate procedures in which the SIJ was injected with local anesthetic. This is likely because of a high false-positive rate, arbitrarily defined as greater than 50% pain relief following first injection but an absence of relief following a second SIJ injection [21].

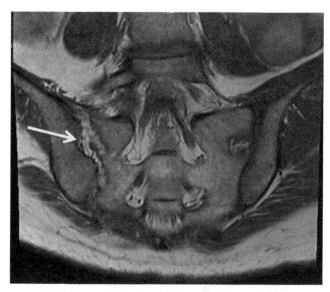

FIGURE 12.15 Coronal magnetic resonance image (MRI) showing disruption of the sacroiliac joint (*arrow*). Image courtesy of Andrea Trescot, MD.

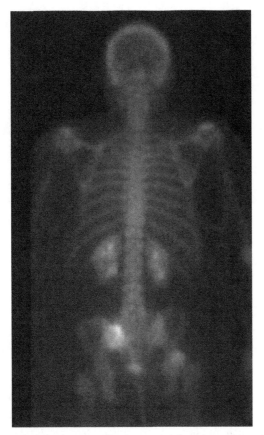

FIGURE 12.16 Nuclear medicine bone scan showing increased uptake at the sacroiliac joint. Image courtesy of Andrea Trescot, MD.

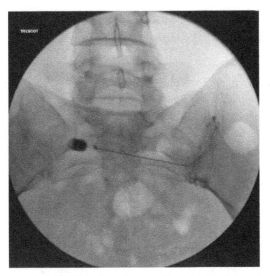

FIGURE 12.17 Fluoroscopic-guided injection of the sacroiliac joint showing contrast in the joint space. Image courtesy of Andrea Trescot, MD.

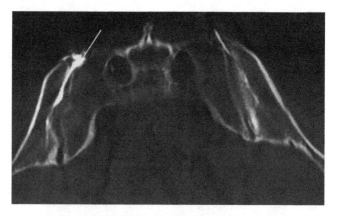

FIGURE 12.18 Computed tomography (CT)-guided injection of the sacroiliac joint showing contrast in the joint space. Image courtesy of Andrea Trescot, MD.

MANAGEMENT OF SIJ PAIN

Conservative Management

As with most pain syndromes, a trial of conservative management of the patient's pain is usually warranted, especially in the acute phase. Medicinally, this may include topical lidocaine or oral nonsteroidal anti-inflammatories (NSAIDs). If pain subsides, efforts should be employed to regain normal mechanics of the joint. Referral to physical therapy for manual medicine techniques for better pelvic stabilization and muscle balance should be considered. Additional options include SIJ belts or pelvic stabilization orthoses, which can include water-resistant tape, cinch-type belts, three-point pelvic stabilization orthoses with trans-iliac fixation, and sophisticated antigravity "leverage" devices [22]. Some patients may respond to a transcutaneous electric nerve stimulation (TENS) unit placed directly over the area causing pain.

Nonconservative Management

Intraarticular steroid injection into the SIJ has long been a treatment of SIJ dysfunction unresponsive to conservative methods. The efficacy of SIJ injections has been reviewed in multiple different studies with variable results. Several prospective case series studies demonstrated 83–92% pain relief after intraarticular steroid injections in patients with spondyloarthropathy for several months [23–25]. In patients without spondyloarthropathies, two randomized-controlled double-blind studies resulted in improved pain scores and physical exam in patients who had received a steroid injection in the SIJ [26,27]. Blind injections are rarely successful; therefore, the use of imaging to ensure proper needle placement is recommended [28].

Regardless the method used for injection, observing the patient for at least 30 minutes for any possible allergic reaction following the procedure is warranted. Other possible complications include bleeding, infection, fever, exacerbation of the pain, nerve damage, transient ipsilateral leg weakness, and difficulty voiding. If the cortical bone is "soft" (as with osteoporosis), it is possible to inject directly into the bone marrow (Figure 12.19). Relative contraindications include uncontrolled diabetes and

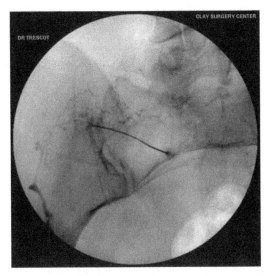

FIGURE 12.19 Fluoroscopic image showing intravascular contrast during sacroiliac injection. Image courtesy of Andrea Trescot, MD.

an allergic reaction (depending on specific reaction) to the prep solution, contract media, local anesthetic, or steroid. An infection in the area and bleeding disorders are considered absolute contraindications to SIJ injection.

Fluoroscopy-Guided SIJ Injection

The injection procedure is performed in the prone position under standard sterile technique. After identifying the joint space on fluoroscopy, the skin and subcutaneous tissue are anesthetized and a 22-guage spinal needle is guided into the joint space. Usually, a change in resistance can be appreciated once in the joint space. Fluoroscopy and contrast can be used to confirm the position in the joint (Figure 12.17). Then, a mixture of steroid with local anesthetic is injected into the joint space; it is critical to limit total injectate to less than 2.5 mL to avoid risk of distention, potentially worsening the pain, and joint rupture [29]. The injectate used is provider-specific but usually consists of a long-acting steroid mixed with a long-acting local anesthetic (i.e., bupivacaine, ropivacaine). The patient should experience almost immediate relief from the local anesthetic but may not begin recognizing the anti-inflammatory effects of the steroids until several days postprocedure.

In patients with degenerative joints, traversing the joint capsule can be difficult. Because intraarticular and extraarticular structures are innervated by nociceptive fibers, periarticular joint injection can also provide pain relief [30]. It is believed that elderly patients most often have bilateral pain arising from within the joint secondary to degenerative changes [21]. In contrast, a younger patient often has unilateral SIJ pain arising from extraarticular structures such as the ligaments, fascia, and muscles [21]. This difference would make it conceivable that the elderly would most benefit from intraarticular injection while the younger patient would benefit most from extraarticular SIJ injection.

Computed Tomography-Guided SIJ Injection

As with the previous technique, this method of injection is completed with the patient in the prone position under standard sterile technique (Figure 12.18). Details regarding this method have been described by Bollow et al. [31], Gevargez et al. [32], and Pulisetti et al. [33] and yield similar results to that of the fluoroscopic method just described. The lack of availability of CT scanners in pain clinics as well as the increased radiation exposure of this imaging method has limited the use of CT-guided SIJ injections.

Ultrasound-Guided SIJ Injection

Radiation exposure in specific patient populations should be considered prior to using fluoroscopy or CT (i.e., pregnant patients). In addition, the radiation exposure to the injectionist is significant [34]. This makes ultrasound-guided SIJ injection an excellent option for the trained practitioner. The procedure is performed in a similar fashion to that of fluoroscopy-guided SIJ injection, with the patient in the prone position and under standard sterile technique (Figure 12.20). Operator experience and injection success rate are directly proportional with this technique [35].

Radiofrequency Lesioning of the SIJ

For patients who experience excellent but short-lived relief from standard SIJ injections, radiofrequency lesioning (RFL) is a viable option for long-term pain relief. The posterior margin of the SIJ is innervated by the L5 dorsal ramus and the lateral branches of S1, S2, and S3, with possible contributions from the L4 dorsal

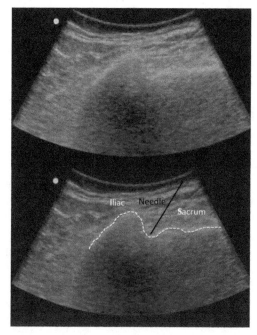

FIGURE 12.20 Ultrasound-guided sacroiliac injection. Image courtesy of Andrea Trescot, MD.

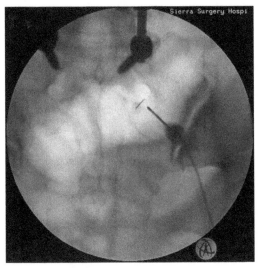

FIGURE 12.21 Fluoroscopic image showing a small gauge needle in the foramen and the cooled radiofrequency (RF) probe at the lateral edge of the foramen. Image courtesy of John DiMuro, DO.

ramus (Figure 12.4) [28]. Similar to lumbar medial branch blocks, L5 and the lateral branches of S1, S2, and S3 can be blocked, thus providing a diagnostic tool for SIJ pain. If successful, these same nerves can be ablated under either traditional thermal techniques or water-cooled RFL ("cooled RF"). With the patient prone and under sterile technique, the target areas are identified and needles guided to the target, usually with fluoroscopy. Because the location of the branches is so variable, one technique involves the placement of a small needle in the foramen (Figure 12.21); an "e"-shaped device (epsilon) can then placed on the skin and cooled RF lesions created at each site (Figure 12.22).

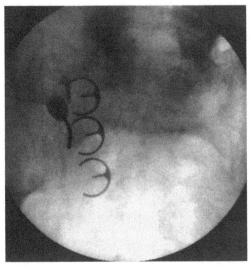

FIGURE 12.22 Fluoroscopic image showing the "epsilon" in place and the cooled radiofrequency (RF) probe at the edge of the lateral edge of the foramen. Image courtesy of Nichelle Renk, MD.

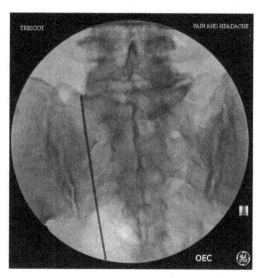

FIGURE 12.23 Fluoroscopic image showing the Simplicity probe in place. Image courtesy of Andrea Trescot, MD.

The efficacy of thermal RFL has been described in several studies, including one in which 88% of patients who underwent thermal RFL of the lateral branches for SIJ dysfunction experienced greater than 50% pain relief for at least 9 months [36]. In another study, 64% of patients had a successful outcome after thermal RFL [37]. Two studies with a combined 66 patients showed significant improvement in pain scores at 3- and 6-month follow-up [38,39]. At least one study has found that cooled RF (SInergy) was associated with a higher success rate than conventional RFL [40]. This is likely due in part to the larger lesions obtained by cooled RFL versus traditional thermal RFL.

An alternative RF technique involves placing a probe underneath the skin over the sacrum, lateral to the sacral foramen and medial to the sacroiliac joint (Figure 12.23). The Simplicity probe uses RF at multiple sites to create a strip lesion. Rea et al. reported the results of 15 patients who underwent a total of 17 Simplicity procedures: 3 patients (17%) noted no relief, but the remaining 14 procedures offered patients greater than 50% relief, with 4 patients noting 100% relief [41].

Cryoneuroablation Lesioning of the SIJ

Less commonly, cryoneuroablation denervation of the SIJ can be used to provide pain relief. The probe is placed at the lateral edge of the foramen, and stimulation is used to identify the location of the nerve (Figure 12.24). Nitrous oxide then passes down the inside of the probe to expand inside the tip, dropping the temperature of the tip of the probe to −70°C, which will kill the nerve but leave the myelin sheath intact. There is no published material on this technique.

SIJ FUSION

If the SIJ is unstable, the patient may be a candidate for a sacroiliac fusion (Figure 12.24). In the past, this fusion required open exposure of the sacrum, but there are now percutaneous techniques for fusion of the SIJ.

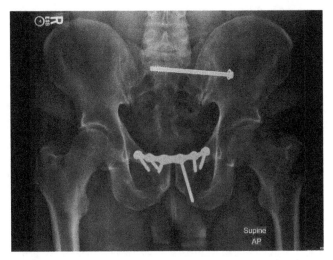

FIGURE 12.24 X-ray showing fusion of the sacroiliac joint. Image courtesy of Andrea Trescot, MD.

CONCLUSION

The SIJ is a significant cause of low back and leg pain, though often under recognized. Several diagnostic tests can help with the differential diagnosis, and injections can confirm the diagnosis. For patients who note good but only temporary relief from the injections, several techniques are available to offer longer relief.

REFERENCES

1. Halderman K, Soto-Hall R. The diagnosis and treatment of sacro-iliac conditions involving injection of procaine (Novocain) *J Bone Joint Surg.* 1938;3:675–685.
2. Norman GF, May A. Sacroiliac conditions simulating intervertebral disk syndrome. *West J Surg Obstet Gynecol.* 1956;64:641–642.
3. Miskew DB, Block RA, Witt PF. Aspiration of infected sacroiliac joints. *J Bone Joint Surg.* 1979;61A:1071–1072.
4. Hendrix RW, Lin PJP, Kane WJ. Brief note. Simplified aspiration or injection technique for the sacroiliac joint. *J Bone Joint Surg.* 1982;64A:1249–1252.
5. Cohen SP. Sacroiliac joint pain: a comprehensive review of anatomy, diagnosis, and treatment. *Anesth Analg.* 2005;101(5):1440–1453.
6. Dijkstra PF, Vleeming A, Stoeckart R. [Complex motion tomography of the sacroiliac joint: an anatomical and roentgenological study] [in German]. *Rofo.* 1989;150:635–642.
7. Ruch WJ. *Atlas of Common Subluxations of the Human Spine and Pelvis.* Boca Raton, FL: CRC Press; 1997.
8. Bernard TN, Kirkaldy-Willis WH. Recognizing specific characteristics of nonspecific low back pain. *Clin Orthop Relat Res.* 1987;217:266–280.
9. Schwarzer A, Aprill C, Bogduk N. The sacroiliac joint in chronic low back pain. *Spine.* 1995;20:31–37.
10. Bogduk N. International Spinal Injection Society guidelines for the performance of spinal injection procedures. Part 1: Zygapophysial joint blocks. *Clin J Pain.* 1997;13(4):285–302.
11. Maigne JY, Aivaliklis A, Pfefer F. Results of sacroiliac joint double block and value of sacroiliac pain provocation tests in 54 patients with low back pain. *Spine (Phila Pa 1976).* 1996;21(16):1889–1892.

12. Slinger PD, Campos JH. In: Miller RD, ed. *Miller's Anesthesia.* 7th ed. Philadelphia: Churchill Livingstone; 2010.

13. Bowen V, Cassidy JD. Macroscopic and microscopic anatomy of the sacroiliac joint from embryonic life until the eighth decade. *Spine.* 1981;6:620–628.

14. Kampen W, Tillman B. Age-related changes in the articular cartilage of human sacroiliac joint. *Anat Embryol.* 1998;198:505–513.

15. Slipman CW, Jackson HB, Lipetz JS, et al. Sacroiliac joint pain referral zones. *Arch Phys Med Rehabil.* 2000;81:334–338.

16. Ostgaard HC, Andersson GBJ, Karlsson K. Prevalence of back pain in pregnancy. *Spine.* 1991;16(5):549–552.

17. van der Wurff P, Buijs EJ, Groen GJ. A multitest regimen of pain provocation tests as an aid to reduce unnecessary minimally invasive sacroiliac joint procedures. *Arch Phys Med Rehabil.* 2006;87:10–14.

18. Fortin JD, Falco FJ. The Fortin finger test: an indicator of sacroiliac pain. *Am J Orthop.* 1997;26(7):477–480.

19. Matlick D, Dressendorfer R. Clinical review: sacroiliac joint dysfunction. *CINAHL Rehabilitation Guide.* 2015;22.

20. Chou LH, Slipman CW, Bhagia SM, et al. Inciting events initiating injection-proven sacroiliac joint syndrome. *Pain Med.* 2004;5(1):26–32.

21. Cohen SP, Chen Y, Neufeld NJ. Sacroiliac joint pain: a comprehensive review of epidemiology, diagnosis and treatment. *Expert Rev Neurother.* 2013;13(1):99–116.

22. Forst SL, Wheeler MT, Fortin JD, Vilensky JA. The sacroiliac joint: anatomy, physiology and clinical significance. *Pain Physician.* 2006;9(1):61–67.

23. Bollow M, Braun J, Taupitz M, et al. CT-guided intraarticular corticosteroid injection into the sacroiliac joints in patients with spondyloarthropathy: indication and follow-up with contrast-enhanced MRI. *J Comput Assist Tomogr.* 1996;20:512–521.

24. Braun J, Bollow M, Seyrekbasan F, et al. Computed tomography guided corticosteroid injection of the sacroiliac joint in patients with spondyloarthropathy with sacroiliitis: clinical outcome and followup by dynamic magnetic resonance imaging. *J Rheumatol.* 1996;23:659–664.

25. Fischer T, Biedermann T, Hermann KG, et al. [Sacroiliitis in children with spondyloarthropathy: therapeutic effect of CT-guided intra-articular corticosteroid injection] [German]. *Rofo.* 2003;175:814–821.

26. Luukkainen R, Nissila M, Asikainen E, et al. Periarticular corticosteroid treatment of the sacroiliac joint in patients with seronegative spondylarthropathy. *Clin Exp Rheumatol.* 1999;17:88–90.

27. Luukkainen RK, Wennerstrand PV, Kautiainen HH, et al. Efficacy of periarticular corticosteroid treatment of the sacroiliac joint in non-spondylarthropathic patients with chronic low back pain in the region of the sacroiliac joint. *Clin Exp Rheumatol.* 2002;20:52–54.

28. Agerson A, Malik K. Sacroiliac joint syndrome: sacroiliac joint injections and block/radiofrequency of the lateral branches. In: Benson H, ed. *Practical Management of Pain.* 5th ed. Philadelphia, PA: Mosby; 2014:866–875.

29. Dreyfuss P, Dreyer SJ, Cole A. Sacroiliac joint pain. *J Am Acad Orthop Surg.* 2004;12:255–265.

30. Szadek KM, Hoogland PV, Zuurmond WW, et al. Nociceptive nerve fibers in the sacroiliac joint in humans. *Reg Anesth Pain Med.* 2008;36:43.

31. Bollow M, Braun J, Taupitz M, et al. CT-guided intraarticular corticosteroid injection into the sacroiliac joints in patients with spondyloarthropathy: indication and follow-up with contrast-enhanced MRI. *J Comput Assist Tomogr.* 1996;20:512–521.

32. Gevargez A, Groenemeyer D, Schirp S. CT-guided percutaneous radiofrequency denervation of the sacroiliac joint. *Eur Radiol.* 2002;12:1360–1365.

33. Pulisetti D, Ebraheim NA. CT-guided sacroiliac joint injections. *J Spinal Disord.* 1999;12:310–312.

34. Botwin KP, Thomas S, Gruber RD, et al. Radiation exposure of the spinal interventionalist performing fluoroscopically guided lumbar transforaminal epidural steroid injections. *Arch Phys Med Rehabil.* 2002;83(5):697–701.

35. Pekkafahli MZ, Kiralp MZ, Basekim CC, et al. Sacroiliac joint injections performed with sonographic guidance. *J Ultrasound Med.* 2003;22:553–559.

36. Barolat G. A prospective multicenter study to assess the efficacy of spinal cord stimulation utilizing a multi-channel radio-frequency system for the treatment of intractable low back and lower extremity pain. *Neuromodulation.* 1999;2:179–183.

37. Yin W, Willard F, Carreiro J, Dreyfuss P. Sensory stimulation-guided sacroiliac joint radiofrequency neurotomy: technique based on neuroanatomy of the dorsal sacral plexus. *Spine.* 2003(28):2419–2425.

38. Karaman H, Kavak GO, Tufek A, et al. Cooled radiofrequency application for treatment of sacroiliac joint pain. *Acta Neurochir.* 2011;153(7):1461–1468.

39. Patel N, Gross A, Brown L. A randomized, placebo-controlled study to assess the efficacy of lateral branch neurotomy for chronic sacroiliac joint pain. *Pain Med.* 2012;13:383–398.

40. Cohen SP, Strassels SA, Kurihara C, et al. Outcome predictors for sacroiliac joint (lateral branch) radiofrequency denervation. *Reg Anesth Pain Med.* 2009;34:206–214.

41. Rea W, Karur S, Mutagi H. Radiofrequency neurotomy of the sacroiliac joint using the Simplicity III probe: a case series. *Reg Anesth Pain Med.* 2011 Conference Paper 36(5). January 2011; New Orleans, LA.

13 Sympathetic Pain Syndromes

Kenneth D. Candido and Teresa M. Kusper

INTRODUCTION

Sympathetically maintained pain (SMP) is a distinct entity influenced and perpetuated by an aberrant activity of the sympathetic efferent pathways responding to sympatholytic interventions. Sympathetic pain syndromes (SPS) might arise in response to a pathologic condition, such as autoimmune, connective tissue, or vasculitic disease or after viral infection with varicella zoster virus. In many instances, SPSs are preceded by an injury or traumatic event. Certain surgical procedures are linked with the development of SPS, wherein certain preventative measures can be undertaken to decrease the likelihood of triggering the pain syndrome.

This chapter is a brief overview of the major SPSs and their clinical characteristics, treatment, and preventative measures. Efforts have been made to provide the reader with a concise overview of distinguishing characteristics, pathogenetic mechanisms, and available treatment options for major SPSs. A substantial portion of the chapter has been dedicated to the information pertaining to complex regional pain syndrome (CRPS) and the influence of specific surgical procedures on the development of this syndrome. Risk factors and pathogenetic mechanisms related to the emergence of CRPS after orthopedic and spine surgeries have been analyzed, as well as therapies and practices used preemptively to prevent new CRPS and worsening of chronic pain and disability in the affected limb. Finally, possible therapies for the postsurgical period are discussed to facilitate rehabilitation and speed up recovery after orthopedic and spinal surgeries in this patient population.

COMPLEX REGIONAL PAIN SYNDROME

CRPS is a well-known representative of SPSs characterized by persistent incapacitating pain and/or significant limb dysfunction (Table 13.1). The estimated incidence of CRPS is 5.46–26.2 per 100,000 person years [1,2]. CRPS is broken down into types

Table 13.1 Summary of distinguishing characteristics, pathogenetic mechanisms, and available treatments related to major sympathetic pain syndromes

Comparison and contrast of major sympathetic pain syndromes

Complex regional pain syndrome	Phantom limb pain	Post-herpetic neuralgia	Raynaud's syndrome	Erythromelalgia
Clinical characteristics				
Sensory changes:	Painful sensation arising from	Constant burning	Intermittent episodic color	Triad of intense
Paresthesia, dysesthesia, allodynia,	the amputated body part	pain with allodynia,	changes in response to cold	burning pain,
hyperalgesia	Pain might be of varying	dysesthesia and	exposure or stress	increased
Autonomic:	quality	hyperalgesia	Features of sweating and coolness	temperature and
Temperature difference, color asymmetry,	Lack of feeling in the middle of		Burning pain	severe redness in the
swelling/edema, sweating asymmetry	the missing limb and illusion		Allodynia	extremities, face or
Motor changes:	that the amputated limb is		Hyperalgesia	trunk
Weakness, limited range of motion, joint	shorter than its counterpart		Cold intolerance	Edema generally not
stiffness	("telescoping")		Might be followed by trophic	present
Trophic changes:			skin changes	
Altered nail and hair growth, skin atrophy				
Unique characteristics				
Nondermatomal	Vascular disease most common	Dermatomal	Idiopathic or associated with	Bilateral symmetric
Initiating noxious event	cause of amputation	Thoracic dermatome	other diseases	involvement
Pain disproportionate to the inciting event	Higher prevalence of limb loss	(T6) most common	Initial symptom of many	Lower > Upper
Fracture leading cause	in diabetic population	Unilateral	connective tissue diseases	extremities
Median nerve (UE) and sciatic nerve (LE)		Follows infection with		Inherited and
injured most in CRPS type II		herpes zoster		sporadic forms
Might arise after orthopedic and spine		Increased age number		Reduced basal skin
surgery		one risk factor		perfusion
Females > Males				
Upper > Lower extremity				

(continued)

Table 13.1 Continued

Comparison and contrast of major sympathetic pain syndromes

	Complex regional pain syndrome	Phantom limb pain	Post-herpetic neuralgia	Raynaud's syndrome	Erythromelalgia
Pathogenesis	Peripheral inflammation and sensitization	Aberrant activity within the SNS	Activation of the dormant herpes zoster virus in the dorsal root (sensory) ganglia during stress, or immunosuppression	Deficient vasodilatory substances	SCN9A gene mutation
	Altered sympathetic nervous system function	Catecholamine sensitivity		Increased release of vasoconstrictors	Postganglionic sympathetic nervous system dysfunction
	Upregulation of adrenergic receptors	Upregulation of sodium channels		Impaired control of vascular tone	Attenuated vasoconstrictor responses
	Exaggerated response to circulating catecholamines	Spinal plasticity		Changes within blood vessel wall	Increased adrenergic vasomotor activity
	Central sensitization	↑ activity of NMDA receptors		Upregulation of adrenoreceptors	Adrenergic receptor hypersensitivity
	Brain plasticity	Sprouting of Aβ afferents		Platelet activation	
	Genetic predisposition	Central sensitization		Impaired fibrinolysis	
	Psychological factors	Cerebral reorganization (1° somatosensory cortex, subcortex and thalamus)		Increased viscosity	
				Oxidant stress	
Treatment	*Medications*: gabapentin, TCAs, clonidine, steroids, ketamine, dextromethorphan, vitamin C, phenoxybenzamine, bisphosphonates.	*Medications*: gabapentin, opioids, ketamine, dextromethorphan	*Medications*: AEDs, TCAs, opioids, lidocaine patch, topical capsaicin	*Medications*: CCBs, reserpine, guanethidine, α adrenergic blockers, ACE inhibitors, statins, antiplatelet therapy, antioxidants	*Medications*: TCAs, gabapentin, CCBs, opioids, prostacyclins, local anesthetic, mexiletine
	Sympathetic blocks	Sympathetic blocks	Sympathetic blocks	Sympathetic blocks	Sympathetic blocks
	Rehabilitation	Trigger point injections	Transforaminal ESI	Botulinum toxin	Neuromodulation
	Neuromodulation	Rehabilitation	Neuromodulation	Physical therapy	
		Complementary options		Neuromodulation	
		Mirror therapy			
		Brain stimulation			
		Neuromodulation			

ACE, angiotensin converting enzyme; AED, antiepileptic drugs; CCB, calcium channel blocker; NMDA, N-methyl-D-aspartate; TCA, tricyclic antidepressants.

I and II, formerly known as reflex sympathetic dystrophy (RSD) and causalgia, respectively. *Causalgia* was first described by a physician, Silas Weir Mitchell, in 1872 after observing the pain in soldiers with traumatic limb injuries during the American Civil War [3]. In 1900, German surgeon Sudeck reported patchy osteoporotic changes (hence the name *Sudeck's dystrophy*), and, in 1936, Rieder provided an account of dystrophic changes in the tissues of affected limbs, giving rise to the term *reflex sympathetic dystrophy* [4]. CRPS I and CRPS II taxonomy was introduced in 1994 by the International Association for the Study of Pain (IASP) [5].

The onset of CRPS is typically precipitated by some type of insult or traumatic event, such as fracture, sprain/strain, crush injury, or surgery [6,7]. Limb fracture is the most common inciting traumatic event (44–46%), followed by sprain (17.6%), elective surgery (12.2%), and tendon injury (5.5%) [1]. Distal radius fractures are most frequently implicated [8], with the incidence of CRPS ranging from 1% to 37% [9–12]. In many cases, however, the onset of the syndrome might be spontaneous [8]. The pain is disproportionate to the inciting event and is nondermatomal in character. Both CRPS types I and II are characterized by a constellation of sensory, autonomic, trophic, and motor changes (Figure 13.1A–D). The distinguishing factor between the two is the

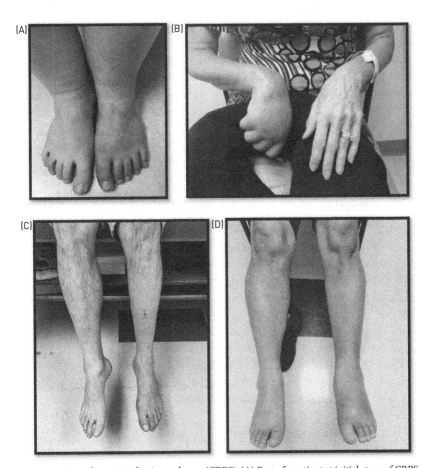

FIGURE 13.1 Complex regional pain syndrome (CRPS). (A) Feet of a patient at initial stage of CRPS with prominent swelling, edema, and discoloration. (B) Upper extremity with advanced CRPS with atrophy and contracture. (C,D) Feet of patients with advanced CRPS with evident calf atrophy, skin discoloration, and hair growth changes. Images courtesy of Kenneth D. Candido, MD.

history of nerve injury present in the CRPS type II syndrome. Median nerve injury accounts for more than 50% of CRPS type II cases in the upper extremity, whereas approximately 60% of cases in the lower extremity are due to sciatic nerve injury [13]. The term "reflex sympathetic dystrophy" (RSD) was originally developed in response to an observation that, in many cases, the sympathetic nervous system efferent fibers were somehow involved in perpetuating the condition. However, over time, it became apparent that many if not a majority of pain sufferers who met clinical criteria for RSD, did not in fact respond to sympatholysis using chemical agents. As such, the designations "sympathetically mediated" and "sympathetically independent" were suggested to differentiate these two types of clinical scenarios in otherwise identical presentations.

Pathophysiology

Several theories have been postulated to explain the emergence of CRPS, although the exact pathophysiological processes are still poorly understood (Table 13.1). It is possible that multiple mechanisms within the central and peripheral nervous systems come into play to trigger and maintain CRPS. An initial insult incites an inflammatory cascade, which sensitizes peripheral nociceptors and decreases the threshold of firing of those nociceptors [14]. The process of central sensitization ensues whereby nociceptive fibers increase firing in response to repeated noxious stimuli [15]. α_1 Adrenoreceptors have been implicated in inducing the pain by stimulating nociceptors located in the peripheral tissues. This theory is supported by the evidence showing that topical application of the α_2 agonist, clonidine, relieves hyperalgesia, whereas injection of the α_1 agonist, phenylephrine, increases pain and hyperalgesia at the site of the injection [16]. Brain plasticity, genetic susceptibility, autoimmunity, and psychological factors also appear to influence the development of CRPS [14].

CRPS After Orthopedic and Spine Surgeries

Orthopedic surgery is a known trigger of CRPS. Cases of the syndrome have been described after carpal tunnel release [17], open reduction and internal fixation (ORIF) for limb fracture [18], and foot and ankle surgery [19]. The incidence of postsurgical CRPS varies between different procedures and different publications: 2.3–4% after knee arthroscopy, 0.8–13% after knee arthroplasty, 2.1–5% after carpal tunnel surgery, 7–37% after wrist surgery, 4.5–40% after repair of Dupuytren's contracture, and 13.6% after ankle surgery [20]. The variability between different reports is attributed to similarity between the signs and symptoms of CRPS and those that might classically be observed in patients recovering from a successful orthopedic surgery. Risk factors associated with the rise of CRPS after orthopedic surgery are multifactorial and can be divided into patient-, injury-, and treatment-related factors (Table 13.2) [21].

Cases of CRPS have also been reported after surgeries of the cervical and lumbar spine involving various techniques: posterior hemilaminotomy, microdiscectomy, foraminal decompression, artificial disc replacement, traditional posterior fusion, and lateral lumbar interbody fusion [26–31]. In many instances, first signs and symptoms manifested within 2 weeks after the surgery; in others, weeks after the surgery. Disease progression resembles that of patients with CRPS from other etiologies [26]. CRPS

Table 13.2 Summary of different factors examined in the studies and their association with the emergence of complex regional pain syndrome (CRPS)

Risk factors for CRPS development in the orthopedic patients		
Positive association	No association	Debatable association
Female gender	Body mass index (BMI)	Age
High baseline pain and	Comorbidities: diabetes, high	Psychiatric issues
functional impairment days	cholesterol, arthritis	Social life events
after fracture	Smoking and alcohol addiction	Education level
Distal radius fracture	Severity of the bone injury	Intraarticular
Comminuted fractures	Radiographic changes	involvement
Motor nerve injury	Regional anesthesia	Severity of the fracture
High-energy injury	Type of surgery	Reduction of displaced
Long duration of the surgery		fracture
Hypovitaminosis C		

References 8, 9, 22–25.

has also been documented in patients with discogenic nerve compression and spine disease [32–35].

Possible reasons for the emergence of CRPS after spinal surgery involve injury to the sympathetic chain or other surrounding neural structures during the retraction [29,31]. Mobilization of the sympathetic trunk is one of the necessary steps during artificial disc implantation, and this frequently produces temporary hyperthermia of the ipsilateral lower extremity lasting between 3 and 4 months [29]. Some have hypothesized that "motion" between the L4 and L5 level may serve as the inciting painful stimulus and that the L5 nerve root is the peripheral-nerve mediator for the changes within the nervous system leading to the development of CRPS [30–32,36]. Afferent sensory stimuli might be in turn carried to the posterior rami containing postganglionic sympathetic fibers by the sinuvertebral nerves [30]. It is also likely that patients with psychiatric illnesses or under great stress might be at higher risk of developing CRPS postoperatively [37].

In relation to the cervical spine, a number of neural structures lie in close proximity to the surgical field and are at risk of being severed during surgical interventions: rami communicantes, sympathetic ganglia, sinuvertebral nerves, and vertebral nerves [28]. Despite inherent challenges in distinguishing the pain syndrome from other surgical complications, early detection of possible CRPS is paramount to ensure timely management leading to improved prognosis and symptom resolution. CRPS should be suspected in any patient developing new pain (particularly if there is tactile allodynia present or hyperalgesia to deep digital pressure), paresthesias, swelling, or other symptoms consistent with CRPS. Early treatment of CRPS is necessary to minimize tissue swelling and prevent progression of the condition due to the presence of tissue lactic acidosis [38].

Preventative Measures

Different methods for reducing the probability of developing CRPS after orthopedic and spinal surgeries have been outlined, and these can be implemented in the presurgical, perioperative, and postsurgical periods. The optimal timeline before surgical interventions can be undertaken in patient with CRPS has not been established. A consensus between authors is not to operate on patients with acute CRPS but to postpone surgical procedures until a sufficient healing period has passed to allow the symptoms to subside and the condition to stabilize [20]. Veldman and Goris state that operating on a cold and edematous extremity is contraindicated [39]. During the waiting period, the patients should be treated with analgesic agents, sympatholytic agents, peripheral vasodilators, serial sympathetic blocks, and physical therapy to minimize derangements, increase perfusion, and optimize functioning of the affected limb.

General anesthetic technique has been associated with an increased risk of recurrence and/or development of CRPS after surgical procedures [40]. Regional anesthesia might then be the more appropriate anesthetic choice for this patient population because it provides perioperative postganglionic sympathectomy, which might prevent CRPS development postoperatively [41,42]. Perioperative sympatholysis can also be achieved with intravenous regional blocks using local anesthetic lidocaine and the α_2 receptor agonist clonidine, an approach shown to decrease the rates of recurrence after surgery [20]. Epidural administration of clonidine (1 µg/kg) has shown promise in reducing the incidence and reducing the flare-up of CRPS postsurgery and has been recommended for patients with lower extremity CRPS undergoing surgery [20,43]. Additional intraoperative measures include minimizing the duration of surgery, reducing the time of tourniquet application, care and caution during instrumentation in close vicinity of the neural structures, and avoidance of nerve traction [44,45]. Adequate control of the pain after the initial injury and increased postsurgical monitoring need to be emphasized because a greater pain level preoperatively has been linked with a higher probability of postsurgical CRPS [46]. Moreover, use of multimodal analgesia before, during, and after surgery has been suggested as a preventative analgesic technique that has shown efficacy in preventing CRPS emergence [47].

Certain supplements and pharmacological agents have demonstrated benefits in preventing CRPS after limb fracture and/or surgical procedures. Ascorbic acid is a natural antioxidant and scavenger of toxic free radicals. A dose of 500 mg of vitamin C is administered to patients on the day of their surgery and continued for 50 days. A systematic review and meta-analysis of randomized placebo-controlled trials ($n = 875$) showed level II evidence in support of the vitamin C supplementation in reducing the risk of CRPS development [48]. The analgesic and anti-inflammatory properties of calcitonin and its application in prevention of CRPS have been examined in patients with and without a history of CRPS, but the studies conducted yielded conflicting results [49,50]. Early anti-inflammatory medications, such as steroids, may be of value in reducing the inflammatory processes leading to CRPS [51]. Perioperative intravenous infusion of the serotonin type 2 receptor antagonist ketanserin or an infusion of 1,000 mL of 10% mannitol have also been studied and might potentially provide some benefit in reducing CRPS after orthopedic surgery [39,52].

Treatment Options

The main goal of treatment is to minimize pain and improve the function of the affected extremity. Three pillars of CRPS management include medical interventions, psychological interventions, and physiotherapy [25]. Multiple pharmacological agents commonly used for neuropathic pain syndromes have been tried in the treatment of CRPS, including gabapentin [53], tricyclic antidepressants (TCAs) [54], clonidine [55,56], systemic steroids [57], phenoxybenzamine [63], bisphosphonates [58], and the NMDA receptor antagonists, ketamine and dextromethorphan [59–61]. An application of ketamine in the treatment of CRPS has been widely investigated and described by different studies. Two separate randomized controlled trials (RCTs) demonstrated significant decrease in pain scores after intravenous ketamine infusion [62,63]. However, two independent systematic reviews assessed the effectiveness of ketamine and concluded that there is only weak evidence supporting the efficacy of ketamine in CRPS treatment [59,60].

Interventional strategies including stellate ganglion (Figure 13.2A,B) and lumbar sympathetic blocks (Figure 13.2C,D) are proven and effective techniques that should be incorporated into the treatment regimen early on to reduce symptoms, decrease the pain, and halt the progression and induce remission of the syndrome if pain is indeed "sympathetically mediated." Meaningful clinical outcomes of long-term pain reduction and improved quality of life have been demonstrated after spinal cord stimulator (SCS) placement (Figure 13.2E,F) [64–66].

Rehabilitation with physical, occupational, and/or cognitive-behavioral therapy is a critical aspect of the recovery to restore functionality and enable timely return to daily activities in this patient population. Engagement in the therapy, however, may be problematic. Continuous regional anesthesia may be used to reduce the pain, minimize fear-avoidant responses, and facilitate participation in high-intensity rehabilitation of pediatric and adult patients with CRPS, although evidence in favor of these techniques is based on a small series of retrospective studies and is largely anecdotal [67]. Pediatric patients with CRPS ($n = 102$) given continuous epidural or peripheral perineural local anesthetic infusions during their inpatient rehabilitation showed marked improvements in pain scores, function, and disability in a retrospective study [67]. Clinically significant pain reduction and improved functionality was demonstrated in 56% and 40% of patients, respectively.

PHANTOM LIMB PAIN

Postamputation pain is a debilitating and exceedingly challenging to treat pain entity arising after amputation of a limb or body part (Figure 13.3A,B). Ambrose Parè, a French military surgeon, provided a first written account of this condition in the 16th century [68]. Silas Weir Mitchell introduced the name of *phantom limb pain* (PLP) and provided a detailed description of the syndrome in the 19th century [69]. PLP syndrome is an umbrella term, which includes *phantom sensation, phantom pain*, and *stump pain*. PLP (postamputation pain) is characterized by an experience of pain, frequently agonizing, perceived in the missing body part. Phantom limb sensation denotes a feeling of nonpainful sensations emanating from the amputated area, while stump pain represents a painful sensation experienced in the retained body part.

Prevalence of PLP ranges from 44.6% to 79.9% [70–73] and reported incidence at 8 days, 6 months, and 2 years after the amputation is 72%, 65%, and 59%, respectively [74]. Vascular disease is the number one cause of nonmilitary amputations (82%), followed by trauma (16.4%), cancer (0.9%), and congenital anomalies (0.8%) [75]. Amputations in the diabetic population far exceed those in nondiabetic patients: 3.83 amputations per 1,000 individuals versus 0.38 per 1,000 [76]. In the military

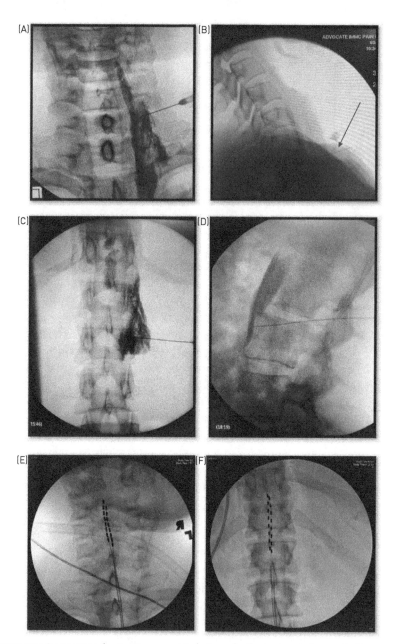

FIGURE 13.2 Interventional pain management techniques for the treatment of sympathetic pain syndromes. (A) Stellate ganglion block anterior approach; fluoroscopic anteroposterior (AP) view of needle located at the transverse process of the C7 and injected contrast extending along the cervical and upper thoracic vertebra. (B) Stellate ganglion block anterior approach; fluoroscopic lateral view of the needle approaching the transverse process of C7 and contrast injected. (C) Lumbar paravertebral sympathetic block; fluoroscopic AP view of needle localized at the lateral aspect of the second lumbar vertebra and contrast along the lumbar vertebral bodies. (D) Lumbar paravertebral sympathetic block; fluoroscopic lateral view demonstrating needle placement at L2 vertebra and linear spread of the injected contrast dye along the anterolateral aspect of the lumbar vertebral bodies. (E) Spinal cord stimulator used to treat complex regional pain syndrome of the upper extremities; fluoroscopic lateral view of two Octrode cervical leads with the proximal most contract at the C2–C3 vertebral interspace. (F) Spinal cord stimulator; fluoroscopic AP view of two cervical Octrode leads. Images courtesy of Kenneth D. Candido, MD.

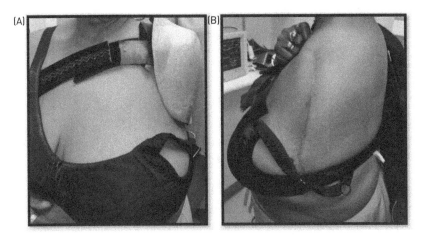

FIGURE 13.3 (A,B) A patient with complete left upper extremity amputation at the shoulder joint who subsequently developed chronic phantom limb pain. Image courtesy of Kenneth D. Candido, MD.

community, PLP was reported by 78% of 2,750 surveyed military veterans [77], which corresponds with a data from surveys from the Vietnam War ($n = 298$) and Operation Iraqi Freedom/Operation Enduring Freedom (OIF/OEF) veterans ($n = 283$) who reported prevalences of 72.2% and 76%, respectively [78].

Pathogenesis and Clinical Presentation

Phantom pain has been described after loss of an extremity, but also in other parts of the body: breast [79,80], tongue [81], digestive tract [82], and urinary tract [83]. PLP can be described as sharp, throbbing, dull, squeezing, piercing, tingling, burning, or cramping (Table 13.1). Some patients report lack of sensation in the middle portion of the affected extremity and an illusion of discrepancy in the length of the extremities, a concept known as "telescoping."[84] Risk factors predisposing to PLP include pain in the affected body part prior to the amputation, presence of stump pain or phantom sensations after the amputation, stump pain, prosthesis use, and increased time interval from the amputation [85]. Different theories have been developed to explain the emergence of phantom limb pain that involve mechanisms within the peripheral, spinal, and supraspinal neural pathways (Table 13.1). The interplay of various mechanisms explains the fact that single therapy is rarely effective in treating the pain, and agents from different groups might be necessary to bring the pain under control [86].

Prevention of Phantom Limb Pain

A preemptive analgesia regime with regional anesthesia has been utilized pre- and postoperatively to diminish noxious stimuli triggering the abnormal processes responsible for neural sensitization at the stump site. The benefits of perioperative perineural and epidural analgesia in preventing PLP has been widely investigated but the results have been largely dichotomous [87–89]. Because of the disparity of the results, the clinical value of this approach is still in question. Infusion of ketamine, an NMDA receptor antagonist, during the perioperative period and continued for 72 hour postoperatively has shown benefit in reducing the incidence of phantom pain at 6 months post surgery [90] and pain reduction in amputees during the postoperative course [91,92].

Treatment of Phantom Limb Pain

The task of formulating an effective treatment plan for PLP using pharmacological agents is difficult to execute. Evidence from placebo RCTs is limited and offers little direction in addressing phantom pain [93]. A 2016 Cochrane review conducted by Alviar et al. demonstrates favorable outcomes after therapy with morphine, gabapentin, ketamine, and dextromethorphan, but not after the treatment with memantine, amitriptyline, or botulinum toxin [94]. Short-term relief has been noted after oral and intravenous morphine [95,96]. In a randomized double-blind placebo-controlled crossover trial, 32 subjects with stump and/or phantom pain were given either treatment with intravenous morphine and lidocaine or placebo (diphenhydramine) for 3 consecutive days [96]. Significant reduction in stump pain was observed after both morphine and lidocaine, whereas phantom pain was only relieved by morphine therapy. Pain relief was also noted in separate reports after tramadol [97] and methadone administration [98].

Although nerve blocks and trigger point injections are frequently employed in the management of phantom pain, available evidence is insufficient to establish a long-term benefit of the therapy [99–101]. A Cochrane review by Alviar et al. demonstrated no improvement in pain intensity after infiltration with botulinum toxin [94]. A case report exists describing blockade of femoral and sciatic nerves, which provided 80% pain reduction in both phantom and stump pain at 1, 3, and 6 months [102].

Support for the effectiveness of complementary modalities comes mostly from case reports. Although some reports show approximately 50% pain reduction after the use of transcutaneous electrical nerve stimulation (TENS) [103,104], a recent Cochrane review found no good-quality RCTs to confirm the effectiveness of the device in treating PLP [105]. Mirror therapy has been used to treat postamputation pain since 1996. The goal of the therapy is to help amputees eliminate the visual-proprioceptive dissociation in their brains and block pain perception in the phantom limb [106–108]. This approach has been validated by a RCT with 22 patients allocated to a mirror, a covered mirror, and mental visualization groups for 4 weeks, which showed pain reduction in the uncovered mirror group compared to the other two groups [109]. Other available noninvasive treatment options include transcranial magnetic stimulation (TMS) [110], electroconvulsive therapy (ECT) [111], acupuncture [112], biofeedback [113], and behavioral therapy [114].

Invasive treatment options are generally reserved for those patients who failed to respond to conservative treatment options. Brain stimulation has been investigated as treatment option for refractory PLP. Deep brain stimulation (DBS) of the periventricular gray and somatosensory thalamus has been assessed in three patients with PLP who reported 55–70% pain reduction [115]. Comparable outcomes have been demonstrated after the use of motor cortex stimulation (MCS) of the precentral gyrus in three amputee patients with treatment-resistant PLP [116]. Neuromodulation with SCS devices is a frequently performed intervention in the management of PLP (Figure 13.4E–F).

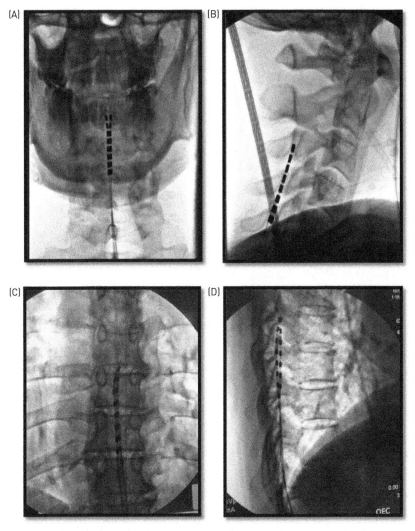

FIGURE 13.4 Fluoroscopic images of the octrode spinal cord stimulation leads placed within the epidural space used for the treatment of phantom limb pain; (A) A-P view of cervical leads; (B) Lateral view of cervical leads; (C) A-P view of thoracolumbar leads; (D) Lateral view of thoracolumbar leads. Image courtesy of Kenneth D. Candido, MD.

In different reports, SCS has been shown to provide excellent pain relief to amputee patients, ranging from 50–80% [117,118].

POSTHERPETIC NEURALGIA

Postherpetic neuralgia (PHN) is a pain syndrome precipitated by shingles infection due to reactivation of the dormant varicella zoster virus (VZV). PHN is characterized by intense, constant burning pain with an intermittent lancinating component associated with evoked allodynia, dysesthesias, and hyperalgesia in a unilateral dermatomal distribution, which persist after the resolution of the infection and disappearance of the vesicular skin eruptions (Table 13.1) [119]. The thoracic dermatome (T6) is the

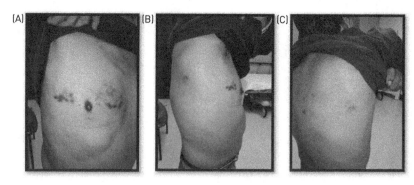

FIGURE 13.5 (A,B,C) Clusters of vesicular eruption in a thoracic dermatomal pattern characteristic of acute phase of herpes zoster infection. Images courtesy of Kenneth D. Candido, MD.

most frequently affected site (45%), followed by the cervical dermatomes (23%) and the ophthalmic division (V_1) of the trigeminal nerve [120].

Zoster sine herpete represents similar neuropathic pain in a dermatomal pattern that is not preceded by the painful herpetic skin lesions. The initial symptoms of acute herpes zoster infection include pain (41%), itching (27%), and paresthesias (12%) [120]. The acute phase might be heralded by the prodromal symptoms of headache, malaise, sensitivity to light, and fever. A painful maculopapular rash emerges within 1–2 days in a unilateral dermatomal pattern and progresses into fluid filled vesicles that crust over after 7–10 days and resolve within 3–4 weeks (Figure 13.5A–C). Changes in skin pigmentation or scars might be visible after the rash heals.

Epidemiology and Pathogenesis

The estimated incidence of PHN ranges from 120,000 to 200,000 cases per year [121]. A majority of cases of herpes zoster infection are reported in the population between the ages of 50 and 79 [122]. Increased age (leading risk factor), female gender, prodromal symptoms prior to active infection, greater rash severity and pain intensity during the HZ infection, use of immunosuppressive therapy, history of malignancy, organ transplantation, and HIV or other diseases resulting in diminished cell-mediated immunity have been listed as risk factors predisposing to PHN [123,124]. The virus remains dormant in the dorsal root (sensory) ganglia for years after the primary HZ infection (chicken pox), which takes place in childhood. The virus is reactivated under the conditions of increased stress, immunosuppression, or decreased cell-mediated immunity, at which time it travels to the epidermis to cause the acute phase of the shingles infection. Separate theories have been put forth to explain the pathogenesis of PHN (Table 13.1).

Prevention of Herpes Zoster and Postherpetic Neuralgia

The best preventative measure is the live attenuated varicella zoster vaccine, which is approved by the US Food and Drug Administration (FDA) for individuals older than 50 years [125]. The Shingles Prevention Study reports 51.2% and 66.5% effectiveness in preventing HZ and PHN, respectively [126]. A drop in incidence by 39%

has been noted after the HZ vaccination [127]. Routine vaccination is recommended by the Advisory Committee on Immunization Practices (ACIP) for all individuals above the age of 60, unless contraindicated [127]. Antiviral medications (acyclovir, famciclovir, or valacyclovir) are considered first-line treatment option for acute HZ infection. Initiated within the first 72 hours after rash formation, the antivirals speed the healing process and decrease pain during the active phase of the infection [128–130]. It is possible that early administration of antivirals might protect against PHN, although studies show conflicting results [131–133]. In one study involving 85 patients with PHN, neuropathic pain was reported 6 months after the acute infection by 18.6% of patients who had foregone the antiviral treatment compared to 2.6% in the group treated with the antiviral therapy [134]. Winnie et al. examined the relationship between the timing of treatment during the acute phase of shingles infection and prevention of PHN in 122 patients who received sympathetic blocks at different time points after symptom presentation [135]. Sympathetic blocks administered within the first 2 months after acute infection prevented PHN in 80% of individuals. After the 2-month window, the effectiveness of the blocks diminished markedly, and repeated injections were necessary to achieve clinically meaningful response. The authors suggested that early blocks prevent PHN by restoring intraneural blood flow before irreversible ischemic damage and demise of large nerve fibers ensues.

Treatment of Postherpetic Neuralgia

A multifaceted approach is necessary to maximize benefits in the treatment of PHN. Pharmacotherapy is the main component of this approach. The use of TCAs, antiepileptic drugs (AEDs), opioids, lidocaine transdermal patches, and topical capsaicin has been supported by a meta-analysis of 35 RCTs [136]. TCAs and AEDs are used as the first-line treatment options, whereas opioid medications are utilized for breakthrough pain. The efficacy of gabapentin and pregabalin in the treatment PHN has been demonstrated by independent RCTs [137–139]. The value of opioid medications in the management of neuropathic pain is debatable [140,141], although some showed notable improvements in PHN patients with this treatment option [142–144]. Raja et al. showed greater pain relief after opioids compared to TCAs in 76 patients diagnosed with PHN (38% vs. 32%) [142]. Transdermal lidocaine and topical capsaicin are viable alternatives of proven effectiveness in reducing PHN [145,146].

Sympathetic nerve blocks have been used to treat pain related to acute HZ infection and PHN. Significant analgesia during the acute HZ phase has been reported by different studies [147,148]. Sympathetic nerve blocks may help to reduce the incidence of PHN if administered early [135]. They might alleviate the pain from PHN, although the response appears to be transient [147]. The evidence in favor of transforaminal epidural steroid injections (TESI) for PHN is inconclusive; Mehta et al. described significant pain relief lasting for several weeks after TESI at T10 [149], but a randomized trial comparing standard therapy (antivirals and analgesics) with the treatment group (epidural injection with standard therapy) in 598 patients by Opstelten et al. has not corroborated those results [150].

SCS implantable devices have been investigated in patients with PHN refractory to the conservative treatment and/or interventional approaches. In a prospective study of 28 patients with intractable pain due to PHN, long-lasting pain relief with a median decrease from 9 to 1 on the visual analog scale was shown in 82% patients [151].

SCS of the dorsal root ganglion shows great promise in treating neuropathic pain of various etiologies in the lower extremity, including that secondary to PHN. A positive outcome was observed in a trial with 51 subjects, 76.5% of whom reported substantial pain relief of an average of 74.2% after a 12-month period [152].

RAYNDAUD'S DISEASE

Raynaud's phenomenon (RP) refers to a condition characterized by intermittent episodic skin changes in the digits in response to cold temperatures or stressful stimuli (Table 13.1). Usually, the discoloration progresses from white to purple to red as the tissue goes from hypoxia to reperfusion. RP can be idiopathic or secondary to other underlying conditions [141], and it is commonly seen in conjunction with connective or autoimmune diseases [153]. In fact, it is listed as the most common initial symptom of many connective diseases in 50% of cases [154]. It is distinguished from *Raynaud's disease*, a vasospastic condition that includes features of sweating and coolness in addition to the color changes seen in the former state [155] not associated with other pathologic entities [153]. Burning pain accompanied by allodynia, hyperalgesia, painful paresthesias, cold intolerance, and color changes in the extremities is the hallmark of the syndrome.

The clinical picture varies depending on the severity of the disease (Figure 13.6A–D) as the degree of cyanosis depends on metabolic activity and the speed of blood flow in the affected tissues [156]. Vasospasm is usually confined to the digital

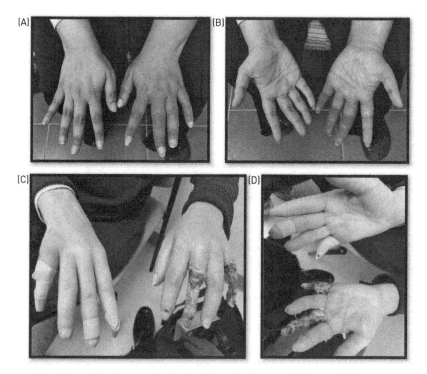

FIGURE 13.6 Raynaud's phenomenon. (A,B) Visible color change purplish over the dorsal and palmar aspects of the left hand. (C,D) Severe form of the disease complicated by vascular insufficiency and dry gangrene. Image courtesy of Kenneth D. Candido, MD.

arterioles rather than larger diameter vessels and occurs below a critical temperature, which varies on a case-to-case basis. The digits feel numb as the temperature descends below the critical temperature, whereas a burning sensation might be experienced with rewarming of the affected phalanges. These might be accompanied by hyperhidrosis, although excessive sweating is rarely present in the advanced stages [156]. In the early phases of the syndrome, peripheral vessels retain their normal architecture, but, as the disease progresses, the microvascular appearance changes, at which point responsiveness to stellate ganglion block diminishes [156]. These structural alterations might be followed by trophic changes, giving rise to skin ulceration or dry gangrene in advanced stages that may even result in amputations of the affected body part (Figure 13.6C,D).

Pathogenesis of Raynaud's Phenomenon

Several pathogenetic mechanisms have been proposed in the literature (Table 13.1). They include deficient release of the vasodilatory chemical calcitonin gene-related peptide (CGRP); increased release of vasoconstricting substances such as catecholamines, endothelin-1, and 5-hydroxytryptamine; overactivity of the sympathetic nervous system encompassing α_2 adrenoreceptor upregulation; increased reactivity of smooth muscle adrenoreceptors to circulating catecholamines; changes related to blood vessel wall architecture, such as intimal thickening; and impaired neurogenic control of the vascular tone [157–159]. Additional mechanisms involve platelet activation, impaired fibrinolysis, increases viscosity, and oxidant stress [158].

Treatment of Raynaud's Phenomenon

Therapeutic considerations include medication therapy, sympathetic blocks, physical and/or occupational therapy, and surgical interventions. Calcium channel blockade is considered the first-line treatment option, although a Cochrane review of 296 RCTs showed only minimal effectiveness in the treatment of RP [160]. Intraarterial reserpine and guanethidine have been employed with variable reductions in symptoms [153]. Other agents with questionable efficacy include α adrenergic receptor blockers, angiotensin- converting enzyme inhibitors, statins, antiplatelet therapy, and antioxidants [161]. Sympathetic blockade is used for therapeutic purposes and/or as a prognostic indicator prior to sympathectomy procedure [156]. Therapeutic stellate ganglion and lumbar sympathetic blocks may minimize the paresthesias and hyperhidrosis in the extremities, and, if repeated at regular intervals, facilitate healing of the ulcerative or gangrenous skin lesions. Moreover, they may also increase the intervals between attacks. Lumbar sympathetic blocks have been documented [153]. Some have tried injections with botulinum toxin, but insufficient evidence exists to assess its efficacy [162,163]. The use of SCS has been described in treatment of pain due to different connective tissue diseases such as scleroderma [164,165], medication-induced vasculitis [164], Sjögren syndrome [166], and thromboangiitis obliterans (Buerger's disease) [167,168]. It has also been successfully used to treat severe microcirculatory insufficiency in patients with Raynaud's phenomenon, who showed improved microcirculation, reduced symptoms of the disease, and reduced pain [165,169–171].

ERYTHROMELALGIA

Another rare member of the SPS family is an autosomal dominant condition known as *erythromelalgia*, characterized by intense chronic neuropathic pain with bilateral and symmetrical involvement of feet or less frequently hands, and sporadic facial or trunk involvement (Table 13.1) [172]. The reported incidence ranges from 0.36 to 1.1 per 100,000 persons [155], with female gender more commonly affected [153,156]. Silas Weir Mitchell, a pioneer in neurology (see earlier discussion on CRPS and phantom limb pain), was first to describe the syndrome in 1878 [173]. The distinguishing feature of this condition, initially known as *Mitchell disease*, is severe warmth and redness in the extremities (Figure 13.7A,B). A report describing a long-term follow-up of 46 patients diagnosed with erythromelalgia shows that burning was present in 96%, heat in 93%, pain in 87%, redness in 83%, swelling in 65%, and numbness in 54% the patients examined [172]. Symptoms appear to be intensified by heat, exercise, dependency of the extremities, and during the night [172,174,175], whereas cooling and elevation of the extremities improved the symptoms [172].

Pathogenesis of Erythromelalgia

A gain-of-function mutation in the SCN9A gene encoding the α subunit of the $Na_v1.7$ protein of the sodium channel has been implicated in the formation of primary erythromelalgia, which results in the prolonged opening of the channel and hyperexcitability of the small-diameter sensory neurons in dorsal root ganglia in response to small stimuli [176–178]. Cases of secondary erythromelalgia have been reported in patients with myeloproliferative diseases, connective tissue diseases (Raynaud's, Sjögren's, systemic sclerosis), blood disorders (polycythemia vera),

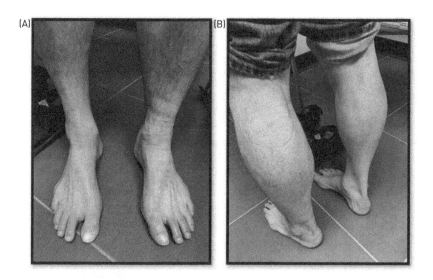

FIGURE 13.7 Lower extremities of a patient diagnosed with erythromelalgia; red discoloration is evident over the right limb characteristic of the condition. Image courtesy of Kenneth D. Candido, MD.

neurologic disorders (multiple sclerosis), paraneoplastic disease, and diabetes mellitus and after exposure to certain medications. Inherited primary erythromelalgia manifests itself usually early in the patient's life, whereas the acquired secondary erythromelalgia might have more delayed onset [179]. Dysfunction of the postganglionic sympathetic peripheral fibers, impaired vasomotor reflexes, and microvascular arteriovenous shunting leading to disturbances in microvascular perfusion during tissue hypoxia have been documented as the pathogenetic mechanism underlying the development of erythromelalgia [180–183] (Table 13.1). The theory has been confirmed with neurophysiologic perfusion testing in patients with erythromelalgia who exhibited attenuated vasoconstrictor responses to Valsalva's maneuver and cold challenge, as well as lower flow on laser Doppler flowmetry signifying impaired neurogenic vasoconstrictor reflexes and diminished basal skin perfusion indicative of sympathetic nerve dysfunction [181].

Treatment of Erythromelalgia

Multimodal treatment involving pharmacological agents, interventional blocks, physical therapy, and neuromodulating devices have been used in the treatment of erythromelalgia, with varying success. Pharmacotherapy including gabapentinoids, TCAs, calcium channel blockers, and opioid medications is a critical component of the multimodal approach. The synthetic prostacyclin analogue iloprost provides pain relief and improves sympathetic dysfunction in selected cases [172,184]. Sodium channel blockers, such as local anesthetics, have been used and offer short-term benefits [185]. Mexiletine, an antiarrhythmic agent that is comparable to lidocaine, has also showed promise in certain patients [186,187].

As with the other SMP syndromes, the challenge in the management of erythromelalgia-related pain lies in the fact that the pain is highly refractory to conservative therapies. In those instances, other more invasive approaches, such as neuromodulation, need to be attempted. Graziotti and Goucke [188] applied neuromodulation technology for the management of erythromelalgia pain in 1993. This was followed by other case reports describing the successful use of SCS treatment after failed therapy with conventional management [189,190]. Now, the number of similar reports continues to grow, and it is reasonable to expect an expansion of SCS use in the clinical practice in upcoming years.

CONCLUSION

SPSs are commonly encountered pain states in many pain clinics. Nevertheless, common as they seem, the syndromes are still exceedingly challenging to treat. One of the traits shared among these syndromes is their poor response to conventional management, typically requiring combinations of pharmacologic, interventional pain management procedures, and aggressive physical therapy approaches. Despite the many available strategies, the treatment of the pain in many cases remains highly unsatisfactory. A superb knowledge of the typical characteristics of each of these syndromes and proper assessment is invaluable in the timely recognition of the syndromes and initiation of appropriate treatment strategies.

REFERENCES

1. de Mos M, de Bruijn AG, Huygen FJ, et al. The incidence of complex regional pain syndrome: a population-based study. *Pain*. 2007;129(1-2):12–20.

2. Sandroni P, Benrud-Larson LM, McClelland RL, et al. Complex regional pain syndrome type I: incidence and prevalence in Olmsted county, a population-based study. *Pain*. 2003;103(1-2):199–207.

3. Weir MS. *Injuries of the Nerves and Their Consequences*. Philadelphia, PA: J. B. Lippincott & Co;1872.

4. Veldman PH. *Clinical Aspects of Reflex Sympathetic Dystrophy*. Doctoral Thesis. Nijmegen, 1995:107–115.

5. Merskey H, Bogduk M. *Classification of Chronic Pain: Descriptions of Chronic Pain Syndromes and Definitions of Pain Terms*. Seattle, WA: IASP Press; 1994.

6. Harden RN, Bruehl S, Galer BS, et al. Complex regional pain syndrome: are the IASP diagnostic criteria valid and sufficiently comprehensive? *Pain*. 1999;83(2):211–219.

7. Allen G, Galer BS, Schwartz L. Epidemiology of complex regional pain syndrome: a retrospective chart review of 134 patients. *Pain*. 1999;80(3):539–544.

8. Veldman PH, Reynen HM, Arntz IE, et al. Signs and symptoms of reflex sympathetic dystrophy: prospective study of 829 patients. *Lancet*. 1993;342(8878):1012–1016.

9. Jellad A, Salah S, Ben Salah Frih Z. Complex regional pain syndrome type I: incidence and risk factors in patients with fracture of the distal radius. *Arch Phys Med Rehabil*. 2014;95(3):487–492.

10. Atkins RM, Duckworth T, Kanis JA. Features of algodystrophy after Colles' fracture. *J Bone Joint Surg Br*. 1990;72(1):105–110.

11. Dijkstra PU, Groothoff JW, ten Duis HJ, et al. Incidence of complex regional pain syndrome type I after fractures of the distal radius. *Eur J Pain*. 2003;7(5):457–462.

12. Beerthuizen A, Stronks DL, Van't Spijker A, et al. Demographic and medical parameters in the development of complex regional pain syndrome type 1 (CRPS1): prospective study on 596 patients with a fracture. *Pain*. 2012;153(6):1187–1192.

13. Hassantash SA, Afrakhteh M, Maier RV. Causalgia: a meta-analysis of the literature. *Arch Surg*. 2003;138(11):1226–1231.

14. Yaguda B, Shekane P, Gharibo C. Complex regional pain syndrome: pathophysiology, diagnosis, and treatment. *Pain Medicine News*. 2014.

15. Gracely RH, Lynch SA, Bennett GJ. Painful neuropathy: altered central processing maintained dynamically by peripheral input. *Pain*. 1992;51(2):175–194.

16. Raja SN, Davis KD, Campbell JN. The adrenergic pharmacology of sympathetically-maintained pain. *J Reconstr Microsurg*. 1992;8(1):63–69.

17. da Costa VV, de Oliveira SB, Fernandes Mdo C, et al. Incidence of regional pain syndrome after carpal tunnel release. Is there a correlation with the anesthetic technique? *Rev Bras Anestesiol*. 2011;61(4):425–433.

18. Sumitani M, Yasunaga H, Uchida K, et al. Perioperative factors affecting the occurrence of acute complex regional pain syndrome following limb bone fracture surgery: data from the Japanese Diagnosis Procedure Combination database. *Rheumatology (Oxford)*. 2014;53(7):1186–1193.

19. Rewhorn MJ, Leung AH, Gillespie A, et al. Incidence of complex regional pain syndrome after foot and ankle surgery. *J Foot Ankle Surg*. 2014;53(3):256–258.

20. Reuben SS. Preventing the development of complex regional pain syndrome after surgery. *Anesthesiology*. 2004;101(5):1215–1224.

21. Roh YH, Lee BK, Noh JH, et al. Factors associated with complex regional pain syndrome type I in patients with surgically treated distal radius fracture. *Arch Orthop Trauma Surg*. 2014;134(12):1775–1781.

22. Moseley GL, Herbert RD, Parsons T, et al. Intense pain soon after wrist fracture strongly predicts who will develop complex regional pain syndrome: prospective cohort study. *J Pain.* 2014;15(1):16–23.

23. Demir SE, Ozaras N, Karamehmetoglu SS, et al. Risk factors for complex regional pain syndrome in patients with traumatic extremity injury. *Ulus Travma Acil Cerrahi Derg.* 2010;16(2):144–148.

24. Dilek B, Yemez B, Kizil R, et al. Anxious personality is a risk factor for developing complex regional pain syndrome type I. *Rheumatol Int.* 2012;32(4):915–920.

25. Stanton-Hicks M, Janig W, Hassenbusch S, et al. Reflex sympathetic dystrophy: changing concepts and taxonomy. *Pain.* 1995;63(1):127–133.

26. Wolter T, Knoller SM, Rommel O. Complex regional pain syndrome following spine surgery: clinical and prognostic implications. *Eur Neurol.* 2012;68(1):52–58.

27. Chae SU, Kim TK, Shim DM, et al. Is complex regional pain syndrome a cause of postoperative syndrome in the lumbar spine?—a case report. *Asian Spine J.* 2009;3(2):101–105.

28. Weisz GM, Houang M, Bogduk N. Complex regional pain syndrome associated with cervical disc protrusion and foraminotomy. *Pain Med.* 2010;11(9):1348–1351.

29. Knoeller SM, Ehmer M, Kleinmann B, et al. CRPS I following artificial disc surgery: case report and review of the literature. *Eur Spine J.* 2011;20(Suppl 2):S278–S283.

30. Sachs BL, Zindrick MR, Beasley RD. Reflex sympathetic dystrophy after operative procedures on the lumbar spine. *J Bone Joint Surg Am.* 1993;75(5):721–725.

31. Morr S, Kanter AS. Complex regional pain syndrome following lateral lumbar interbody fusion: case report. *J Neurosurg Spine.* 2013;19(4):502–506.

32. Bernini PM, Simeone FA. Reflex sympathetic dystrophy associated with low lumbar disc herniation. *Spine (Phila Pa 1976).* 1981;6(2):180–184.

33. Condon F, Kenny PJ, Griffin JG, et al. Reflex sympathetic dystrophy associated with extraforaminal disc herniation at the L5-S1 level. *J Spinal Disord.* 1998;11(5):448–451.

34. Gunn CC. "Prespondylosis" and some pain syndromes following denervation supersensitivity. *Spine (Phila Pa 1976).* 1980;5(2):185–192.

35. Ballard EM, Ellenberg M, Chodoroff G. Reflex sympathetic dystrophy syndrome secondary to L5 radiculopathy. *Arch Phys Med Rehabil.* 1991;72(8):595–597.

36. Carlson DH, Simon H, Wegner W. Bone scanning and diagnosis of reflex sympathetic dystrophy secondary to herniated lumbar disks. *Neurology.* 1977;27(8):791–793.

37. Pak TJ, Martin GM, Magness JL, et al. Reflex sympathetic dystrophy. Review of 140 cases. *Minn Med.* 1970;53(5):507–512.

38. Birklein F, Weber M, Ernst M, et al. Experimental tissue acidosis leads to increased pain in complex regional pain syndrome (CRPS). *Pain.* 2000;87(2):227–234.

39. Veldman PH, Goris RJ. Surgery on extremities with reflex sympathetic dystrophy. *Unfallchirurg.* 1995;98(1):45–48.

40. Rocco AG. Sympathetically maintained pain may be rekindled by surgery under general anesthesia. *Anesthesiology.* 1993;79(4):865.

41. Viel EJ, Pelissier J, Eledjam JJ. Sympathetically maintained pain after surgery may be prevented by regional anesthesia. *Anesthesiology.* 1994;81(1):265–266.

42. Reuben SS. Sympathetically maintained pain and the use of regional anesthesia. *Anesthesiology.* 1994;81(6):1548.

43. Cramer G, Young BM, Schwarzentraub P, et al. Preemptive analgesia in elective surgery in patients with complex regional pain syndrome: a case report. *J Foot Ankle Surg.* 2000;39(6):387–391.

44. Marx C, Wiedersheim P, Michel BA, et al. Preventing recurrence of reflex sympathetic dystrophy in patients requiring an operative intervention at the site of dystrophy after surgery. *Clin Rheumatol.* 2001;20(2):114–118.

45. Zyluk A. Complex regional pain syndrome type I. Risk factors, prevention and risk of recurrence. *J Hand Surg Br.* 2004;29(4):334–337.

46. Harden RN, Bruehl S, Stanos S, et al. Prospective examination of pain-related and psychological predictors of CRPS-like phenomena following total knee arthroplasty: a preliminary study. *Pain.* 2003;106(3):393–400.

47. Kehlet H, Dahl JB. The value of "multimodal" or "balanced analgesia" in postoperative pain treatment. *Anesth Analg.* 1993;77(5):1048–1056.

48. Aim F, Klouche S, Frison A, et al. Efficacy of vitamin C in preventing complex regional pain syndrome after wrist fracture: a systematic review and meta-analysis. *Orthop Traumatol Surg Res.* 2017;103(3):465–470.

49. Perez RS, Kwakkel G, Zuurmond WW, et al. Treatment of reflex sympathetic dystrophy (CRPS type 1): a research synthesis of 21 randomized clinical trials. *J Pain Symptom Manage.* 2001;21(6):511–526.

50. Kissling RO, Bloesch AC, Sager M, et al. Prevention of recurrence of Sudeck's disease with calcitonin [in German]. *Rev Chir Orthop Reparatrice Appar Mot.* 1991;77(8):562–567.

51. Goris RJ, Leixnering M, Huber W, et al. Delayed recovery and late development of complex regional pain syndrome in patients with an isolated fracture of the distal radius: prediction of a regional inflammatory response by early signs. *J Bone Joint Surg Br.* 2007;89(8):1069–1076.

52. Hanna MH, Peat SJ. Ketanserin in reflex sympathetic dystrophy. A double-blind placebo controlled cross-over trial. *Pain.* 1989;38(2):145–150.

53. Mellick GA, Mellick LB. Reflex sympathetic dystrophy treated with gabapentin. *Arch Phys Med Rehabil.* 1997;78(1):98–105.

54. McQuay HJ, Tramer M, Nye BA, et al. A systematic review of antidepressants in neuropathic pain. *Pain.* 1996;68(2-3):217–227.

55. Rauck RL, Eisenach JC, Jackson K, et al. Epidural clonidine treatment for refractory reflex sympathetic dystrophy. *Anesthesiology.* 1993;79(6):1163–1169; discussion 27A.

56. Borg PA, Krijnen HJ. Long-term intrathecal administration of midazolam and clonidine. *Clin J Pain.* 1996;12(1):63–68.

57. Christensen K, Jensen EM, Noer I. The reflex dystrophy syndrome response to treatment with systemic corticosteroids. *Acta Chir Scand.* 1982;148(8):653–655.

58. Chevreau M, Romand X, Gaudin P, et al. Bisphosphonates for treatment of Complex Regional Pain Syndrome type 1: a systematic literature review and meta-analysis of randomized controlled trials versus placebo. *Joint Bone Spine.* 2017;84(4):393–399.

59. Connolly SB, Prager JP, Harden RN. A systematic review of ketamine for complex regional pain syndrome. *Pain Med.* 2015;16(5):943–969.

60. Azari P, Lindsay DR, Briones D, et al. Efficacy and safety of ketamine in patients with complex regional pain syndrome: a systematic review. *CNS Drugs.* 2012;26(3):215–228.

61. Weinbroum AA, Ben-Abraham R. Dextromethorphan and dexmedetomidine: new agents for the control of perioperative pain. *Eur J Surg.* 2001;167(8):563–569.

62. Schwartzman RJ, Alexander GM, Grothusen JR, et al. Outpatient intravenous ketamine for the treatment of complex regional pain syndrome: a double-blind placebo controlled study. *Pain.* 2009;147(1-3):107–115.

63. Sigtermans MJ, van Hilten JJ, Bauer MC, et al. Ketamine produces effective and long-term pain relief in patients with Complex Regional Pain Syndrome Type 1. *Pain.* 2009;145(3):304–311.

64. Turner JA, Loeser JD, Deyo RA, Sanders SB. Spinal cord stimulation for patients with failed back surgery syndrome or complex regional pain syndrome: a systematic review of effectiveness and complications. *Pain.* 2004;108(1-2):137–147.

65. Grabow TS, Tella PK, Raja SN. Spinal cord stimulation for complex regional pain syndrome: an evidence-based medicine review of the literature. *Clin J Pain.* 2003;19(6):371–383.

66. Kemler MA, De Vet HC, Barendse GA, et al. The effect of spinal cord stimulation in patients with chronic reflex sympathetic dystrophy: two years' follow-up of the randomized controlled trial. *Ann Neurol.* 2004;55(1):13–18.

67. Donado C, Lobo K, Velarde-Alvarez MF, et al. Continuous regional anesthesia and inpatient rehabilitation for pediatric Complex Regional Pain Syndrome. *Reg Anesth Pain Med.* 2017;42(4):527–534

68. Weinstein SM. Phantom limb pain and related disorders. *Neurol Clin.* 1998;16(4): 919–936.

69. Louis ED, York GK. Weir Mitchell's observations on sensory localization and their influence on Jacksonian neurology. *Neurology.* 2006;66(8):1241–1244.

70. Ehde DM, Czerniecki JM, Smith DG, et al. Chronic phantom sensations, phantom pain, residual limb pain, and other regional pain after lower limb amputation. *Arch Phys Med Rehabil.* 2000;81(8):1039–1044.

71. Ephraim PL, Wegener ST, MacKenzie EJ, et al. Phantom pain, residual limb pain, and back pain in amputees: results of a national survey. *Arch Phys Med Rehabil.* 2005;86(10):1910–1919.

72. Kooijman CM, Dijkstra PU, Geertzen JH, et al. Phantom pain and phantom sensations in upper limb amputees: an epidemiological study. *Pain.* 2000;87(1):33–41.

73. Schley MT, Wilms P, Toepfner S, et al. Painful and nonpainful phantom and stump sensations in acute traumatic amputees. *J Trauma.* 2008;65(4):858–864.

74. Jensen TS, Krebs B, Nielsen J, et al. Immediate and long-term phantom limb pain in amputees: incidence, clinical characteristics and relationship to pre-amputation limb pain. *Pain.* 1985;21(3):267–278.

75. Dillingham TR, Pezzin LE, MacKenzie EJ. Limb amputation and limb deficiency: epidemiology and recent trends in the United States. *South Med J.* 2002;95(8):875–883.

76. Wrobel JS, Mayfield JA, Reiber GE. Geographic variation of lower-extremity major amputation in individuals with and without diabetes in the Medicare population. *Diabetes Care.* 2001;24(5):860–864.

77. Sherman RA, Sherman CJ, Parker L. Chronic phantom and stump pain among American veterans: results of a survey. *Pain.* 1984;18(1):83–95.

78. Reiber GE, McFarland LV, Hubbard S, et al. Service members and veterans with major traumatic limb loss from Vietnam war and OIF/OEF conflicts: survey methods, participants, and summary findings. *J Rehabil Res Dev.* 2010;47(4):275–297.

79. Jamison K, Wellisch DK, Katz RL, et al. Phantom breast syndrome. *Arch Surg.* 1979;114(1):93–95.

80. Rothemund Y, Grusser SM, Liebeskind U, et al. Phantom phenomena in mastectomized patients and their relation to chronic and acute pre-mastectomy pain. *Pain.* 2004;107(1-2):140–146.

81. Hanowell ST, Kennedy SF. Phantom tongue pain and causalgia: case presentation and treatment. *Anesth Analg.* 1979;58(5):436–438.

82. Fingren J, Lindholm E, Carlsson E. Perceptions of phantom rectum syndrome and health-related quality of life in patients following abdominoperineal resection for rectal cancer. J Wound Ostomy Continence Nurs. 2013;40(3):280–286.

83. Biley FC. Phantom bladder sensations: a new concern for stoma care workers. Br J Nurs. 2001;10(19):1290–1296.

84. Jensen TS, Krebs B, Nielsen J, et al. Phantom limb, phantom pain and stump pain in amputees during the first 6 months following limb amputation. *Pain.* 1983;17(3):243–256.

85. Manchikanti L, Singh V. Managing phantom pain. *Pain Physician.* 2004;7(3):365–375.

86. Le Feuvre P, Aldington D. Know pain know gain: proposing a treatment approach for phantom limb pain. *J R Army Med Corps.* 2014;160(1):16–21.

87. Borghi B, Bugamelli S, Stagni G, et al. Perineural infusion of 0.5% ropivacaine for successful treatment of phantom limb syndrome: a case report. *Minerva Anestesiol.* 2009;75(11):661–664.

88. Nikolajsen L, Ilkjaer S, Christensen JH, et al. Randomised trial of epidural bupivacaine and morphine in prevention of stump and phantom pain in lower-limb amputation. *Lancet.* 1997;350(9088):1353–1357.

89. Pinzur MS, Garla PG, Pluth T, et al. Continuous postoperative infusion of a regional anesthetic after an amputation of the lower extremity. A randomized clinical trial. *J Bone Joint Surg Am.* 1996;78(10):1501–1505.

90. Hayes C, Armstrong-Brown A, Burstal R. Perioperative intravenous ketamine infusion for the prevention of persistent post-amputation pain: a randomized, controlled trial. *Anaesth Intensive Care.* 2004;32(3):330–338.

91. Nikolajsen L, Hansen CL, Nielsen J, et al. The effect of ketamine on phantom pain: a central neuropathic disorder maintained by peripheral input. *Pain.* 1996;67(1):69–77.

92. Eichenberger U, Neff F, Sveticic G, et al. Chronic phantom limb pain: the effects of calcitonin, ketamine, and their combination on pain and sensory thresholds. *Anesth Analg.* 2008;106(4):1265–1273.

93. Halbert J, Crotty M, Cameron ID. Evidence for the optimal management of acute and chronic phantom pain: a systematic review. *Clin J Pain.* 2002;18(2):84–92.

94. Alviar MJ, Hale T, Dungca M. Pharmacologic interventions for treating phantom limb pain. *Cochrane Database Syst Rev.* 2016;10:CD006380.

95. Huse E, Larbig W, Flor H, et al. The effect of opioids on phantom limb pain and cortical reorganization. *Pain.* 2001;90(1-2):47–55.

96. Wu CL, Tella P, Staats PS, et al. Analgesic effects of intravenous lidocaine and morphine on postamputation pain: a randomized double-blind, active placebo-controlled, crossover trial. *Anesthesiology.* 2002;96(4):841–848.

97. Wilder-Smith CH, Hill LT, Laurent S. Postamputation pain and sensory changes in treatment-naive patients: characteristics and responses to treatment with tramadol, amitriptyline, and placebo. *Anesthesiology.* 2005;103(3):619–628.

98. Bergmans L, Snijdelaar DG, Katz J, et al. Methadone for phantom limb *Pain. Clin J Pain.* 2002;18(3):203–205.

99. Borghi B, D'Addabbo M, Borghi R. Can neural blocks prevent phantom limb pain? *Pain Manag.* 2014;4(4):261–266.

100. Lierz P, Schroegendorfer K, Choi S, et al. Continuous blockade of both brachial plexus with ropivacaine in phantom pain: a case report. *Pain.* 1998;78(2):135–137.

101. Reiestad F, Kulkarni J. Role of myofascial trigger points in post-amputation pain: causation and management. *Prosthet Orthot Int.* 2013;37(2):120–123.

102. Zeng Y, Wang X, Guo Y, et al. Coblation of femoral and sciatic nerve for stump pain and phantom limb pain: a case report. *Pain Pract.* 2016;16(2):E35–E41.

103. Giuffrida O, Simpson L, Halligan PW. Contralateral stimulation, using TENS, of phantom limb pain: two confirmatory cases. *Pain Med.* 2010;11(1):133–141.

104. Mulvey MR, Radford HE, Fawkner HJ, et al. Transcutaneous electrical nerve stimulation for phantom pain and stump pain in adult amputees. *Pain Pract.* 2013;13(4):289–296.

105. Johnson MI, Mulvey MR, Bagnall AM. Transcutaneous electrical nerve stimulation (TENS) for phantom pain and stump pain following amputation in adults. *Cochrane Database Syst Rev.* 2015;8:CD007264.

106. Ramachandran VS, Rogers-Ramachandran D. Synaesthesia in phantom limbs induced with mirrors. *Proc Biol Sci.* 1996;263(1369):377–386.

107. Ramachandran VS, Rogers-Ramachandran D. Sensations referred to a patient's phantom arm from another subjects intact arm: perceptual correlates of mirror neurons. *Med Hypotheses.* 2008;70(6):1233–1234.

108. Rossi S, Tecchio F, Pasqualetti P, et al. Somatosensory processing during movement observation in humans. *Clin Neurophysiol.* 2002;113(1):16–24.

109. Chan BL, Witt R, Charrow AP, et al. Mirror therapy for phantom limb pain. *N Engl J Med.* 2007;357(21):2206–2207.

110. Andre-Obadia N, Peyron R, Mertens P, et al. Transcranial magnetic stimulation for pain control. Double-blind study of different frequencies against placebo, and correlation with motor cortex stimulation efficacy. *Clin Neurophysiol.* 2006;117(7):1536–1544.

111. Rasmussen KG, Rummans TA. Electroconvulsive therapy for phantom limb pain. *Pain.* 2000;85(1-2):297–299.

112. Bradbrook D. Acupuncture treatment of phantom limb pain and phantom limb sensation in amputees. *Acupunct Med.* 2004;22(2):93–97.

113. Harden RN, Houle TT, Green S, et al. Biofeedback in the treatment of phantom limb pain: a time-series analysis. *Appl Psychophysiol Biofeedback.* 2005;30(1):83–93.

114. MacIver K, Lloyd DM, Kelly S, et al. Phantom limb pain, cortical reorganization and the therapeutic effect of mental imagery. *Brain.* 2008;131(Pt 8):2181–2191.

115. Bittar RG, Otero S, Carter H, et al. Deep brain stimulation for phantom limb pain. *J Clin Neurosci.* 2005;12(4):399–404.

116. Sol JC, Casaux J, Roux FE, et al. Chronic motor cortex stimulation for phantom limb pain: correlations between pain relief and functional imaging studies. *Stereotact Funct Neurosurg.* 2001;77(1-4):172–176.

117. Viswanathan A, Phan PC, Burton AW. Use of spinal cord stimulation in the treatment of phantom limb pain: case series and review of the literature. *Pain Pract.* 2010;10(5):479–484.

118. Krainick JU, Thoden U, Riechert T. Pain reduction in amputees by long-term spinal cord stimulation. Long-term follow-up study over 5 years. *J Neurosurg.* 1980;52(3):346–350.

119. Dworkin RH, Gnann JW, Jr., Oaklander AL, et al. Diagnosis and assessment of pain associated with herpes zoster and postherpetic neuralgia. *J Pain.*2008;9(1 Suppl 1):S37–S44.

120. Goh CL, Khoo L. A retrospective study of the clinical presentation and outcome of herpes zoster in a tertiary dermatology outpatient referral clinic. *Int J Dermatol.* 1997;36(9):667–672.

121. Shakir A, Kimbrough DA, Mehta B. Postherpetic neuralgia involving the right C5 dermatome treated with a cervical transforaminal epidural steroid injection: a case report. *Arch Phys Med Rehabil.* 2007;88(2):255–258.

122. Insinga RP, Itzler RF, Pellissier JM, et al. The incidence of herpes zoster in a United States administrative database. *J Gen Intern Med.* 2005;20(8):748–753.

123. Dworkin RH, Johnson RW, Breuer J, et al. Recommendations for the management of herpes zoster. *Clin Infect Dis.* 2007;44(Suppl 1):S1–26.

124. Jung BF, Johnson RW, Griffin DR, et al. Risk factors for postherpetic neuralgia in patients with herpes zoster. *Neurology.* 2004;62(9):1545–1551.

125. U.S. Food and Drug Administration. FDA approves Zostavax vaccine to prevent shingles in individuals 50 to 59 years of age 2011. https://www.fda.gov/BiologicsBloodVaccines/Vaccines/QuestionsaboutVaccines/ucm070418.htm

126. Oxman MN, Levin MJ, Johnson GR, et al. A vaccine to prevent herpes zoster and postherpetic neuralgia in older adults. *N Engl J Med*. 2005;352(22):2271–2284.

127. Harpaz R, Ortega-Sanchez IR, Seward JF; Advisory Committee on Immunization Practices Centers for Disease Control and Prevention. Prevention of herpes zoster: recommendations of the Advisory Committee on Immunization Practices (ACIP). *MMWR Recomm Rep*. 2008;57(RR-5):1-30; quiz CE2–4.

128. Tyring SK, Beutner KR, Tucker BA, et al. Antiviral therapy for herpes zoster: randomized, controlled clinical trial of valacyclovir and famciclovir therapy in immunocompetent patients 50 years and older. *Arch Fam Med*. 2000;9(9):863–869.

129. Tyring S, Barbarash RA, Nahlik JE, et al. Famciclovir for the treatment of acute herpes zoster: effects on acute disease and postherpetic neuralgia. A randomized, double-blind, placebo-controlled trial. Collaborative Famciclovir Herpes Zoster Study Group. *Ann Intern Med*. 1995;123(2):89–96.

130. Wood MJ, Kay R, Dworkin RH, Soong SJ, Whitley RJ. Oral acyclovir therapy accelerates pain resolution in patients with herpes zoster: a meta-analysis of placebo-controlled trials. *Clin Infect Dis*. 1996;22(2):341–347.

131. Gnann JW, Jr., Whitley RJ. Clinical practice. Herpes zoster. *N Engl J Med*. 2002;347(5):340–346.

132. Alper BS, Lewis PR. Does treatment of acute herpes zoster prevent or shorten postherpetic neuralgia? *J Fam Pract*. 2000;49(3):255–264.

133. High KP. Preventing herpes zoster and postherpetic neuralgia through vaccination. *J Fam Pract*. 2007;56(10 Suppl A):51A–7A; quiz 8A.

134. Pica F, Gatti A, Divizia M, et al. One-year follow-up of patients with long-lasting postherpetic neuralgia. *BMC Infect Dis*. 2014;14:556.

135. Winnie AP, Hartwell PW. Relationship between time of treatment of acute herpes zoster with sympathetic blockade and prevention of post-herpetic neuralgia: clinical support for a new theory of the mechanism by which sympathetic blockade provides therapeutic benefit. *Reg Anesth*. 1993;18(5):277–282.

136. Hempenstall K, Nurmikko TJ, Johnson RW, et al. Analgesic therapy in postherpetic neuralgia: a quantitative systematic review. *PLoS Med*. 2005;2(7):e164.

137. Rowbotham M, Harden N, Stacey B, et al. Gabapentin for the treatment of postherpetic neuralgia: a randomized controlled trial. *JAMA*. 1998;280(21):1837–1842.

138. Sabatowski R, Galvez R, Cherry DA, et al. Pregabalin reduces pain and improves sleep and mood disturbances in patients with post-herpetic neuralgia: results of a randomised, placebo-controlled clinical trial. *Pain*. 2004;109(1–2):26–35.

139. Freynhagen R, Strojek K, Griesing T, et al. Efficacy of pregabalin in neuropathic pain evaluated in a 12-week, randomised, double-blind, multicentre, placebo-controlled trial of flexible- and fixed-dose regimens. *Pain*. 2005;115(3):254–263.

140. Arner S, Meyerson BA. Lack of analgesic effect of opioids on neuropathic and idiopathic forms of pain. *Pain*. 1988;33(1):11–23.

141. Portenoy RK, Foley KM, Inturrisi CE. The nature of opioid responsiveness and its implications for neuropathic pain: new hypotheses derived from studies of opioid infusions. *Pain*. 1990;43(3):273–286.

142. Raja SN, Haythornthwaite JA, Pappagallo M, et al. Opioids versus antidepressants in postherpetic neuralgia: a randomized, placebo-controlled trial. *Neurology*. 2002;59(7):1015–1021.

143. Watson CP, Babul N. Efficacy of oxycodone in neuropathic pain: a randomized trial in postherpetic neuralgia. *Neurology*. 1998;50(6):1837–1841.

144. Hollingshead J, Duhmke RM, Cornblath DR. Tramadol for neuropathic pain. *Cochrane Database Syst Rev*. 2006;(3):CD003726.

145. Wolff RF, Bala MM, Westwood M, et al. 5% lidocaine-medicated plaster vs other relevant interventions and placebo for post-herpetic neuralgia (PHN): a systematic review. *Acta Neurol Scand.* 2011;123(5):295–309.

146. Derry S, Lloyd R, Moore RA, et al. Topical capsaicin for chronic neuropathic pain in adults. *Cochrane Database Syst Rev.* 2009(4):CD007393.

147. Colding A. Treatment of pain: organization of a pain clinic: treatment of acute herpes zoster. *Proc R Soc Med.* 1973;66(6):541–543.

148. Riopelle JM, Naraghi M, Grush KP. Chronic neuralgia incidence following local anesthetic therapy for herpes zoster. *Arch Dermatol.* 1984;120(6):747–750.

149. Mehta P, Maher P, Singh JR. Treatment of postherpetic neuralgia using a thoracic transforaminal epidural steroid injection. *PM R.* 2015;7(4):443–446.

150. Opstelten W, van Wijck AJ, Moons KG, et al. Treatment of patients with herpes zoster by epidural injection of steroids and local anaesthetics: less pain after 1 month, but no effect on long-term postherpetic neuralgia--a randomised trial [in Dutch]. *Ned Tijdschr Geneeskd.* 2006;150(48):2649–2655.

151. Harke H, Gretenkort P, Ladleif HU, et al. Spinal cord stimulation in postherpetic neuralgia and in acute herpes zoster pain. *Anesth Analg.* 2002;94(3):694–700.

152. Liem L, Russo M, Huygen FJ, et al. One-year outcomes of spinal cord stimulation of the dorsal root ganglion in the treatment of chronic neuropathic pain. *Neuromodulation.* 2015;18(1):41–48; discussion 8–9.

153. Skeehan TM, Cory PC, Jr. Neurolytic lumbar sympathetic block in the treatment of Raynaud's phenomenon. *Anesthesiology.* 1986;64(1):119–120.

154. Ungprasert P, Crowson CS, Chowdhary VR, et al. Epidemiology of mixed connective tissue disease, 1985-2014: a population-based study. *Arthritis Care Res (Hoboken).* 2016;68(12):1843–1848.

155. Moore DC. Raynaud's phenomenon. In: *Stellate Ganglion Block: Techniques, Indications, Uses.* Springfield, IL: Charles C. Thomas;1954:152.

156. Moore DC. Raynaud's disease. In: *Stellate Ganglion Block: Techniques, Indications, Uses.* Springfield, IL: Charles C Thomas; 1954:147–151.

157. Turton EP, Kent PJ, Kester RC. The aetiology of Raynaud's phenomenon. *Cardiovasc Surg.* 1998;6(5):431–440.

158. Herrick AL. Pathogenesis of Raynaud's phenomenon. *Rheumatology (Oxford).* 2005;44(5):587–596.

159. Cooke JP, Marshall JM. Mechanisms of Raynaud's disease. *Vasc Med.* 2005;10(4):293–307.

160. Ennis H, Hughes M, Anderson ME, et al. Calcium channel blockers for primary Raynaud's phenomenon. *Cochrane Database Syst Rev.* 2016;2:CD002069.

161. Hughes M, Herrick AL. Raynaud's phenomenon. *Best Pract Res Clin Rheumatol.* 2016;30(1):112–132.

162. Zhang X, Hu Y, Nie Z, et al. Treatment of Raynaud's phenomenon with botulinum toxin type A. *Neurol Sci.* 2015;36(7):1225–1231.

163. Zebryk P, Puszczewicz MJ. Botulinum toxin A in the treatment of Raynaud's phenomenon: a systematic review. *Arch Med Sci.* 2016;12(4):864–870.

164. Raso L, Deer T. Spinal cord stimulation in the treatment of acute and chronic vasculitis: clinical discussion and synopsis of the literature. *Neuromodulation.* 2011;14(3):225–228; discussion 8.

165. Provenzano DA, Nicholson L, Jarzabek G, et al. Spinal cord stimulation utilization to treat the microcirculatory vascular insufficiency and ulcers associated with scleroderma: a case report and review of the literature. *Pain Med.* 2011;12(9):1331–1335.

166. Moro-Velasco C, Cuesta-Agudo MJ, Sannorberto L, et al. Sjogren syndrome and spinal cord stimulation: a case report. *Neuromodulation.* 2005;8(2):100–104.

167. Manfredini R, Boari B, Gallerani M, et al. Thromboangiitis obliterans (Buerger disease) in a female mild smoker treated with spinal cord stimulation. *Am J Med Sci.* 2004;327(6):365–368.

168. Swigris JJ, Olin JW, Mekhail NA. Implantable spinal cord stimulator to treat the ischemic manifestations of thromboangiitis obliterans (Buerger's disease). *J Vasc Surg.* 1999;29(5):928–935.

169. Benyamin R, Kramer J, Vallejo R. A case of spinal cord stimulation in Raynaud's Phenomenon: can subthreshold sensory stimulation have an effect? *Pain Physician.* 2007;10(3):473–478.

170. Wolter T, Kieselbach K. Spinal cord stimulation for Raynaud's syndrome: long-term alleviation of bilateral pain with a single cervical lead. *Neuromodulation.* 2011;14(3):229–233; discussion 233–234.

171. Sibell DM, Colantonio AJ, Stacey BR. Successful use of spinal cord stimulation in the treatment of severe Raynaud's disease of the hands. *Anesthesiology.* 2005;102(1):225–227.

172. Parker LK, Ponte C, Howell KJ, et al. Clinical features and management of erythromelalgia: long term follow-up of 46 cases. *Clin Exp Rheumatol.* 2017;35(1):80–84.

173. Mitchell SW. On a rare vasomotor neurosis of the extremities and on maladies with which it may be confounded. *Am J Med Sci.* 1878;76:2–36.

174. Berlin AL, Pehr K. Coexistence of erythromelalgia and Raynaud's phenomenon. *J Am Acad Dermatol.* 2004;50(3):456–460.

175. Cohen JS. Erythromelalgia: new theories and new therapies. *J Am Acad Dermatol.* 2000;43(5 Pt 1):841–847.

176. Waxman SG. Nav1.7, its mutations, and the syndromes that they cause. *Neurology.* 2007;69(6):505–507.

177. Hoeijmakers JG, Faber CG, Merkies IS, et al. Painful peripheral neuropathy and sodium channel mutations. *Neurosci Lett.* 2015;596:51–59.

178. Yang Y, Wang Y, Li S, et al. Mutations in SCN9A, encoding a sodium channel alpha subunit, in patients with primary erythermalgia. *J Med Genet.* 2004;41(3):171–174.

179. Tang Z, Chen Z, Tang B, et al. Primary erythromelalgia: a review. *Orphanet J Rare Dis.* 2015;10:127.

180. Kazemi B, Shooshtari SM, Nasab MR, et al. Sympathetic skin response (SSR) in erythromelalgia. *Electromyogr Clin Neurophysiol.* 2003;43(3):165–168.

181. Mork C, Kalgaard OM, Kvernebo K. Impaired neurogenic control of skin perfusion in erythromelalgia. *J Invest Dermatol.* 2002;118(4):699–703.

182. Sandroni P, Davis MD, Harper CM, et al. Neurophysiologic and vascular studies in erythromelalgia: a retrospective analysis. *J Clin Neuromuscul Dis.* 1999;1(2):57–63.

183. Littleford RC, Khan F, Belch JJ. Impaired skin vasomotor reflexes in patients with erythromelalgia. *Clin Sci (Lond).* 1999;96(5):507–512.

184. Kalgaard OM, Mork C, Kvernebo K. Prostacyclin reduces symptoms and sympathetic dysfunction in erythromelalgia in a double-blind randomized pilot study. *Acta Derm Venereol.* 2003;83(6):442–444.

185. Davis MD, Sandroni P. Lidocaine patch for pain of erythromelalgia: follow-up of 34 patients. *Arch Dermatol.* 2005;141(10):1320–1321.

186. Iqbal J, Bhat MI, Charoo BA, et al. Experience with oral mexiletine in primary erythromelalgia in children. *Ann Saudi Med.* 2009;29(4):316–318.

187. Choi JS, Zhang L, Dib-Hajj SD, et al. Mexiletine-responsive erythromelalgia due to a new Na(v)1.7 mutation showing use-dependent current fall-off. *Exp Neurol*. 2009;216(2):383–389.

188. Graziotti PJ, Goucke CR. Control of intractable pain in erythromelalgia by using spinal cord stimulation. *J Pain Symptom Manage*. 1993;8(7):502–504.

189. Patel N, Chen E, Cucchiaro G. The complexity of pain management in patients with erythromelalgia. *A Case Rep*. 2015;5(9):151–153.

190. Matzke LL, Lamer TJ, Gazelka HM. Spinal cord stimulation for treatment of neuropathic pain associated with erythromelalgia. *Reg Anesth Pain Med*. 2016;41(5):619–620.

14 Comprehensive Review of Discography in Spinal Pain

Graham R. Hadley, Matthew Novitch,
Mark R. Jones, Vwaire Orhurhu,
Alan D. Kaye, and Sudhir A. Diwan

BACKGROUND

Discography dates back to the late 1920s, when Dandy and Schmorl adopted the procedure of injecting oil contrast into the peri spinal space as a rudimentary means to investigate back pain. Lindblom, a Swedish radiologist, was the first to introduce contrast dye into the intervertebral disc to identify the source of back discomfort. The practice of modern discography has not changed significantly since it was brought to the United States in the early 1950s by Wise and Weiford [1–2].

The aim of discography involves determination of the morphology of the nucleus pulposus and annulus fibrosus of the intervertebral disc. The knowledge of structural integrity of the disc is the fundamental principle in determining whether the neck or back pain is discogenic in nature. A spinal needle is inserted into the nucleus pulposus of the disc of interest under fluoroscopic guidance. Once the location of the needle is confirmed in the center of the disc, dye is injected into the disc to study its morphology, intradiscal pressure, and response of the patient to the chemical reaction caused by injection. The elicited pain response, or lack thereof, to the provocation is then judged and compared to asymptomatic control discs. The test is considered positive if the disc in question elicits a painful response and this response is similar or concordant with the patient's baseline symptoms. If pain is not elicited, then it is likely that the particular disc is not the source of pain. The pain is reproduced by provocative discography in two ways: first by causing chemical irritation of sensitive tissue and, second, by increasing the intradiscal pressure related to volume and stretching of the annular fibers of the disc. Moreover, a positive test may be a representation of the associated innervation. More than one protocol exists which standardizes its utiliza-tion, and the operator is encouraged to adhere to one that reduces false-positive rates.

Numerous researchers have studied the safety profile and diagnostic utility of dis-cography over the past half-century, and much controversy still remains over its clin-ical use. Its application has been both praised and discouraged by clinicians spanning several decades, and the following subsections will discuss such topics with respect to the cervical, thoracic, and lumbar spinal regions.

CERVICAL DISCOGRAPHY

Overview and Epidemiology

Neck pain is quite common in the adult population, with 10% of adults experiencing neck pain at any one point in time. It is a common cause of disability and socio-economic burden, with an annual prevalence rate of between 15% and 50% [3–5]. Common pain generators include the cervical intervertebral discs, facet joints, and atlantoaxial joints, and several pathophysiologic processes affect these anatomical structures. Neck pain does not result in as much lost time from work as low back pain, nor is it associated with as many neurological deficits. A number of methods are used to diagnose neck pain, but cervical provocation discography remains controver-sial related to insufficient validation and controlled outcome studies. However, it is still commonly used to assist in diagnosing and treating neck pain. Its usefulness, clinical implications, and current recommendations are discussed here.

Approximately half of all individuals will experience a clinically relevant episode of neck pain in their lifetime [5]. Back pain, depression, arthralgia, and neck pain are the four leading causes of years lost to disability, which highlights the socioeconomic impact of neck pain on the general population [4,6]. The prevalence rates range from 15% to 50%, with one systematic review reporting a mean rate of 37.2% across sev-eral studies [6]. Risk factors include female sex, age, genetic predisposition, smoking, sedentary lifestyle, sleep disorders, and obesity [7–11]. Obesity itself has been studied widely, and several reasons have been proposed as to why obesity is a risk for neck pain. Chronic systemic inflammation, deleterious structural changes, increased me-chanical stress, and psychosocial issues are common factors [12]. There are several common comorbidities associated with neck pain, most often headache, back pain, arthralgias, and depression [6]. Last, those with unique occupations that may lead to trauma, such as football players and construction workers, have a higher incidence. By contrast, those in less physically demanding situations, like office workers, computer workers, and healthcare workers, have a higher incidence of neck pain, as do those with low job satisfaction and self-reported poor workplace environments [13].

Anatomy

The cervical spine is composed of seven vertebrae. The first two vertebrae, the atlas and axis, allow for a significant percentage of the range of motion in the neck. The atlantooccipital joint, composed of the occiput and first cervical vertebra, allows for one-third of flexion and one-half of lateral bending of the neck. Rotational motion is attributed largely to the atlantoaxial joint, the space between the first and second cervical vertebrae. Injuries most commonly occur between C4 and C7, which house nerve roots

C5, C6, and C7 passing through the intervertebral foramina. Articulations of Luschka are present in the C3–C7 spinal segments, which are not true synovial joints but can hypertrophy and are associated with disc degeneration and narrowing of the intervertebral foramina. Compression of nerve roots may result in cervical radiculopathy [14–16].

The musculature surrounding the cervical spine provides support and facilitates movement as well as alignment for the head and neck. A secondary function is protection of the spinal cord and spinal nerves when the spinal column is under stress. The normal curvature of the cervical spine is slight lordosis, which can be decreased in patients with degenerative changes.

There are eight cervical spinal nerves, C1–C8, each of which arises from the spinal cord by a ventral and dorsal spinal root. The spinal nerves divide into a dorsal primary ramus and ventral primary ramus, which divide and supply the posterior and anterior neck structures. The cervical sinuvertebral nerves have been found to have an upward course into the vertebral canal, supplying each disc at its level of entry and the disc above. Branches of the vertebral nerve supply the lateral aspects of the cervical discs. Histologic studies have shown that the presence of nerve fibers can extend as deeply as the outer third of the annulus fibrosus, providing evidence for the use of provocation discography [16].

The intervertebral discs lie between the cervical vertebrae, linking them together. The disc is supplied hemodynamically by the cartilaginous endplates and neurologically via the sinuvertebral nerves. The main components of the disc are the nucleus pulposus, annulus fibrosus, and cartilaginous superior and inferior end plates. The disc is made up biochemically of collagen fibers, elastin fibers, and aggrecan. Osmotic pressure can be lost in the nucleus as disc degeneration occurs, and the disc may lose height. Nociceptive nuclear material tracks and leaks through the outer rim of the annulus, which is the main source of discogenic pain [16].

Pathophysiology

Several pathophysiological conditions may result in neck pain. The most common cause of neck pain is of degenerative origin, but it may also arise from systemic diseases such as rheumatoid arthritis, spondyloarthritis, bone metastases, and polymyalgia rheumatica [8]. Trauma, whiplash syndrome, facet joint abnormalities, and congenital defects are other sources of neck pain. Neck pain may be categorized into four grades. Grade 1 includes no signs of major pathology and little interference with daily activities. Grade 2 is described by no signs of major pathology but impacts daily activities. Grade 3 is neck pain with neurologic signs or symptoms such as radiculopathy, and grade 4 is neck pain with major pathology such as fracture, myelopathy, neoplasm, and spinal infection [4,8].

Cervical discogenic pain is perhaps the most common cause of neck pain and is most often caused by cervical degenerative disc disease. Discogenic pain refers to derangement in the architecture of the disc that results in mechanical neck pain regardless of the presence of inflammation. Degenerative disc disease results in the inability to effectively distribute pressures between the disc, the vertebral endplates, and the facet joints. Axial neck pain is more common in degenerative disc, while extremity or radicular extremity pain is more common in herniated or bulging discs. Severe axial neck pain with radicular pain exists simultaneously in herniated or bulging disc associated with disc degeneration [17–19].

Cervical provocative discography is used to identify a painful cervical intervertebral disc and produce an image of internal derangements of that disc [19,20]. The use of discography is advantageous related to the ability to directly diagnose discogenic pain without disc herniation and radiculitis for which history, physical exam, neurophysiologic assessment, and imaging studies are nondiagnostic [21–23]. However, a major concern exists related to cervical discography because a positive response is a subjective perception of the patient's pain levels. Variations in criteria exist for a positive response, and several investigators have found a lack of correlation between morphology and pain reproduction of discogenic origin [20,24–29].

False-positive rates are high, there is a lack of standardization, and there are discrepancies regarding the need for control levels of pain in the use of provocative discography [24–28].

Upon review, the validity of cervical provocative discography has been exemplified by disc stimulation symptom mapping in patients with pain and asymptomatic volunteers [30–32]. One particular study found a significant relationship between imaging and symptom provocation [32]. Vilkari-Juntura et al. have demonstrated the value of discography in that it provides additional information regarding structural changes not available by other noninvasive methods of examination [28]. Similarly, Parfenchuck and Janssen found that although the magnetic resonance imaging (MRI) is a useful additional examination to cervical discography, some MRI patterns should not be considered pathologic, and discography is necessary to identify a painful disc and definitely determine discogenic pain [24]. Multiple systematic reviews have found that evidence is limited for the use of discography [19,25–29].

Overall, despite extensive affirmation of discogenic pain in the literature and correlations of discogenic pain and discographic techniques, the conclusion is that there is a lack of diagnostic criteria and uniform terminology and limited evidence for discographic techniques [18].

Technique

First introduced in 1957, cervical discography is an invasive procedure with several steps. The patient is first positioned supine with support of the lower neck in order to improve access to the upper and mid-cervical regions of the neck. The neck may be maneuvered, often extended and slightly turned to the right [33–35]. An anterolateral approach is used to avoid injury to vital structures, such as the spinal cord, airway, and vertebral artery. Using fluoroscopy, a 23-gauge 3.5-inch spinal needle is inserted between the carotid pulse, esophagus, and trachea, which are deviated medially by manual displacement. Using great care not to puncture the carotid, the right anterior portion of the disc is entered and contrast is injected: 0.3–0.5 mL of nonionic contrast should be injected into the cervical discs without high resistance [35].

This test is performed without sedation or analgesics in order to avoid masking the patient's pain sensation. A positive test is defined by predominantly axial pain that persists for a substantial duration without improvement after conservative measures. Each disc is evaluated by the amount of pain provoked, the pressure measured within the disc, the volume of contrast injected, and the imaging findings. Positive pain reports must be confirmed minutes after the first report of discomfort. If pain is provoked between 15 and 50 psi, the disc is classified as mechanically sensitive. If between 51 and 90 psi, other sources of pain should be investigated rather than further consideration of discogenic pain. If no pain is provoked by 90 psi, the disc is considered negative [35]. Last, immediately following the discography, a computed tomography (CT) scan is performed to confirm contrast injection into the nucleus pulposus. This may also be used to assess annular degeneration and annular disruption [35,36].

Complications

Complications with discography are rare, with an estimated rate of 0.6% for cervical spine discograms [37]. Most commonly, transient exacerbations of pain, infectious discitis, and epidural abscess complicate discography, however, this is more common in lumbar than cervical techniques [37–39]. Epidural, subdural, or retropharyngeal abscesses or neural injury may also occur in cervical discograms, as well as the very rare spinal cord injury. Only a few case reports have been published regarding these complications, and these describe radicular pain and C5 tetraplegia [40–42].

The most common complication in cervical discography is discitis, ranging from 1:30 to 1:50. *Staphylococcus aureus* and *S. epidermidis* are the most likely culprits of infectious processes, and these are due to needle contamination, inadequate skin preparation, and inadvertent puncture of the esophagus [40–42]. Signs of discitis include significant increases in neck or back pain with elevated sedimentation rate. Cervical discitis resolves in 6–7 weeks, and risk factors include male gender and presence of a beard or a thick neck. There is currently not enough evidence in the literature to suggest the prophylactic use of antibiotics [40–42].

THORACIC DISCOGRAPHY

Overview and Epidemiology

Discussions surrounding the prevalence of thoracic back pain are limited due to the relatively small number of studies compared to the other spinal regions, and the true epidemiological values may be entirely unknown. Yet, despite thoracic spinal pain being reported as less common than cervical and lumbar back pathology, recent meta-data suggest that its lifetime prevalence is between 54% and 80%, and its incidence is highest especially during adolescence—most likely due to its association with backpacks. Of those that suffer from this condition in young adulthood, up to 10% are so debilitated by its disease course that it begins to interfere with school and extracurricular activities. Certain external factors contribute to thoracic spinal pain in youth and include chair height, female sex, the use of backpacks and their associated weight, sports, and even psychosocial elements such as poor mental health [43–46]. Internal factors thought to play a role include vertebral fractures, bone loss, kyphosis, ankylosing spondylitis, arthritis, and referred pain from the cardiopulmonary, gastrointestinal, and renal systems—especially in the setting of neoplastic disorders [43,47–52].

The adult population is affected by thoracic spinal pain at a rate of anywhere between 3% and 55% according to Briggs et al [43–46]. Common triggers of thoracic pain for adults between the third and fifth decades of life include discogenic pain and herniation, facet joint destruction, nerve root impingement, and tendinopathies, with males found to be affected 50% more than females [46]. Of these, multiple studies have highlighted that thoracic facet joint destruction and intervertebral disc pathologies such as annular tears with or without disc avulsion (Scheuermann's disease and Schmorl's nodes) contribute disproportionately to pain compared with other etiologies [43,53–57]. For this reason, thoracic discography has the potential to play a crucial role in identifying and confirming this varying etiologies in adult patients complaining of pain.

Anatomy

The thoracic spine is responsible for axial loading and support and is functionally unique in holding the rib cage and protecting the heart and lungs. The range of motion of this vertebral area is considered limited due to the angle of contact of the facet joints being greater than the cervical, but less than the lumbar. The discs of the thoracic spine are distinctive in that they have smaller volumes than their lumbar disc counterparts, have a more central location, and are encased by a thick annulus fibrosus consisting of a meshwork of collagen fibers. The thorax is largely responsible for the kyphotic curvature of the spine due to the asymmetry in height between the anterior and posterior borders of the intervertebral discs, with the more dorsal portions being shorter. The shape of the discs also varies greatly, with the more cephalad portions taking on more of an elliptical shape, becoming more triangular, and then reverting back to being elliptical. These anatomic variants account for the difference in technique that is required during discography and interventional procedures [46].

Applications

The indications for discography are similar to those for the cervical and lumbar regions. As previously discussed, the most common causes of thoracic pain include musculoskeletal and referred visceral pain. Since the two can often mislead clinicians with respect to the origin of a patient's pain, discography can be an essential tool for any interventionist, especially when taking into consideration that the thoracic spine is responsible for the majority of "silent" disc herniations. Several studies have published data on the use of discography, leading to mixed recommendations. Schellhas et al. was one of the first to author on the use of discography for thoracic pain and advised clinicians to use it as a third-line tool to correlate abnormal MRIs with back pain. In his retrospective analysis, patients reported pain 75% of the time when discs with intrinsic degeneration, annular tears, or vertebral body endplate infarctions were injected with dye. Confounding factors included the provocation of extraspinal pain such as that located in the chest wall or abdomen [43,51–52]. Wood et al. revealed through their study that patients who had Schmorl's nodes (protrusions of the nucleus pulposus through the vertebral body endplate), regardless if they had chronic thoracic pain or not, reported pain with discography, although this pain was nonconcordant. These authors also showed that MRI was only successful in identifying abnormal discs 56% of the time and was not sensitive in detecting discs with annular pathology. The most detected derangement was when a patient had Scheurmann's disease, a nonprotruding disc disease found in juvenile osteochondrosis patients. The bulk of data surrounding the use of thoracic discography originate from several decades ago, and the authors of the two landmark studies in existence related to this area, Schellhas et al., failed to provide critical statistical information such as true-positive, true-negative, and false-negative rates. Therefore, it is difficult to ascertain whether their techniques are accurate. Additionally, they assert that discography only identifies the pattern of pain associated with its respective innervation and not necessarily its source or structure, arguing that it is imperative for the clinician to rule out other causes affecting similar spinal levels, such as facet joint pain. Since current guidelines are heavily impacted by the limited aforementioned studies, the recommendation for using discography to diagnose thoracic discogenic back pain remains poor [52–58].

Technique

Performing discography near the thoracic spine carries with it the inherent risk of puncturing the anterolaterally located pleural space, potentially causing pneumothorax and spinal cord trauma. The upper thoracic spine contains discs that are closer in proximity to one another, along with more acute angles between the ribs and costovertebral joints. Thus, the clinician may be challenged in finding adequate access points for injection above the T5–T6 level. Other variables that affect access include deformations of the spine such as scoliosis, extreme kyphosis, and osteophyte formation. Preparation begins by first properly positioning the patient in the prone position and mapping the discs of interest fluoroscopically. Of course, the appropriate needle length and gauge will depend on anatomy and body habitus. Typically, a 23- or 25-gauge, 3.5-inch spinal needle will suffice for most adults, and the operator has the option to use a 5-inch, 22-gauge for larger individuals. As with cervical and lumbar discography, the particular disc of interest is marked along with an adjacent asymptomatic disc for comparison. Once placement of needle is confirmed in the disc under fluoroscopy, 0.5–1.0 mL nonionic contrast is injected and morphology and patient's response to injection and intradiscal pressure noted [54–59].

Complications

The technical aspects of thoracic discography exceeds that of cervical or even lumbar discography, and a variety of anatomical factors influence this disparity. A fundamental difference arises from the aforementioned narrow disc space unique to this region. In addition to the narrow disc space, the rib head attachment to the transverse process and the proximity of the pleura can cloud the operator's view and accessibility to such a degree that the potential risks of the procedure may outweigh its benefits. These anatomical hurdles can be mitigated; however, the onus is on the operator to compensate for the elevated level of difficulty via foundational techniques like carefully directed needle advancement. Failure to do so can lead to complications like pneumothorax and spinal cord trauma. It is important to recognize that complications such as pneumothorax or damaged thoracic cavity structures may not manifest until the point of recovery. Typical postprocedure complications inclusive of other spinal discography procedures also apply, such as contrast spillage resulting in headaches. Tallroth et al. documented this occurrence in as many as 10% of those receiving discography [58].

Overview and Epidemiology

Low back pain is a common complaint among the aging population and has a considerable socioeconomic impact. According to the Global Burden of Disease 2010 study, low back pain is the leading disability in the world and ranked sixth with respect to global burden. In the United States alone, chronic low back pain has an economic cost of nearly $100 billion. Recent research suggests that the percentage of adults affected for the first time in a 1-year time span ranges anywhere between 6% and 15%, with recurrence rates as high as 24–80%. Surprisingly, those in their 20s have the highest incidence of low back pain, and prevalence reaches a peak in the seventh decade of life. Similar to the cervical and thoracic spine, lumbar back pain has several risk factors including smoking, obesity, age, female gender, strenuous work, sedentary work, psychologically strenuous work, job dissatisfaction, and depression [60–68].

Anatomy

The lumbar spine is composed of five vertebrae which are separated by intervertebral discs connected by a network of ligaments and supported by dense musculature. The vertebral column, particularly the lumbar spine, provides basic structural support and protects the spinal cord, which projects to L2 and then progresses as the cauda equina. The lumbar back supports the majority of the torso's weight, and, as one progresses down the spine, each intervertebral disc bears more load than the one above it. Therefore, the last two intervertebral discs are subject to high rates of injury, usually in the form of degradation. Due to the same processes, most thoracolumbar injuries as a whole happen between T11and L4. In contrast to the thoracic spine, the lumbar spine is responsible for the lordotic shape of the vertebral column. The vertebral bodies in this area have a larger horizontal length than vertical height, and the transverse processes do not make contact with any of the ribs [68].

There are five lumbar spinal nerves, L1–L5, each of which arises from the spinal cord by a ventral and dorsal spinal root. The spinal nerves divide into a dorsal primary ramus and ventral primary ramus, which divide and supply the posterior and anterior structures in the lumbar region [69]. Just as in the cervical spine, histologic studies have shown that the presence of nerve fibers can extend as deeply as the outer third of the annulus fibrosus in the lumbar spine, providing evidence for the use of provocation discography. Interestingly, severely degenerated lumbar discs have been shown to have more extensive innervation than normal discs. Furthermore, these nerves have been shown to be substance P immunoreactive, further supporting the idea of discogenic pain and an indication for discography [70].

Pathophysiology

The most common diagnosis made at acute presentation of low back pain is nonspecific low back pain. Greater than 85% of cases result in the diagnosis of back pain without a specific underlying condition that can be reliably identified [61–73]. Most

of these patients improve within a few weeks. Less than 1% of these patients have serious etiologies such as metastatic cancer, spinal infection, or cauda equine syndrome
[74,75]. Only 3–4% of these patients have symptomatic disc herniation or spinal stenosis [75,76]. If a patient presents with radiculopathy, clinicians should consider L5 or
S1 nerve root compression as more than 90% of radiculopathies are of that origin [77].

Lumbar spine stenosis is a common cause of chronic low back pain, most often
affecting patients greater than 60 years of age. Pseudoclaudication is a common clinical sign of lumbar spine stenosis, exemplified as sitting forward or leaning forward
to reduce pain radiating to the legs. Most of these patients have stable symptoms
over time, or symptoms may congruently progress as their arthritic disease worsens.
Conservative, nonsurgical treatment is the initial therapy for most patients [77]. Other
etiologies include ankylosing spondylitis, osteoarthritis, scoliosis, kyphosis, psychological distress, and, rarely pancreatitis, nephrolithiasis, pyelonephritis, abdominal
aortic aneurysm, or herpes zoster [72,78].

Applications

Lumbar spine discography is an interventional diagnostic imaging technique in which
contrast dye is injected into the nucleus of an intervertebral disc under fluoroscopy.
Diagnostic criteria depend on the patient's response to dye injection and the resulting
imaging done immediately following injection. Discography is thus controversial because a positive test relies partially on a subjective report of pain [78–80].

A recent systematic review showed limited evidence supporting functional anesthetic discography or provocation discography with local anesthetic injection due
to possible masking of symptoms. Upon accuracy testing, the prevalence of internal
disc disruption was estimated at 39% and 42% in a cohort of younger and heteroge-
neous populations with low back pain, respectively [81–83]. The systematic review
concluded that the evidence for provocation discography was acceptable based on
three well-performed accuracy studies but mentioned the ongoing debate due to lack
of outcome parameters. The indicated strength of evidence for the diagnostic accuracy
of lumbar provocation discography was thus considered fair and subject to interpretation by the clinician due to unsettled diagnostic criteria, lack of standardization, and
dependence subjective reports [84].

Technique

As with any interventional procedure, it is critical that the patient is positioned correctly. Technicians prefer their patients positioned at 45 degrees as this opens the
space between adjacent vertebrae and avoids the needle contacting the iliac crest.
The lower lumbar discs tend to be hidden by the iliac crest when using fluoroscopy
due to the oblique position of the fluoroscopic C-arm. After proper positioning,
the needle should be introduced parallel to the coronal plane of the L3–L4 disc and
slightly angled up for the L2–L3 disc. A local anesthetic is infiltrated into the skin
and musculature, but the superior articular process should be avoided to prevent
anesthetizing the area of diagnostic interest and thus creating a false-negative result.

An 18-gauge 3.5-inch needle is then used to infiltrate the musculature, striking
the superior articular process, walked slightly laterally and then placed at a midpoint

between the endplates. The stylet is removed and a 22-gauge, 6-inch-long needle is inserted via the introducer needle. The needle passes lateral to the superior articular process yet medial to the exiting nerve root, directly through the annulus fibrosis. The patient may experience pain during this process, and lancinating pain into the extremity is a sign of nerve root penetration, indicating the needle should be redirected. Once the disc is penetrated, anteroposterior and lateral images of the disc are obtained via fluoroscopy to confirm that the needle is in the center of the disc space. Deviation leads to the risk of annular injection of contrast, compromising the result of the test. Contrast is then injected, along with intradiscal antibiotics at the discretion of the clinician. A pressure syringe may be used to gather information about opening pressure, pressure at the onset of pain, and maximum pressure. An incompetent disc will lose pressure rapidly because of a leakage in contrast, and a typical or nonpainful lumbar disc should be able to hold a pressure of at least 90 mm H_2O.

Diagnostic criteria should be investigated systematically. If there are reports of pain, the clinician must inquire about the location, intensity, severity, and quality of the pain. Guarding or autonomic behaviors indicating pain should also be noted. Disc morphological characteristics upon imaging should then be evaluated. The presence of tears, either complete or partial, or any epidural spread of contrast should be considered as injury to the disc and part of a pathological process. If multiple discs are being evaluated, it is important to not inject anesthetic into previously evaluated discs due to the risk of compromising future reports of pain and resulting in a possible false-negative result [85].

Complications

Discitis, nerve root injury, disc herniation, subarachnoid puncture, epidural abscess, allergic contrast reaction, and other side effects are potential complications for lumbar discography [86–92]. Approximately 1 in 1,000 cases result in discitis, which is regarded as one of the worst outcomes as a result of poor technique or contamination of the needle tip. Meticulous technique, double-needle technique, and prophylactic antibiotics have been recommended as preventative measures against discitis [93,94]. Discitis usually presents as severe back pain 2–4 weeks postprocedure, with associated fever and chills. This presentation warrants MRI and sedimentation rates to rule out early discitis [95,96].

Intravascular uptake of contrast is another common result of lumbar discography, once estimated at 14.3% prevalence. Last, it has been shown that needle puncture of intervertebral discs may accelerate or produce disc degeneration. The size of the needle and depth of penetration correlated with the degree of histological changes in one study, with the authors recommending that discography benefits be weighed against the risks of the procedure and the potential for exacerbating patient symptoms [97,98].

CONCLUSION

Back pain related to discogenic sources is common and of significant socioeconomic detriment. Discogenic pain is difficult to diagnose; however, discography can be a useful technique to specifically identify pathological discs. Presently, there is strong evidence in support of using discography for the lumbar spine more than the cervical and thoracic regions. The technique has been solidified for decades, and its complication rate is low, although it is variable depending on the diagnostician. Although some have argued that it provides valuable diagnostic information that MRI and other imaging techniques cannot, its high false-positive rate, subjective diagnostic criteria, and lack of standardization brings its functional utility into question.

REFERENCES

1. Walker J, El Abd O, Isaac Z, Muzin S. Discography in practice: a clinical and historical review. *Curr Rev Musculoskel Med*. 2008;1(2):69–83. doi: 10.1007/s12178-007-9009-9.
2. Wise RE, Weiford EC. X-ray visualization of the intervertebral disc. *Cleve Clin Med*. 1951;18:127–130 [PubMed]
3. Hoy DG, Protani M, De R, Buchbinder R. The epidemiology of neck pain. *Best Pract Res Clin Rheumatol*. 2010;24(6):783–792. doi: 10.1016/j.berh.2011.01.019.
4. Murray CJL, Atkinson C, Bhalla K, et al. The state of US health, 1990-2010: burden of diseases, injuries, and risk factors. *JAMA*. 2013;310(6):591–608. doi: 10.1001/jama.2013.13805.
5. Brooks P, Blyth F, Buchbinder R, Hoy D. (2010). The epidemiology of low back pain. *Best Pract Res Clin Rheumatol*. 2010;24(6): 769–781.
6. Fejer R, Kyvik KO, Hartvigsen J. The prevalence of neck pain in the world population: a systematic critical review of the literature. *Eur Spine J*. 2006;15(6):834–848. doi: 10.1007/s00586-004-0864-4.
7. Hogg-Johnson S, van der Velde G, Carroll LJ, et al. The burden and determinants of neck pain in the general population. *Spine (Phila Pa 1976)*. 2008;33(Supplement):S39–S51. doi: 10.1097/BRS.0b013e31816454c8.
8. Binder AI. Neck pain. *BMJ Clin Evid*. 2008;2008. http://www.ncbi.nlm.nih.gov/pubmed/19445809. Accessed August 4, 2017.
9. Nilsen TIL, Holtermann A, Mork PJ. Physical exercise, body mass index, and risk of chronic pain in the low back and neck/shoulders: longitudinal data from the Nord-Trondelag Health Study. *Am J Epidemiol*. 2011;174(3):267–273. doi: 10.1093/aje/kwr087.
10. Kääriä S, Laaksonen M, Rahkonen O, Lahelma E, Leino-Arjas P. Risk factors of chronic neck pain: a prospective study among middle-aged employees. *Eur J Pain*. 2012;16(6):911–920. doi: 10.1002/j.1532-2149.2011.00065.x.
11. Son KM, Cho NH, Lim SH, Kim HA. Prevalence and risk factor of neck pain in elderly Korean community residents. *J Korean Med Sci*. 2013;28(5):680–686. doi: 10.3346/jkms.2013.28.5.680.
12. Vincent HK, Adams MCB, Vincent KR, Hurley RW. Musculoskeletal pain, fear avoidance behaviors, and functional decline in obesity: potential interventions to manage pain and maintain function. *Reg Anesth Pain Med*. 2013;38(6):481–491. doi: 10.1097/AAP.0000000000000013.
13. Côté P, van der Velde G, Cassidy JD, et al. The burden and determinants of neck pain in workers. *J Manipulative Physiol Ther*. 2009;32(2):S70–S86. doi: 10.1016/j.jmpt.2008.11.012.
14. Bogduk N. Functional anatomy of the spine. In: *Handbook of Clinical Neurology*. Masdeu JC, González RG, eds. Newcastle: Elsevier; Vol. 136; 2016:675–688. doi: 10.1016/B978-0-444-53486-6.00032-6.

15. Holck P. Cervikalcolumnas anatomi. *Tidsskr Den Nor legeforening*. 2010;130(1):29–32. doi: 10.4045/tidsskr.09.0296.

16. Bogduk N, Windsor M, Inglis A. The innervation of the cervical intervertebral discs. *Spine (Phila Pa 1976)*. 1988;13(1):2–8. http://www.ncbi.nlm.nih.gov/pubmed/3381132. Accessed August 4, 2017.

17. Raj PP. Intervertebral disc: anatomy-physiology-pathophysiology-treatment. *Pain Pract*. 2008;8(1):18–44. doi: 10.1111/j.1533-2500.2007.00171.x.

18. Malik KM, Cohen SP, Walega DR, Benzon HT. Diagnostic criteria and treatment of discogenic pain: a systematic review of recent clinical literature. *Spine J*. 2013;13(11):1675–1689. doi: 10.1016/j.spinee.2013.06.063.

19. Singh V. The role of cervical discography in interventional pain management. *Pain Physician*. 2004;7(2):249–255. http://www.ncbi.nlm.nih.gov/pubmed/16868599. Accessed August 4, 2017.

20. Willems PC. Provocative diskography: safety and predictive value in the outcome of spinal fusion or pain intervention for chronic low-back pain. *J Pain Res*. 2014;7:699–705. doi: 10.2147/JPR.S45615.

21. Bogduk N, McGuirk B. *Management of Acute and Chronic Neck Pain : An Evidence-Based Approach*. Edinburgh: Elsevier; 2006.

22. Modic MT, Masaryk TJ, Mulopulos GP, Bundschuh C, Han JS, Bohlman H. Cervical radiculopathy: prospective evaluation with surface coil MR imaging, CT with metrizamide, and metrizamide myelography. *Radiology*. 1986;161(3):753–759. doi: 10.1148/radiology.161.3.3786728.

23. Boden SD, McCowin PR, Davis DO, Dina TS, Mark AS, Wiesel S. Abnormal magnetic-resonance scans of the cervical spine in asymptomatic subjects. A prospective investigation. *J Bone Joint Surg Am*. 1990;72(8):1178–1184. http://www.ncbi.nlm.nih.gov/pubmed/2398088. Accessed August 4, 2017.

24. Parfenchuck TA, Janssen ME. A correlation of cervical magnetic resonance imaging and discography/computed tomographic discograms. *Spine (Phila Pa 1976)*. 1994;19(24):2819–2825. http://www.ncbi.nlm.nih.gov/pubmed/7899985. Accessed August 4, 2017.

25. Onyewu O, Manchikanti L, Falco FJE, et al. An update of the appraisal of the accuracy and utility of cervical discography in chronic neck pain. *Pain Physician*. 15(6):E777–E806. http://www.ncbi.nlm.nih.gov/pubmed/23159976. Accessed August 4, 2017.

26. Shah R V, Everett CR, McKenzie-Brown AM, Sehgal N. Discography as a diagnostic test for spinal pain: a systematic and narrative review. *Pain Physician*. 2005;8(2):187–209. http://www.ncbi.nlm.nih.gov/pubmed/16850074. Accessed August 4, 2017.

27. Buenaventura RM, Shah R V, Patel V, Benyamin R, Singh V. Systematic review of discography as a diagnostic test for spinal pain: an update. *Pain Physician*. 2007;10(1):147–164. http://www.ncbi.nlm.nih.gov/pubmed/17256028. Accessed August 4, 2017.

28. Viikari-Juntura E, Raininko R, Videman T, Porkka L. Evaluation of cervical disc degeneration with ultralow field MRI and discography. An experimental study on cadavers. *Spine (Phila Pa 1976)*. 1989;14(6):616–619. http://www.ncbi.nlm.nih.gov/pubmed/2749378. Accessed August 4, 2017.

29. Manchikanti L, Abdi S, Atluri S, et al. An update of comprehensive evidence-based guidelines for interventional techniques in chronic spinal pain. Part II: guidance and recommendations. *Pain Physician*. 2013;16(2 Suppl):S49–283. http://www.ncbi.nlm.nih.gov/pubmed/23615883. Accessed August 4, 2017.

30. Sasso RC, Anderson PA, Riew KD, Heller JG. Results of cervical arthroplasty compared with anterior discectomy and fusion: four-year clinical outcomes in a

prospective, randomized controlled trial. Chutkan NB, ed. *Orthopedics.* 2011;34(11):889. doi: 10.3928/01477447-20110922-24.

31. Schellhas KP, Smith MD, Gundry CR, Pollei SR. Cervical discogenic pain. Prospective correlation of magnetic resonance imaging and discography in asymptomatic subjects and pain sufferers. *Spine (Phila Pa 1976).* 1996;21(3):300–11-2. http://www.ncbi.nlm. nih.gov/pubmed/8742205. Accessed August 4, 2017.

32. Ohnmeiss DD, Guyer RD, Mason SL. The relation between cervical discographic pain responses and radiographic images. *Clin J Pain.* 2000;16(1):1–5. http://www.ncbi.nlm. nih.gov/pubmed/10741811. Accessed August 4, 2017.

33. Smith GW, Nichols P. The technique of cervical discography. *Radiology.* 1957;68(5):718–720. doi: 10.1148/68.5.718.

34. Walker J, El Abd O, Isaac Z, Muzin S, Muzin S. Discography in practice: a clinical and historical review. *Curr Rev Musculoskelet Med.* 2008;1(2):69–83. doi: 10.1007/s12178-007-9009-9.

35. Fenton DS, Douglas S, Czervionke LF. *Image-Guided Spine Intervention.* Philadelphia, WB: Saunders; 2003.

36. Derby R, Howard MW, Grant JM, Lettice JJ, Van Peteghem PK, Ryan DP. The ability of pressure-controlled discography to predict surgical and nonsurgical outcomes. *Spine (Phila Pa 1976).* 1999;24(4):364–71-2. http://www.ncbi.nlm.nih.gov/pubmed/10065521. Accessed August 4, 2017.

37. Zeidman SM, Thompson K, Ducker TB. Complications of cervical discography: analysis of 4400 diagnostic disc injections. *Neurosurgery.* 1995;37(3):414–417. http://www.ncbi.nlm.nih.gov/pubmed/7501104. Accessed August 4, 2017.

38. Junila J, Niinimäki T, Tervonen O. Epidural abscess after lumbar discography. A case report. *Spine (Phila Pa 1976).* 1997;22(18):2191–2193. http://www.ncbi.nlm.nih.gov/pubmed/9322332. Accessed August 4, 2017.

39. Guyer RD, Ohnmeiss DD. Lumbar discography. Position statement from the North American Spine Society Diagnostic and Therapeutic Committee. *Spine (Phila Pa 1976).* 1995;20(18):2048–2059. http://www.ncbi.nlm.nih.gov/pubmed/8578384. Accessed August 4, 2017.

40. Connor PM, Darden B V. Cervical discography complications and clinical efficacy. *Spine (Phila Pa 1976).* 1993;18(14):2035–2038. http://www.ncbi.nlm.nih.gov/pubmed/8272955. Accessed August 4, 2017.

41. Laun A, Lorenz R, Agnoli AL. Complications of cervical discography. *J Neurosurg Sci.* 25(1):17–20http://www.ncbi.nlm.nih.gov/pubmed/7328431. Accessed August 4, 2017.

42. Guyer RD, Ohnmeiss DD, Mason SL, Shelokov AP. Complications of cervical discography: findings in a large series. *J Spinal Disord.* 1997;10(2):95–101. http://www.ncbi.nlm.nih.gov/pubmed/9113607. Accessed August 4, 2017.

43. Singh V, Manchikanti L, Onyewu O, et al. An update of the appraisal of the accuracy of thoracic discography as a diagnostic test for chronic spinal pain. *Pain Physician.* 2012;15(6):E757–E775.

44. Briggs AM, Smith AJ, Straker LM, Bragge P. Thoracic spine pain in the general population: prevalence, incidence and associated factors in children, adolescents and adults. A systematic review. *BMC Musculoskel Dis.* 2009;10:77. doi: 10.1186/1471-2474-10-77.

45. Grimmer K, Nyland L, Milanese S. Repeated measures of recent headache, neck and upper back pain in Australian adolescents. *Cephalalgia.* 2006 Jul;26(7):843–851.

46. Singh V. Thoracic discography. *Pain Physician.* 2004;7:451–458.

47. Mixter WJ, Barr JS. Rupture of the intervertebral disc with involvement of the spinal canal. *N Eng J Med.* 1934;211:210–215.

48. Ohnmeiss DD, Vanharanta H, Ekholm J. Degree of disc disruption and lower extremity pain. *Spine*. 1997;22:1600–1605.

49. Wheeler AH, Murrey DB. Chronic lumbar spine and radicular pain: pathophysiology and treatment. *Curr Pain Headache Rep*. 2002;6:97–105.

50. Falco FJ, Zhu J, Irwin L, Onyewu CO, Kim D. Thoracic discography. In: Manchikanti L, Singh V, eds., *Interventional Techniques in Chronic Spinal Pain*. Paducah, KY: ASIPP Publishing; 2007: 553–566.

51. Simmons EH, Segil CM. An evaluation of discography in the localization of symptomatic levels in discogenic disease of the spine. *Clin Orthop*. 1975;108:57–69

52. Schellhas KP, Pollei SR, Dorwart RH. Thoracic discography. A safe and reliable technique. *Spine*. 1994;19:2103–2109.

53. Whitecloud TS, Seago RA. Cervical discogenic syndrome: results of operative intervention in patients with positive discography. *Spine*. 1987;12:313–316.

54. Cloward RB. The anterior surgical approach to the cervical spine: the Cloward procedure: past, present, and future. The presidential guest lecture, Cervical Spine Research Society. *Spine*. 1988;13:823–827.

55. Cloward RB. Anterior herniation of a ruptured lumbar intervertebral disk: comments on the diagnostic value of the diskogram. *AMA Arch Surg*. 1952;64:457–463.

56. Lindblom K. Technique and results in myelography and disc puncture. *Acta Radiol*. 1950;34:321–330.

57. Tallroth K, Soini J, Antti-Poika I, et al. Premedication and short term complications in iohexol discography. *Ann Chir Gynaecol*. 1991;80(1):49–53.

58. Wood KB, Schellhas KP, Garvey TA, Aeppli D. Thoracic discography in healthy individuals. A controlled prospective study of magnetic resonance imaging and discography in asymptomatic and symptomatic individuals. *Spine (Phila Pa 1976)*. 1999;24:1548–1555.

59. Walker J, 3rd, El Abd O, Isaac Z, et al. Discography in practice: a clinical and historical review. *Curr Rev Musculoskel Med*. 2008;1:69–83.

60. Steffens D, Ferreira ML, Latimer J, et al. What triggers an episode of acute low back pain? A case-crossover study. *Arthritis Care Res (Hoboken)*. 2015;67(3):403–410. doi: 10.1002/acr.22533.

61. Skovron ML, Szpalski M, Nordin M, Melot C, Cukier D. Sociocultural factors and back pain. A population-based study in Belgian adults. *Spine (Phila Pa 1976)*. 1994;19(2):129–137. http://www.ncbi.nlm.nih.gov/pubmed/8153818. Accessed August 4, 2017.

62. Macfarlane GJ, Thomas E, Papageorgiou AC, Croft PR, Jayson MI, Silman AJ. Employment and physical work activities as predictors of future low back pain. *Spine (Phila Pa 1976)*. 1997;22(10):1143–1149. http://www.ncbi.nlm.nih.gov/pubmed/9160474. Accessed August 4, 2017.

63. Katz JN. Lumbar disc disorders and low-back pain: socioeconomic factors and consequences. *J Bone Joint Surg Am*. 2006;88 Suppl 2(suppl_2):21–24. doi: 10.2106/JBJS.E.01273.

64. Deyo RA, Loeser JD, Bigos SJ. Herniated lumbar intervertebral disk. *Ann Intern Med*. 1990;112(8):598–603. http://www.ncbi.nlm.nih.gov/pubmed/2139310. Accessed August 4, 2017.

65. Croft PR, Papageorgiou AC, Thomas E, Macfarlane GJ, Silman AJ. Short-term physical risk factors for new episodes of low back pain. Prospective evidence from the South Manchester Back Pain Study. *Spine (Phila Pa 1976)*. 1999;24(15):1556–1561. http://www.ncbi.nlm.nih.gov/pubmed/10457575. Accessed August 4, 2017.

66. Croft PR, Papageorgiou AC, Ferry S, Thomas E, Jayson MI, Silman AJ. Psychologic distress and low back pain. Evidence from a prospective study in the general population. *Spine (Phila Pa 1976)*. 1995;20(24):2731–2737. http://www.ncbi.nlm.nih.gov/pubmed/ 8747252. Accessed August 4, 2017.

67. Cassidy JD, Carroll LJ, Côté P. The Saskatchewan health and back pain survey. The prevalence of low back pain and related disability in Saskatchewan adults. *Spine (Phila Pa 1976)*. 1998;23(17):1860–1866;discussion 1867. http://www.ncbi.nlm.nih.gov/ pubmed/9762743. Accessed August 4, 2017.

68. Snell RS, Smith MS. *Clinical Anatomy for Emergency Medicine*. St Louis: Mosby; 1993.

69. Artner J, Cakir B, Reichel H, Lattig F. Bildwandlergestützte Injektionstechniken an der Lendenwirbelsäule. *Orthopade*. 2013;42(4):281–294. doi: 10.1007/ s00132-013-2078-0.

70. Coppes MH, Marani E, Thomeer RT, Groen GJ. Innervation of painful lumbar discs. *Spine (Phila Pa 1976)*. 1997;22(20):2342-9–50. http://www.ncbi.nlm.nih.gov/pubmed/ 9355214. Accessed August 4, 2017.

71. Deyo RA, Weinstein JN. Low back pain. *N Engl J Med*. 2001;344(5):363–370. doi: 10.1056/NEJM200102013440508.

72. Chou R, Qaseem A, Snow V, et al. Diagnosis and treatment of low back pain: a joint clinical practice guideline from the American College of Physicians and the American Pain Society. *Ann Intern Med*. 2007;147(7):478–491. http://www.ncbi.nlm.nih.gov/ pubmed/17909209. Accessed August 4, 2017.

73. Chou R, Qaseem A, Owens DK, Shekelle P, Clinical Guidelines Committee of the American College of Physicians. Diagnostic imaging for low back pain: advice for high-value health care from the American College of Physicians. *Ann Intern Med*. 2011;154(3):181–189. doi: 10.7326/0003-4819-154-3-201102010-00008.

74. Deyo RA, Rainville J, Kent DL. What can the history and physical examination tell us about low back pain? *JAMA*. 1992;268(6):760–765. http://www.ncbi.nlm.nih.gov/ pubmed/1386391. Accessed August 4, 2017.

75. Jarvik JG, Deyo RA. Diagnostic evaluation of low back pain with emphasis on imaging. *Ann Intern Med*. 2002;137(7):586–597. http://www.ncbi.nlm.nih.gov/pubmed/ 12353946. Accessed August 4, 2017.

76. Underwood MR, Dawes P. Inflammatory back pain in primary care. *Br J Rheumatol*. 1995;34(11):1074–1077. http://www.ncbi.nlm.nih.gov/pubmed/8542211. Accessed August 4, 2017.

77. Acute low back problems in adults: assessment and treatment. Agency for Health Care Policy and Research. *Clin Pract Guide Quick Ref Guide Clin*. 1994;(14):iii–iv, 1–25. http://www.ncbi.nlm.nih.gov/pubmed/7987418. Accessed August 4, 2017.

78. Chou R. In the clinic. Low back pain. *Ann Intern Med*. 2014;160(11):ITC6-1. doi: 10.7326/0003-4819-160-11-201406030-01006.

79. Walsh TR, Weinstein JN, Spratt KF, Lehmann TR, Aprill C, Sayre H. Lumbar discography in normal subjects. A controlled, prospective study. *J Bone Joint Surg Am*. 1990;72(7):1081–1088. http://www.ncbi.nlm.nih.gov/pubmed/2384508. Accessed August 4, 2017.

80. Carragee EJ, Tanner CM, Khurana S, et al. The rates of false-positive lumbar discography in select patients without low back symptoms. *Spine (Phila Pa 1976)*. 2000;25(11):1373–1380;discussion 1381. http://www.ncbi.nlm.nih.gov/pubmed/ 10828919. Accessed August 4, 2017.

81. DePalma MJ, Ketchum JM, Saullo T. What is the source of chronic low back pain and does age play a role? *Pain Med*. 2011;12(2):224–233. doi: 10.1111/j.1526-4637.2010.01045.x.

82. Wolfer LR, Derby R, Lee J-E, Lee S-H. Systematic review of lumbar provocation discography in asymptomatic subjects with a meta-analysis of false-positive rates. *Pain*

Physician. 11(4):513–538. http://www.ncbi.nlm.nih.gov/pubmed/18690280. Accessed August 4, 2017.

83. Manchikanti L, Singh V, Pampati V, et al. Evaluation of the relative contributions of various structures in chronic low back pain. *Pain Physician.* 2001;4(4):308–316. http://www.ncbi.nlm.nih.gov/pubmed/16902676. Accessed August 4, 2017.

84. Manchikanti L, Benyamin RM, Singh V, et al. An update of the systematic appraisal of the accuracy and utility of lumbar discography in chronic low back pain. *Pain Physician.* 2013;16(2 Suppl):SE55–SE95. http://www.ncbi.nlm.nih.gov/pubmed/23615887. Accessed August 4, 2017.

85. Tomecek FJ, Anthony CS, Boxell C, Warren J. Discography interpretation and techniques in the lumbar spine. *Neurosurg Focus.* 2002;13(2):E13. http://www.ncbi.nlm.nih.gov/pubmed/15916397. Accessed August 4, 2017.

86. Quero L, Klawitter M, Nerlich AG, Leonardi M, Boos N, Wuertz K. Bupivacaine: the deadly friend of intervertebral disc cells? *Spine J.* 2011;11(1):46–53. doi: 10.1016/j.spinee.2010.11.001.

87. Wang D, Vo N V., Sowa GA, et al. Bupivacaine decreases cell viability and matrix protein synthesis in an intervertebral disc organ model system. *Spine J.* 2011;11(2):139–146. doi: 10.1016/j.spinee.2010.11.017.

88. Willems PC. Provocative diskography: safety and predictive value in the outcome of spinal fusion or pain intervention for chronic low-back pain. *J Pain Res.* 2014;7:699–705. doi: 10.2147/JPR.S45615.

89. Poynton AR, Hinman A, Lutz G, Farmer JC. Discography-induced acute lumbar disc herniation: a report of five cases. *J Spinal Disord Tech.* 2005;18(2):188–192. http://www.ncbi.nlm.nih.gov/pubmed/15800440. Accessed August 4, 2017.

90. Phillips H, Glazebrook JJ, Timothy J. Cauda equina compression post lumbar discography. *Acta Neurochir (Wien).* 2012;154(6):1033–1036. doi: 10.1007/s00701-012-1322-4.

91. Werner BC, Hogan M V., Shen FH. Candida lusitaniae discitis after discogram in an immunocompetent patient. *Spine J.* 2011;11(10):e1–e6. doi: 10.1016/j.spinee.2011.09.004.

92. Gay RE, Ilharreborde B, Zhao KD, Berglund LJ, Bronfort G, An K-N. Stress in lumbar intervertebral discs during distraction: a cadaveric study. *Spine J.* 2008;8(6):982-990. doi: 10.1016/j.spinee.2007.07.398.

93. Fraser RD, Osti OL, Vernon-Roberts B. Discitis after discography. *J Bone Joint Surg Br.* 1987;69(1):26–35. http://www.ncbi.nlm.nih.gov/pubmed/3818728. Accessed August 4, 2017.

94. Willems PC, Jacobs W, Duinkerke ES, De Kleuver M. Lumbar discography: should we use prophylactic antibiotics? A study of 435 consecutive discograms and a systematic review of the literature. *J Spinal Disord Tech.* 2004;17(3):243–247. http://www.ncbi.nlm.nih.gov/pubmed/15167342. Accessed August 4, 2017.

95. Guyer RD, Collier R, Stith WJ, et al. Discitis after discography. *Spine (Phila Pa 1976).* 1988;13(12):1352–1354. http://www.ncbi.nlm.nih.gov/pubmed/3212569. Accessed August 4, 2017.

96. Arrington JA, Murtagh FR, Silbiger ML, Rechtine GR, Nokes SR. Magnetic resonance imaging of postdiscogram discitis and osteomyelitis in the lumbar spine: case report. *J Fla Med Assoc.* 1986;73(3):192–194. http://www.ncbi.nlm.nih.gov/pubmed/3701296. Accessed August 4, 2017.

97. Johnson RG. Does discography injure normal discs? An analysis of repeat discograms. *Spine (Phila Pa 1976).* 1989;14(4):424–426. http://www.ncbi.nlm.nih.gov/pubmed/2718046. Accessed August 4, 2017.

98. Flanagan MN, Chung BU. Roentgenographic changes in 188 patients 10-20 years after discography and chemonucleolysis. *Spine (Phila Pa 1976).* 1986;11(5):444–448. http://www.ncbi.nlm.nih.gov/pubmed/3750081. Accessed August 4, 2017.

15 Open Endoscopic Rhizotomy

Raj J. Gala, Lauren Szolomayer, and James Yue

CONSIDERATIONS

The etiology of axial low back pain is multifactorial and includes pain arising from lumbar facet joints [1,2]. The reported prevalence of facetogenic pain is around 30% in patients with chronic low back pain [3]. The facet joints, capsules, and surrounding tissues are innervated by the medial branches of the dorsal rami. Rhizotomy of these nerves can provide pain relief in patients with lumbar facetogenic pain. It is recommended that the clinician confirm facetogenic pain, either through intraarticular lumbar facet joint injection or through nerve block of the ramus medialis of the ramus dorsalis prior to performing rhizotomy [4].

The medial branch of the dorsal ramus passes through a notch at the base of the transverse process. The nerve is covered by an extension of the intertransverse membrane and mamillo-accessory ligament (Figure 15.1). After passing through the notch, the medial branch splits into several small fibers that enter the facet joint and capsule. Each dorsal ramus provides nerve fibers to at least two facet joints, and each facet joint receives afferent sensation from at least two spinal levels [5].

On examination, patients will often exhibit pain with extension and simultaneous rotation. Pain off the midline in a lateral location often is indicative of facet-mediated pain. Rhizotomy procedures should be reserved for patients with confirmatory medial branch and/or facet injection block testing. Diagnosis is best confirmed using both radiographic (x-rays, computed tomography [CT], and magnetic resonance imaging [MRI]) as well as injection techniques (facet blocks/medial branch blocks). Patients should complain mainly of low back pain with minimal leg pain.

TECHNIQUE

The specific facet joints to target should be determined preoperatively. The patient should be positioned prone on a well-cushioned radiolucent bed. Either general

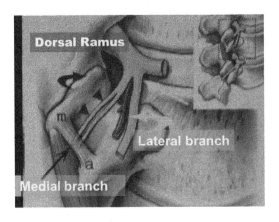

FIGURE 15.1 Diagram of the medial branch (*short arrows*) of the dorsal ramus coursing under the mamillo-accessory ligament (MAL). This osseofibrous tunnel maintains the medial branch in a constant location, allowing for accurate ablation during rhizotomy. Mamillary process (m), accessory process (a), lateral branch (*curved white arrow*).

anesthesia or monitored anesthesia care (MAC) using local anesthetics with mild IV sedation will be sufficient for most cases. The goal is to aim for the junction of the base of the superior articular process (SAP) and the transverse process. The approach is from slightly lateral to the midline. Using anteroposterior (AP) intraoperative fluoroscopy, the midline is marked. Also under AP fluoroscopy, the intersection of the lateral facet and superior medial aspect of the transverse process is marked (Figure 15.2A). A skin marking approximately 1 cm lateral to this intersection line is marked to be used as the incision. If a two-level rhizotomy is to be performed, the incision is marked on the superior level. For example, if a rhizotomy is planned for the L4–L5 and L3–L4 facets, the entry incision is made over the L3 transverse process. If a three-level rhizotomy is to be performed, the incision is made over the middle transverse process, and the scope is angled cephalad and caudad after the middle segment rhizotomy is completed. Alternatively, individual incisions over each transverse process can be made.

Once the incision is made, a small hemostat is used to spread and open the dorsal fascia. A two-hole obturator is placed in the incision and then docked under lateral fluoroscopy onto the superior aspect of the transverse process (Figure 15.2B,C). A beveled working cannula is then placed over the obturator, and the endoscope and

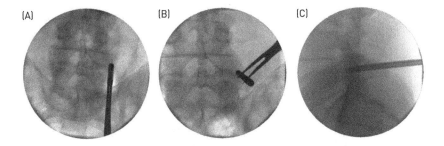

FIGURE 15.2 Intraoperative fluoroscopy demonstrating the landmarks used for endoscopic rhizotomy. (A) The intersection of the lateral facet and superior medial aspect of the transverse process. (B,C) The docking of the obturator onto the superior aspect of the transverse process.

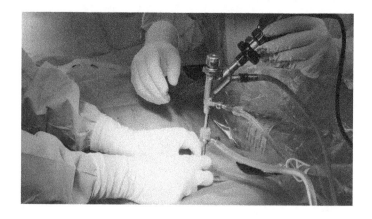

FIGURE 15.3 Setup in the operating room for endoscopic rhizotomy. The camera is placed through a cannula, allowing for inflow and outflow of irrigation. Instruments can be placed through the cannula to perform the rhizotomy. It is paramount to maintain the stability of the cannula so inadvertent injury to surrounding tissues is avoided.

instruments are used to identify the tissue overlying the superior medial aspect of the transverse process. The camera is placed through the cannula to visualize the structures (Figure 15.3). The camera should allow visualization of the medial branch of the dorsal ramus (Figure 15.4A,B). Rhizotomy can be performed using electrocautery devices under camera visualization (Figure 15.4C). A Holmium YAG laser and cauterization can be used to ablate the nerve tissue.

If the L3–L4 facet is degenerative and symptomatic, the nerve over the L4 and L3 transverse process should be ablated. If the L4–L5 and L5–S1 facet joints are degenerative and symptomatic, the L4, L5, and S1 nerves should be ablated. After completion of the rhizotomy, the instruments are removed and the skin incision can be closed with absorbable suture.

COMPLICATIONS

In addition to normal surgical risks such as infection, the patient can infrequently experience transient dysesthesia in a radicular pattern whether or not the more anterior dorsal root ganglion is inadvertently directly irritated. It is hypothesized that the bipolar rhizotomy can induce a retrograde effect on the more proximal nerve elements.

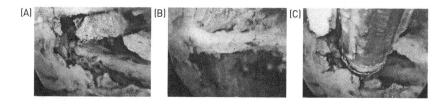

FIGURE 15.4 View during endoscopic rhizotomy. The medial branch of the dorsal ramus is coursing horizontally in these images. (C) An electrocautery device ablating the medial branch.

Care should be taken to confidently dock the scope over the transverse process and not anterior to the posterior aspect of the transverse process.

RESULTS

There are relatively few studies assessing the efficacy of endoscopic lumbar facet rhizotomy. A retrospective study published in 2014 reported on the results of 50 patients who underwent endoscopic facet rhizotomy [6]. The inclusion criteria were patients with lumbar spondylosis and facet arthrosis who had at least 50% pain relief from medial branch nerve block. At 1 year follow-up, all patients were satisfied with their decision to undergo the procedure: 90% of patients improved, 10% of patients had partially regressed, and no patients got worse. Visual Analog Scale (VAS) pain scores decreased from an average of 6.2 to 2.5.

In a 2014 prospective study, 45 patients who underwent endoscopic rhizotomy were compared against 13 patients who underwent conservative treatment with nonsteroidal anti-inflammatory drugs, physical therapy, and cognitive-behavioral therapy [7]. Patients had to experience at least 80% pain relief from two separate lumbar medial branch blocks to be included in this study. The patients were re-examined at 3, 6, and 12 months. The VAS pain scores were not statistically different between the two groups; however, the operative group did report statistically better percentage of pain relief. At 1 year follow-up, the McNab outcomes were statistically better in the operative group as compared to the conservative group.

CONCLUSION

Ideal candidates for endoscopic rhizotomy are patients who have undergone successful and effective needle injection anesthetic blocks and have complementary clinical and radiographic findings. Endoscopic rhizotomy affords the practitioner the ability to directly visualize the medial branch and thereby directly ablate the tissue. Multiple levels can be performed under a single 6 mm incision as an ambulatory procedure. Due to the cross-innervation of the superior medial branch to the inferior facet, consideration for two-level rhizotomy should be assessed in most cases in order to adequately obtain the desired result.

REFERENCES

1. Yue JJ, Long W. Full endoscopic spinal surgery techniques: advancements, indications, and outcomes. *Int J Spine Surg.* 2015;9:17.
2. McLain RF, Pickar JG. Mechanoreceptor endings in human thoracic and lumbar facet joints. *Spine (Phila Pa 1976).* 1998;23(2):168–173.
3. Manchikanti L, Boswell MV, Singh V, Pampati V, Damron KS, Beyer CD. Prevalence of facet joint pain in chronic spinal pain of cervical, thoracic, and lumbar regions. *BMC Musculoskelet Disord.* 2004;5:15.
4. Sehgal N, Dunbar EE, Shah RV, Colson J. Systematic review of diagnostic utility of facet (zygapophysial) joint injections in chronic spinal pain: an update. *Pain Physician.* 2007;10(1):213–228.

5. Pedersen HE, Blunck CF, Gardner E. The anatomy of lumbosacral posterior rami and meningeal branches of spinal nerve (sinu-vertebral nerves); with an experimental study of their functions. *J Bone Joint Surg. Am Vol.* 1956;38-A(2):377–391.

6. Yeung A, Gore S. Endoscopically guided foraminal and dorsal rhizotomy for chronic axial back pain based on cadaver and endoscopically visualized anatomic study. *Int J Spine Surg.* 2014;8.

7. Li ZZ, Hou SX, Shang WL, Song KR, Wu WW. Evaluation of endoscopic dorsal ramus rhizotomy in managing facetogenic chronic low back pain. *Clin Neurol Neurosurg.* 2014;126:11–17.

16 Endoscopically Assisted Lumbar Medial Branch Rhizotomy

Raj J. Gala, Lauren Szolomayer, Raysa Cabrejo, and James Yue

INTRODUCTION: FACET JOINTS AS A CAUSE OF LUMBAR BACK PAIN

A variety of causes for lumbar back pain have been postulated. The concept that facet joints are involved in the etiology of low back pain is attributed to Goldthwait in 1911 and was refined by Ghormley in 1933, who described "Facet syndrome" as a pattern of symptoms whereby patients complain of sudden-onset low back pain, usually brought on by twisting or a rotation motion that strains the lumbosacral region.

It has seemed to me that many of the aches and pains which are known as "backache" are true pains of the joints. They represent the same type of pain as that seen in arthritis of the knee or hip, and the accompanying changes are characteristic of degeneration or traumatic arthritis. [1]

Axial back pain has been attributed to the facet joints or zygapophysial joints in anywhere from 15% to 40% of cases [2]. Despite this association of back pain to the facet joints, we have not yet developed well-studied methods for treating this pain. A selective dorsal rhizotomy has emerged as an option for treatment for this variety of lumbar back pain. Selective dorsal rhizotomy has been most commonly used in applications to control pain and spasticity in children with cerebral palsy (CP). This procedure gained popularity in the 1980s and then was tailored for improved outcomes. Mostly for children with spastic diplegia, this procedure can treat both pain and spasticity for these children and help to improve their gait. When the effects of dorsal rhizotomy were studied, there was a trend toward decreased tone and improved gait in children with

CP who were walkers [3]. The concepts behind this treatment were later expanded to include treatment of trigeminal neuralgia and lumbar facet pain.

Rees and Shealy are credited with some of the first uses of selective rhizotomy to treat lumbar back pain [4,5]. Rees used a knife cut in an open surgical procedure around the area of the facet joint to provide pain relief. In a study of more than 200 patients, results showed 79% relief of lumbar back pain in patients who had not been previously treated with surgery. A similar procedure was introduced to North America by Shealy, with the alteration of using radiofrequency (RF) coagulation in the region of the nerve near the facet joint in order to avoid the complication of hematomas seen in the open procedure [6]. Over the years, it was difficult to replicate their results in providing substantial pain relief as it was believed that the sources of axial back pain were from a variety of causes.

Use of diagnostic injection can help determine the relative contributions of facet joint pain to overall axial back pain. The diagnosis of facet joint pain is considered when there is at least 50–75% relief of the targeted pain after local anesthetic blockade of the medial branches of the posterior rami of the spinal nerves that supply the painful joint(s). Usually facet joint pain is diagnosed after two separate occasions of a medial branch block provide relief, as it was shown that relief from a single injection has a high false-positive rate [7]. Intraarticular blocks and medial branch blocks are generally performed in a procedure room with computed tomography (CT)- or fluoroscopy-guided injection and are considered nonsurgical options for treatment of axial lumbar back pain. These injections typically produce a limited duration of relief of pain but may provide helpful diagnostic information.

ANATOMY OF DORSAL RAMI MEDIAL BRANCH

Pain arising from this area can be reduced with blockade or neurotomy due to the specific innervation of the facet joint. A common dorsal ramus exits from the spinal cord through the vertebral foramen and then divides into two branches: a medial and a lateral branch, which contain both sensory and motor fibers [8]. The medial sensory branch then runs inferiorly in a groove between the superior articulating process of the facet joint and the base of the transverse process. Figure 16.1. It then innervates the facet joint capsule, and a smaller branch continues caudally to innervate the facet joint one level below [8,9].

The facet joint is therefore innervated by the medial branch of dorsal ramus at that level and one level above it. To successfully treat pain arising from a facet joint, the medial branch one level above the target needs to be ablated as well [9].

INDICATIONS AND WORKUP

Indications for performing lumbar medial branch rhizotomy include single or multi-level lumbar spondylosis, chronic low back pain without leg pain. Symptoms are typically unilateral and are exacerbated by lumbar extension or rotation. The pain may radiate to the ipsilateral low back or buttock region as referred pain but does not typically travel to the legs as in radicular pain. Patients may also present with paraspinal muscle spasms [8].

Patients with facet-generated pain typically have already had a magnetic resonance imaging (MRI) study prior to presentation. These will show facet joint arthropathy—loss of cartilage, hypertrophy of the joint, osteophytes, joint space narrowing, sclerosis

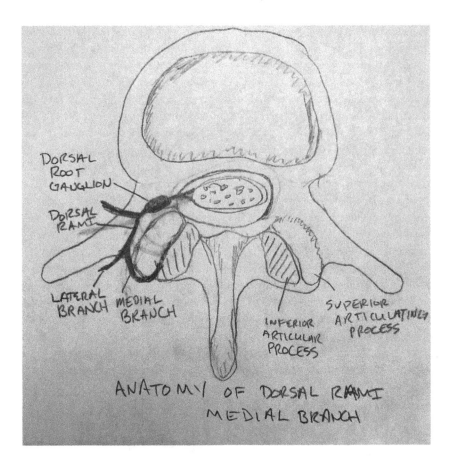

FIGURE 16.1 Dorsal Medial Branch Anatomy Medial branch as it exits the dorsal rami in a groove in transverse process between superior articulating process before inserting at facet joint.

or edema. Other imaging studies to identify these characteristics include standing anteroposterior (AP) and lateral lumbar spine radiographs. A CT scan may help to delineate bony issues that may be present, cysts, or facet arthropathy, but it is not essential.

As mentioned previously, corticosteroid injections to the lumbar facets or medial branch blocks have both diagnostic and therapeutic properties. If these injections provide temporary relief of pain, these patients may get better relief from rhizotomy. Current observation is that patients who report total pain relief showed greater pain reduction after an RF lumbar facet denervation compared with patients who reported only good pain relief [10]. Most practitioners require diagnostic relief from injection prior to treatment via surgical ablation. Jeong reported on diagnostic screening of two medial branch blocks performed on separate occasions to rule out false-positive results; if the patient was responsive to both medial branch blocks, endoscopic radiofrequency ablation was performed. Responsiveness to medial branch block was defined as 50% or more alleviation of pain [9].

PROCEDURE

While this procedure is sometimes performed with use of CT-guided placement of an RF probe, the author's preferred treatment is endoscopically assisted dorsal rhizotomy.

The advantages of percutaneous treatment with endoscopy are that this method allows direct visualization of the nerve root after its location is identified with fluoroscopic imaging. The facet joint is innervated by the medial branch of the dorsal ramus at the level and one level above it. Therefore, to successfully treat pain arising from a facet joint, the medial branch one level above the target needs to be ablated as well. The dorsal ramus also gives off a lateral branch and sometimes an intermediate branch, and while they do not primarily innervate the facet joints, they provide iliolumbar musculature and cutaneous innervation and may contribute to the generation of back pain. As discussed in the anatomy section, the target point for ablation is the junction of the transverse process and the base of the superior articular process [9].

The patient is given perioperative antibiotics and placed under general anesthesia. The patient is then placed in prone position on the table. All pressure points are well padded and protected. The most medial aspect of the transverse process of the affected lumbar vertebrae of the affected sides (left right or bilateral) is marked under AP fluoroscopic imaging. The patient is then sterilely prepped and draped in the usual fashion.

A single incision is made approximately 6 mm in length just off the region where the medial border of the transverse process was marked for the middle of the affected levels. Two level rhizotomies can be performed through the same incision. A hemostat is used to dissect through the deep fascia and a two-hole endoscopic obturator is then placed, docking it on top of the affected transverse process at the medial superior aspect. Figure 16.2 shows the endoscopic setup. The position is then confirmed under

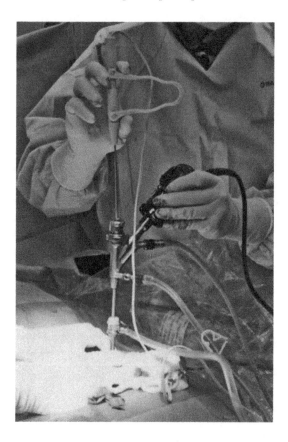

FIGURE 16.2 Surgical setup including port, suction, water irrigation, endoscopic camera, and radio frequency ablator.

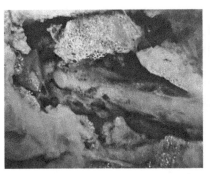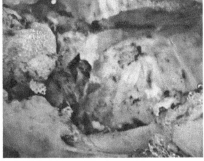

FIGURE 16.3 (A) Medial branch nerve visible in picture from endoscopic camera. (B) Transverse process after ablation of the medial branch nerve.

lateral fluoroscopic imaging. Sequential dilators are then used over the tube obturator, and then under direct visualization a rhizotomy is performed a using bipolar cauterization at the superior aspect of the transverse process, thereby ablating the medial branch. Figure 16.3A shows an endoscopic view of the medial branch of the dorsal ramus, and [Figure 16.3B] shows results after ablation of the nerve, with the superior margin of the transverse process visible at the inferior aspect of the image.

The cannula can then be removed through the same incision, re-placing the two-hole obturator on the superior aspect of the next affected level's transverse process. This continues until all affected levels have had rhizotomy performed. The entire process can then be repeated on the contralateral side. The incisions are then closed with a monofilament absorbable suture, and a small dry sterile dressing is applied. The patient is then placed in the supine position, awakened, extubated, and transferred to the recovery room.

Other authors describe techniques for performing surgery with limited anesthesia such that the patient can respond to questions about his or her pain. The medial branch is first stimulated with an RF probe to determine if the pain generated is concordant with their usual pain. If it is similar, the selective denervation is performed and then the area is restimulated. When no significant similar pain is elicited, the procedure is concluded [9]. In a study on long-term results, 5-year data found that definitive transection of the medial branch provides longer and more complete relief of pain [11]. See Figure 16.4 for procedure details.

POSTOPERATIVE PLAN

Patients are typically discharged to home from the postoperative recovery area with a limited prescription for non-narcotic pain medicine. They are advised to refrain from high-stress, high-impact activities until seen in follow-up, but they may progress to activities as tolerated over the course of 3–4 weeks. No bracing is required. Some patients do feel subjective improvement from physical therapy after the procedure, but it is not required.

RESULTS OF PROCEDURE

There are few studies available detailing the results of pain control with percutaneous rhizotomy and particularly lacking are long-term results covering greater than 1 year.

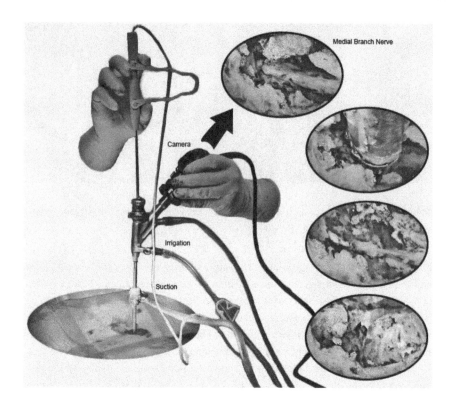

FIGURE 16.4 Endoscopically assisted dorsal rhizotomy procedure.

Yeung compared fluoroscopically guided radiofrequency ablation with an endoscopic technique. Using the same cannula and endoscope, they published a retrospective 1-year follow-up of 50 patients which showed improvement in visual analog scale (VAS) scores from 6.2 to 2.5 and Oswestry Disability Index (ODI) scores from 48 to 28; they also reported approximately 10% of patients who returned at 1- or 2-year follow-up with recurrence of symptoms [12].

Park et al. published a prospective study of 58 patients who underwent similar RF neurotomy on the posterior primary ramus for low back pain of more than 3 months' duration, with or without nonradicular radiation to the buttock and hip. The mean VAS score decreased from 6.57 to 1.48 on the third day after treatment, to 1.79 at 3 months, with a total duration of follow-up of 6 months [13].

Van Kleef et al. presented a randomized, double-blind control trial that included patients with chronic low back pain of more than 12 months' duration and required patients to have at least 50% pain relief from a diagnostic dorsal ramus nerve block prior to undergoing neurotomy or percutaneous RF ablation of the medial dorsal nerve root. In the placebo group, a sham procedure was included in which the electrodes were introduced but no RF generated. Differences in effect on the VAS scores (4.1 points), global perceived effect, and the Oswestry disability scale were statistically significant between the groups and favored denervation [10].

Jeong presented a retrospective study of 52 consecutive patients undergoing endoscopic RF ablation of the medial branch in cases with chronic low back pain originating from facet joints. They determined that patients had improved VAS scores and reduced ODI scores 26.5% to 7.7% postoperatively, and 80% of patients reported being satisfied with the procedure at a 24-month follow-up. They did not report any complications [9].

In 2005, there were three randomized controlled trials evaluating RF neurotomy, two showing improvement with treatment and one showing no difference but noting that these studies differed in patient selection criteria and RF ablation techniques, as well as in measured outcome [14].

In one retrospective cohort study, a total of 42 patients (25 women and 17 men) were followed for an average of 3.5 years. These patients had clinical signs of zygapophysial joint involvement, had failed conservative treatment, and had a favorable response to a diagnostic medial branch block or zygapophysial joint injection [15]. Patients had symptom durations ranging from 5 months to 45 years. The identified subjects underwent RF denervation from 1998 to 2006. Fifty-two percent of patients reported a successful outcome with improved function at a minimum follow-up period of 2 years (mean 3.5 years, range 2–8.8 years). Patients in the failure group were more likely to be older and have moderate to severe neuroforaminal stenosis (77.8%) compared to patients in the success group (24.2%). From this information, the authors concluded that RF denervation in selected patients with chronic zygapophysial joint-mediated low back pain provides long-term reduction in pain and improved function with minimum morbidity. In order to truly evaluate the effectiveness of this method, we need additional randomized control trials, ideally with a sham procedure as control.

Complications of dorsal rhizotomy can include the theoretical development of a "Charcot-type" facet joint, weakness of the multifidus paraspinal musculature, muscle soreness, progressive thoracolumbar kyphosis, infection, or recurrence of axial back pain at the same or adjacent levels. These complications are not well-quantified in the literature.

Ideally, the use of endoscopically assisted dorsal rhizotomy could be expanded for additional applications, including pain at other levels in the spine or sacroiliac joint pain. The short- and long-term results need better characterization and identification of complications through larger studies and, ideally, randomized controlled trials comparing conservative therapy, medial branch blocks, and endoscopically assisted dorsal rhizotomy.

REFERENCES

1. Ghormley R. Low back pain with special reference to the articular facets with presentation of an operative procedure. *JAMA*. 1933;101:10773–10777.
2. Manchikanti L, Singh V, Vilims BD, Hansen HC, Schultz DM, Kloth DS. Medial branch neurotomy in management of chronic spinal pain: systematic review of the evidence. *Pain Physician*. 2002;5(4):405–418.
3. McLaughlin JF, Bjornson KF, Astley SJ, et al. Selective dorsal rhizotomy: efficacy and safety in an investigator-masked randomized clinical trial. *Dev Med Child Neurol*. 1998;40(4):220–232.
4. Rees WS. Multiple bilateral percutaneous rhizolysis. *Med J Aust*. 1975;1(17):536–537.
5. Shealy CN. Percutaneous radiofrequency denervation of spinal facets. Treatment for chronic back pain and sciatica. *J Neurosurg*. 1975;43(4):448–451.
6. McCulloch JA. Percutaneous radiofrequency lumbar rhizolysis (rhizotomy). *Appl Neurophysiol*. 1976;39(2):87–96.

7. Schwarzer AC, Derby R, Aprill CN, Fortin J, Kine G, Bogduk N. The value of the provocation response in lumbar zygapophyseal joint injections. *Clin J Pain.* 1994;10(4):309–313.

8. Zhou LCDS, Zhenai Shao. Anatomy of dorsal ramus nerves and its implications in lower back pain. *Neurosci Med.* 2012;3:192–201.

9. Jeong SY, Kim JS, Choi WS, Hur JW, Ryu KS. The effectiveness of endoscopic radiofrequency denervation of medial branch for treatment of chronic low back pain. *J Korean Neurosurg Soc.* 2014;56(4):338–343.

10. van Kleef M, Barendse GA, Kessels A, Voets HM, Weber WE, de Lange S. Randomized trial of radiofrequency lumbar facet denervation for chronic low back pain. *Spine (Phila Pa 1976).* 1999;24(18):1937–1942.

11. Siddiqi FMJAR, Victor Hayes, MD, Casey O'Donnell. Long-term results of endoscopic dorsal ramus rhizotomy and anatomic variations of the painful lumbar facet joint. *Spine J.* 2013;13(9):S161.

12. Yeung A, Gore S. Endoscopically guided foraminal and dorsal rhizotomy for chronic axial back pain based on cadaver and endoscopically visualized anatomic study. *Int J Spine Surg.* 2014;8.

13. Park SJ, Ji C, Kwon JY, Ha KY. The effect of radiofrequency neurotomy on chronic low back pain. *Asian Spine J.* 2007;1(2):88–90.

14. Hooten WM, Martin DP, Huntoon MA. Radiofrequency neurotomy for low back pain: evidence-based procedural guidelines. *Pain Med.* 2005;6(2):129–138.

15. Manejias EM, Hu J, Tatli Y, Lutz GE. Lumbar zygapophysial joint radiofrequency denervation: a long-term clinical outcome study. *HSS J.* 2008;4(2):180–187.

17 Advances in Dorsal Column Stimulation

Chirag D. Shah and Maunak V. Rana

INTRODUCTION

Low back pain with or without prior surgical intervention is a disease process that plagues much of the population. It is estimated that 84% of adults experience low back pain at some point in their lives [1,2]. This condition is often self-limited; however, in some cases, it can persist for longer than 12 weeks and become a chronic illness. As a potential cure for this debilitating condition, electrical stimulation of the dorsal column of the spinal cord for pain relief was first used on humans in 1967 [3]. There have been many theories that postulate the mechanism by which spinal cord stimulation (SCS) is effective for pain relief since the presentation of the hypothetical gate theory in 1965 by Melzack and Wall [4]. Despite a clear understanding of its mechanism of action, the use of SCS has continued to grow with evidence grade B for failed back surgery (FBBS) and grade A for complex regional pain syndrome type I (CRPS), as well as ischemic pain either due to peripheral vascular or coronary artery disease [5–7]. Additionally, SCS has been successful in treating other chronic pain conditions such as diabetic neuropathy, postherpetic neuralgia, chronic angina, visceral abdominal pain from chronic pancreatitis [8–11], and other gastrointestinal entities as seen in Table 17.1.

HISTORY OF SPINAL CORD STIMULATION

It was initially suggested that a "gate" existed in the dorsal horn of the spinal cord that regulated the perception and transmission of pain, according to the theory of Melzack and Wall [4]. Noxious stimuli from the skin, muscles, joints, and internal organs are recorded at peripheral pain receptors and traverse to the dorsal root ganglion (DRG). Here, the peripheral nerves converge to become the wide dynamic range neuron. Activation of small fibers in the peripheral nervous system (PNS) open the "gate," whereas activation of large fibers close the "gate." More specifically, stimulation of myelinated Aβ fibers inhibit pain transmission whereas stimulation of thinly

Table 17.1 Select pain syndromes treated with spinal cord stimulation

Indications

Neuropathic Pain	Visceral Pain	Vascular Pain	Potential Indications
Failed back surgery syndrome	Chronic Pancreatitis	Angina pectoris	Brachial plexus injury
Complex regional pain syndrome I and II	Irritable bowel syndrome	Peripheral arterial disease	Spinal cord injury
Radicular pain			Polyneuropathy
Nerve root pain			Postaneurysmal subarachnoid hemorrhage
Postherpetic neuralgia			
Peripheral nerve injury pain			
Intercostal neuralgia			
Phantom limb pain			
Occipital neuralgia			

myelinated Aδ and unmyelinated C fibers enhance pain transmission [12]. Using this theory, investigators began implanting spinal cord stimulators to selectively excite large-diameter fibers and ultimately reduce the perception of pain by masking the nociceptive sensation. This theory, however, had several drawbacks that became apparent as the technology evolved. For example, both acute and chronic pain should be affected by SCS, but only chronic pain appears to improve with treatment. In addition, this theory does not fully explain why there is continuous pain relief with periods of stimulation cessation. There are likely other factors, including neurochemical modulation of glutamate, γ-aminobutyric acid (GABA), and acetylcholine that are affected by SCS. Finally, supraspinal centers likely also play a role in chronic pain relief [12]. Further investigation into the mechanism of action is needed and warranted.

ANATOMIC BASIS FOR SPINAL CORD STIMULATION

Once it was discovered that the spinal cord was able to send messages from the brain to the peripheral muscles and back via a loop pathway, it was only a matter of time before theories and experiments began on how to control and modulate those signals. In a preliminary clinical report, Shealy noted that peripheral nerve stimulation led to a focal analgesic effect in an animal model [13]. This finding was repeated and confirmed in multiple trials. To determine if this result could be extrapolated to humans, he persuaded a 70-year-old man with inoperable metastatic bronchogenic cancer and intractable right lower chest and upper abdominal pain to undergo an experimental spinal cord stimulator trial. After successful implantation, the patient was noted to be pain free, but with the presence of paresthesias. Periodic adjustments in the frequency of the stimulator provided better analgesic coverage. Unfortunately, the patient died

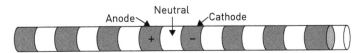

FIGURE 17.1 Depiction of SCS electrode lead where current flows from cathode to anode. Image courtesy of Abbott (formerly St. Jude).

2 days later from a left-sided embolic stroke due to undiagnosed subacute endocarditis. The blessing in the unfortunate outcome of this case report was the realization that pain could be modulated by spinal cord stimulation without affecting other sensory inputs [13].

From a mathematical perspective, Holsheimer used empirical and computer modeling data to describe the recruitment pattern of nerves in the spinal cord after stimulation [14]. He noted that the current between two electrodes placed in the epidural space will flow from cathode to anode and take the path of least resistance, as seen Figure 17.1. After calculating the resistance of the different parts of the spine and concluding that the cerebrospinal fluid (CSF) has the least resistance, he found that 90% of the current will flow via the CSF and 10% via the spinal cord [14]. After quantifying the range of stimulation that could be used to provide paresthesias but not discomfort, he was able to determine the size of the nerves and nerve tracts that would be affected. Generally, large myelinated fibers in the dorsal column and dorsal roots are likely to be targeted by the stimulus, as seen Figure 17.2. This therapeutic stimulus range will likely be limited to a 0.2–0.25 mm of depth into the dorsal layer and affect Aβ fibers [14].

Knowing the optimal stimulus range along with the depth of penetration can help guide clinicians in the placement of SCS electrodes that optimally target the dorsal column of the spinal cord. These dorsal column fibers are organized in a lamellated fashion representing caudal to rostral structures in a medial to lateral pattern [15]. Thus, the sacral and perineal areas have their sensory organization in the most medial

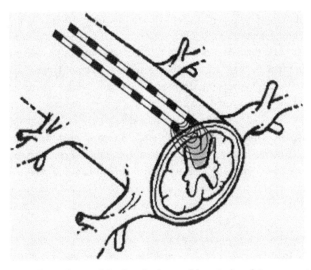

FIGURE 17.2 Targeted stimulation of the dorsal column of the spinal cord. Image courtesy of Abbott (formerly St. Jude).

and caudal aspect of the dorsal column. As nerve fibers progress laterally and rostrally, coverage of more proximal levels occur [15]. The leads are optimally placed midline in the epidural space under radiographic guidance to stimulate the fibers of targeted dermatomes. An appropriately placed lead will reproduce sensation in the targeted ipsilateral and caudal dermatome. An important consideration in lead placement is keeping in mind the morphology of the spinal cord within the spinal canal at a particular level and the amount of CSF surrounding the spinal cord. CSF thickness is least in the cervical spine, peaks at the mid-thoracic level, and then continues to taper down. Furthermore, the spinal cord sits medially in the spinal canal at the upper thoracic level, more ventrally at the mid-thoracic level, and again more medially in the lower thoracic level based on the curvature of the spine. CSF acts as a natural impeder of current so that spinal levels with greater CSF thickness will require greater stimulation. Finally, SCS has been found to be less effective on peripheral nerves [15]. Since the spinal cord generally ends after the level of L1, it would be ill-advised to place leads below that level.

SCS leads are commonly placed between T8 and T11 for low back and leg pain. As noted earlier, the nerve fibers for proximal levels are located medial to the dorsal roots which enter the spinal cord via the dorsolateral sulcus. As stimulation propagates through the CSF laterally, the targeted dorsal column nerve fibers will be activated at essentially the same time as the similarly situated dorsal roots. Since the dorsal roots are larger, they are preferentially targeted. Clinically, the patient will feel an uncomfortable radicular thoracic stimulation rather than the preferred low back paresthesia [16]. To remedy this problem, Strujik and Holsheimer devised a new "transverse tripolar" stimulation paradigm [16]. Laterally placed anodes would hyperpolarize the dorsal roots, making them difficult to activate, while the centrally placed cathode would provide deeper and more medial penetration of the dorsal column [16]. This theoretical model has been proved clinically and used for the treatment of neuropathic pain [17].

SELECT INDICATIONS

Pain is a critically important defense mechanism that alerts the human body against harmful stimuli; however, when nerve pathways become chronically irritated, it can lead to debilitating consequences for the individual. The Spinal Cord Injury Pain Task Force of the International Association of the Study of Pain (IASP) has proposed a taxonomy approach with three tiers to distinguish the different types of pain [18]. The first tier encompasses neuropathic and nociceptive pain. Nociceptive pain results from stimulation of the somatic or visceral system. It is generally associated with trauma or inflammation unrelated to a sensory or motor deficit [19]. Pain is often characterized as dull, aching, or stabbing. In contrast, the IASP defines neuropathic pain as a pain caused by a lesion leading to a dysfunction of the somatosensory system. Thus, this pain is usually associated with sensory disturbances including numbness or paresthesia. Patients will often describe this pain as burning, electric, and shooting. Patients with neuropathic pain are often more negatively impacted with symptoms of insomnia, anxiety, and depression [12].

Barring any contradictions as seen in Table 17.2, SCS constitutes an alternative approach to the treatment pain. SCS has a better impact on pain relief for neuropathic versus nociceptive pain [12]. Regardless of which type of pain is being treated, an SCS trial can still be justified.

Table 17.2 Contraindications to spinal cord stimulation

Contraindications	
Somatic	*Psychiatric*
Sepsis	Psychosis
Coagulopathy	Schizophrenia
Infection	Substance abuse
Inability to understand patient duties in SCS	Severe depression/anxiety
Complete destruction of spinal cord	

Radicular pain secondary to lumbar disc surgery (FBSS) is one of the most common and well-studied indications for SCS [20] FBSS is a common sequelae in roughly 30% of patients after lumbar disc surgery [12]. In the past, FBSS was often treated with reoperation. North et al. set out to determine whether SCS was a better alternative for pain reduction. Fifty patients who would normally undergo reoperation by standardized criteria were randomized between the two groups and prospectively monitored for 3 years [21]. After treatment, they had the option to cross over if they felt that their treatment was unsatisfactory. Of the 90% available for follow-up, there was a statistically significant improvement in pain control within the SCS group over the reoperation group [21]. Furthermore, there was a larger proportion of patients in the reoperation group who crossed over to the SCS group ($P = 0.02$). However, there was no apparent difference in work status or in measures of activities of daily living between the two groups [21].

A randomized trial conducted by Kumar et al. attempted to compare the efficacy of conventional therapy alone versus conventional therapy with SCS for the treatment of FBSS. One hundred patients with predominantly radicular leg pain underwent one of the two options with the ability to cross over after 6 months of treatment [22]. Successful treatment was defined as greater than 50% pain improvement. Forty-eight percent of patients had a successful measure in the SCS group versus 9% in the conventional therapy group alone at 6 months. There was also a higher crossover rate from conventional therapy to SCS at 6 months primarily because of inadequate pain control. SCS has significant therapeutic benefit in the treatment of FBSS [22].

Another well-studied indication for SCS is CRPS I and II. CRPS is a debilitating clinical condition characterized by pain out of proportion to the inciting injury and a variable combination of signs and symptoms: sensory, vasomotor, sudomotor, trophic, and motor dysfunction. CRPS can be a difficult ailment to treat, but the use of SCS provides significant pain reduction in its patients. A systematic review of the literature has shown high-level (randomized control trial) evidence for its use in CRPS in lieu of patient-perceived pain relief, pain score improvement, quality of life, and satisfaction [23]. Evidence for functional status improvement and psychological effects, however, were inconclusive and will require further investigation. Finally, outcomes regarding both sleep hygiene and resolution of CRPS signs emanated from low-quality research, making conclusions difficult [23].

Visceral pain refers to pain from an ongoing insult to internal organs or the tissue that surrounds them. Sometimes poorly localized, the pain is often characterized as deep, aching, cramping, or stabbing. SCS has found promise in treating certain visceral conditions like chronic pancreatitis. A quadripolar SCS electrode was inserted from T8 to T10 in two patients with intractable pain secondary to chronic pancreatitis. At the 7-year follow-up, they endorsed an 80% and 90% reduction in pain as assessed by the visual analogue scale (VAS) [24]. Sphincter of Oddi dysfunction (SOD), sometimes a sequela of chronic pancreatitis, occurs when the pancreaticoduodenal flow is obstructed from scarring or spasm of the sphincter. This condition can manifest itself as abdominal pain that is very difficult to remedy. A patient with intractable abdominal pain from SOD was treated with a spinal cord stimulator implanted from T5 to T7. Follow-up after 6 months showed a reduction in pain according to the VAS and a decrease in opioid medication use [25]. Although encouraging, further long-term and randomized control studies are needed to determine the effectiveness of SCS in these visceral conditions.

In irritable bowel syndrome (IBS) cases where conservative treatment fails, SCS may be a valid consideration. IBS is a disorder commonly affecting bowel transit times in susceptible patients who describe cramping, bloating, abdominal pain, gas, and/or constipation/diarrhea. A tripolar SCS implanted at the T8 level in a 36-year-old man with an 8-year history of sharp abdominal pain compounded by thoracic spine pain secondary to scoliosis led to an abatement of his symptoms [26]. The theory behind this case study was expanded into a randomized crossover study done by Lind et al. They noted that SCS in animal studies reduced bowel distention, which is known to be increased in IBS. Ten patients were implanted with a four-polar electrode at the levels of T5–T8. At the end of the trial, patients with the SCS were found to have reduced pain levels during stimulation, fewer pain attacks, and fewer reported episodes of diarrhea [27]. Thus, SCS may be a minimally invasive treatment option to improve abdominal pain, normalize bowel habits, and improve quality of life in patients suffering from IBS.

When targeting visceral pain, electrodes are generally placed between T5 and T8. Due to the kyphotic curvature of the spine, the spinal cord sits more anteriorly in the spinal canal. Thus, dorsal column stimulation has to travel through more CSF to reach its destination. In lieu of the extra impedance from CSF at this level, higher stimulation intensities are required to achieve analgesia and functional alterations of visceral function. Baranidharan noticed that his patients sometimes had more difficulty tolerating this higher intensity, especially at night when posture and pressure changed the perceived stimulus [28]. His group conducted a retrospective study assessing the benefits of ventral column stimulation for the treatment of visceral neuropathic pain. Since there is animal study evidence that nociceptive visceral information ascends the spinal cord in both the dorsal midline and lateral spinal pathways, they felt that ventral column stimulation may have better access to the latter and result in good pain control. Twenty-six patients were observed in this study with a statistically significant improvement in the visual analogue pain score and a reduction of opioid consumption. Patients reported improvement in functional activities of daily living and quality of life. Of note, there was a lower energy requirement for SCS in the ventral column SCS versus the dorsal column, the circumventing the prior greater energy requirements [28]. Although the authors did not comment on any complications, patients may be subject to dural irritation and increased paresthesias with ventral placement of leads and tonic stimulation.

SCS has successfully been utilized to treat a number of neuropathic pain conditions. Studies investigating its efficacy in postherpetic neuralgia have been encouraging.

A prospective study over 29 months showed 23/28 patients with a 2-year history of intractable pain reporting its near complete resolution [9].

Initial studies for the treatment of painful diabetic polyneuropathy with SCS have had promising results. A systematic review of three prospective case series and one retrospective cohort study revealed a greater than 50% pain reduction in 63% of patients after 1 year of treatment with SCS. Furthermore, no adverse events were noted [29].

Advances in medicine and longer patient lives inevitably lead to more unique medical complications and their sequela. Among them are patients who continue to complain of chest pain secondary to objective cardiac ischemia despite optimal medical and surgical management. Many of these patients are status post revascularization with percutaneous coronary intervention (PCI) or coronary artery bypass graft (CABG), and further procedural intervention for pain control would be futile. These patients are diagnosed with refractory angina pectoris. Studies have shown that SCS is good adjunct therapy to medical management for this population. There is a statistically significant decrease in anginal severity, fewer anginal episodes, and increased exercise threshold and tolerance, as well as a reduction in nitrate use. Furthermore, these benefits are secondary to an antiischemic effect versus placebo [30–32].

The mechanism of action for this anti-ischemic effect is not well understood. However, most theories postulate that SCS causes a vasodilatory effect on vasculature by modulating either phosphodiesterase-5, prostaglandin production, upregulation of nitric oxide, or regulation of the sympathetic nervous system. Many studies have proved the efficacy of using SCS in this way for the treatment of peripheral vascular disease (PVD). This therapy is generally reserved for patients with viable limbs who have end-stage PVD refractory to medical management and are nonamenable to surgery [33]. Vasodilation of the cerebral vessels via cervical SCS has opened up a realm of possibilities. Yin et al. has proposed the use of SCS for the prevention and management of cerebral vasospasm after aneurysmal subacute hemorrhage (SAH). Research shows that the vascular tone changes may be the result of decreased nitric oxide (NO) production. Thus, if SCS leads to increased cerebral blood flow via upregulation of NO, then SCS could logically be an excellent treatment modality [34]. More controlled double-blind and randomized studies, however, are required to demonstrate safety and efficacy for this indication.

INNOVATION

In its simplest form, spinal cord stimulators consist of stimulating electrodes, a pulse generator and its controls, and wires that connect the two. Historically, spinal cord stimulators involved the placement of four contact percutaneous leads in the epidural space. This system was beneficial for treating leg pain, but not axial back pain. Furthermore, single leads were prone to dislodgement with patient movement. Studies showed that using multiple columns of electrodes (paddle leads) produced more comprehensive pain coverage that was less influenced by patient posture and movement. Paddle leads, however, require more invasive surgery (laminotomy or laminectomy) [35]. The procedure has a longer recovery period and is considered more painful than percutaneous lead placement. Certain techniques have now been developed for placement of paddle leads percutaneously to avoid complications from a more invasive approach [35]. Overall, the number of options has dramatically increased with multiple contact leads in a wide array of spacing with both percutaneous and paddle leads, allowing for a variety of programming options.

Traditionally, generators were nonrechargeable and with a relatively short battery life. They have evolved into rechargeable pulse generators with longer battery duration. The benefit of a rechargeable pulse generator is that it can run multiple programs concurrently as well as expend energy for high-intensity stimulation without draining the life span of the battery. Generators have become more than just a power supply. Some now have an embedded accelerometer that monitors a patient's mobility patterns and postural changes. It has been shown that different positions (lying, sitting, standing) lead to changes in stimulation impedances [36]. This results in variable pain coverage. By utilizing this information, generators can automatically modify stimulation intensities and optimize patient preferences [37,38]. Schade conducted a 15-person study that yielded greater patient satisfaction with automatic stimulation versus manual stimulation [36]. A larger 79-person study corroborated these same findings and also noted increased patient convenience with automatic stimulation changes [39].

Having open ports during SCS trials as well as the medical complications inherent with creating a pocket to implant the generator subjects a patient to possible additional failure of a system and/or revision of the generator site after the finite span of the generator function. This time-dependent ending of generator function leads to a future procedure for "swapping" out the battery, which involves an incision to remove the old battery, insert a new battery, and close the prior wound. Using a multicontact lead containing a wireless telemetry unit and energy receiver would bypass the need for an implanted generator [40]. Rather, an externally worn device would serve as the power source for this system, as seen in Figure 17.3. This device has been certified Magnetic Resonance Imaging (MRI) Conditional based on testing with 1.5 and 3 Tesla MRI magnets [41].

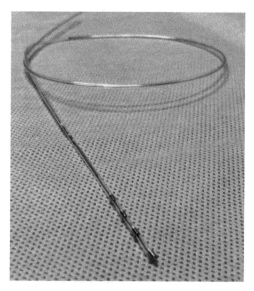

FIGURE 17.3 Multicontact lead containing a wireless telemetry unit and energy receiver. Image courtesy of Stimwave Technologies Incorporated.

TECHNIQUES

Several different SCS platforms have been implemented as the technology has evolved. Electrical stimulation to the spinal cord via an implantable pulse generator (IPG) can utilize two different power sources: constant current (CC) or constant voltage (CV). Having a basic understanding of Ohm's Law (Voltage = I [current] × R [resistance-impedance]) can illuminate the distinction between the two systems. CC supplies a current to the spinal cord by adjusting the voltage based on impedance to flow resulting from scar tissue, lead positioning, or patient posturing. CV supplies a constant current irrespective of impedance, potentially resulting in variable voltage levels sent to the spinal cord [42]. Therefore, changes in impedance can change the stimulation strength during the interstimulus pulse [43]. Depending on what level of impudence is detected when calibrating the device, this can also affect battery life of the SCS as well as effectiveness of the stimulation [44]. How does this translate to the patient? Recent evidence has shown that more patients seem to prefer CC rather than CV stimulation. In Washburn et al., a group of 30 patients were evaluated with the two different systems while measuring patient pain relief, quality of life, and patient satisfaction. This randomized and double-blinded study concluded that both systems produce paresthesias, and both provide significant and comparable pain relief, improved quality of life, and patient satisfaction; however, 70% of the group still preferred the sensation that CC provided to CV stimulation [42]. It should be pointed out that the study was performed by a neuromodulation company whose device is a CC platform system.

Traditional SCS devices are generally capable of delivering pulse frequencies that range from 2 to 1,200 Hz, with most typically set at 40 to 60 Hz [45]. Patients generally perceive pulse frequencies less than 300 Hz as a tingling sensation [46]. The goal of using these low-frequency SCS devices is to produce the aforementioned paresthesia in the specific pain distribution so as to mask the pain perception [45]. In order for traditional SCS devices to be effective, intraoperative paresthesia mapping is required. Here, patients actively provide feedback regarding pain relief and comfort level while adjustment of stimulation location, pulse frequency, pulse width, and pulse amplitude occurs [45]. Thus, SCS success depends on its ability to provide a continuous and adequate stimulation that the patient can tolerate. Some patients may not be able to tolerate this sensation or would prefer not to feel any paresthesias [47].

With this select population in mind, experimentation with a complex rather than monotonous mode began [48]. Research has shown that certain neurons in the central nervous system including the spinal cord fire in bursts followed by periods of latency, whereas others fire continuously [49]. *Burst stimulation* involves neurostimulation that is delivered in quanta of energy rather than tonically. Animal studies showed that burst firing was more powerful than tonic continuous firing in activating the cerebral cortex [49]. In lieu of this, de Riddler et al. used burst stimulation on 12 patients in whom a 40 Hz pulse with 5 spikes at 500 Hz per burst was administered to patients with surgically implanted electrodes. Only 17% of individuals experienced paresthesias under this model rather than 92% with conventional stimulation [49]. Furthermore, there was equivalent if not more analgesic effect with this complex mode [49]. Given the average 2-year follow-up, this was the first step in utilizing a technology that provided long-term paresthesia-free analgesia.

As noted earlier, treatment with burst SCS can provide significant pain relief for SCS naïve patients, but what about patients who have already begun treatment with traditional SCS and are acclimated to paresthesia-conjunct analgesia? De Vos et al. studied 48 patients who had already been treated with at least 6 months of tonic stimulation and who were transitioned to 2 weeks of burst stimulation [50]. The burst parameters utilized pulse trains of five high-frequency pulses delivered at 500 Hz, 40 times per second and with a pulse width of 1 msec. These patients were being treated for painful diabetic neuropathy (PDN), FBSS, and FBSS patients who eventually became poor responders (PR) to SCS. The authors noted that there was statistically significant additional pain relief in 48% of patients with PND and 28% for FBSS. Patients in the PR group benefited less from burst stimulation. Side effects included headaches, dizziness, and the sensation of "heavy legs." Some patients preferred the tonic stimulation because the paresthesias reminded them that the device was working. Overall, 60% of the patients received additional pain relief with burst stimulation over tonic stimulation despite having started with traditional SCS [50]. Thus, good analgesia is achievable for both patients who are naïve to SCS and those who are tolerant to the effects of SCS.

As prior studies have shown, SCS has been proved and used for the treatment of neuropathic pain. Furthermore, the American Society of Anesthesiologists and the American Society of Regional Anesthesia and Pain Medicine recommend it [51]. Animal studies have shown that traditional SCS (50–100 Hz) improves pain-like behavior induced by nerve and muscle injury. There is evidence that even lower frequencies (4 Hz) also reduce pain-like behavior [51]. This begs the question of whether there are different mechanisms of action that provide analgesia at different frequencies. If so, further investigation into each type of frequency for different causes and types of pain may be worthwhile. Gong et al. set out to do just that. They designed an animal study to analyze the effectiveness of different frequencies in the modulation of neuropathic pain with a variety of burst modes. This study corroborated older studies in finding pain relief at 500 and 1,000 Hz (high frequency) but also noted that there was similar paw hyperalgesia at 60 Hz as well. SCS at high pulse frequencies also restored physical activity levels more than tonic stimulation, suggesting the possibility of reduced pain-related disability [51].

There appears to be promise that kilohertz-frequency spinal cord stimulation (KHF-SCS) can provide paresthesia-free treatment for chronic pain [52]. The mechanism of action by which this treatment works, unfortunately, is not fully understood. The objective of the study done by Crosby et al. was to evaluate and quantify the activation and conduction block of the dorsal column axons by high-frequency stimulation across a range of frequencies from 1 to 20 kHz with biphasic or sinusoidal waveforms [52]. This was an animal study in which platinum electrodes delivered SCS to the T10–T11 dorsal columns of anesthetized male Sprague-Dawley rats while researchers recorded single dorsal column axons and compound action potentials to evaluate its evoked activity. Measurements were similar across a range of frequencies (5–20 kHz) and waveforms (biphasic and sinusoidal). Stimulation at 1 kHz evoked more phase-synchronous axonal firing at amplitudes above the motor threshold. The authors asserted that, in lieu of the asynchronous and transient nature of dorsal column activity, the mechanism of analgesia for HF-SCS is likely different from that for persistent and periodic dorsal column activity in tonic stimulation [52].

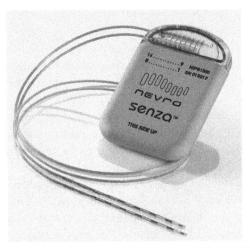

FIGURE 17.4 SENZA SCS system. Image Courtesy of Nevro Corp. SENZA, HF10, Nevro, and the Nevro logo are trademarks of Nevro Corp.

A new SCS system that delivers stimulation up to 10,000 Hz has sparked interest in a new paradigm in SCS. The HF10 therapy system, as seen in Figure 17.4 (Nevro, Redwood City, CA) has been implemented in Europe for several years and has now reached the United States. HF10 therapy delivers short-duration (30 μsec), high-frequency (10 kHz), low-amplitude (1–5 mA) pulses to the T8–T11 (for back and leg pain) spinal epidural space [45]. Results have been promising in that patients obtain relief without the need for paresthesias. The economic benefits of this procedure are evident in that patients have fewer opioid requirements. Furthermore, this eliminates the need for paresthesia mapping as in traditional SCS systems, which may improve the predictability of the implant operative time. In patients with chronic low back pain, previous prospective but nonrandomized studies have shown clinically significant improvement in back and leg pain, functional status, overall sleep, and opioid use reduction that can last for up to 24 months [53]. The objective of this prospective and multicenter study was to determine the long-term efficacy and safety of high-frequency SCS. The study enrolled 82 subjects with chronic low back pain to be implanted with HF-SCS with two leads positioned midline between T8 and T11 without paresthesia mapping. After the trial period, 88% of patients reported significant improvement in pain scores and underwent permanent implantation. There was a statistically significant mean reduction in back pain from 8.4 ± 0.1 cm to 3.3 ± 0.1 cm and leg pain from 5.4 ± 0.1 cm to 2.3 ± 0.1 cm [53]. Furthermore, there was a reduction in opioid use and improvement in sleep disturbances, which may be attributed to HF-SCS being paresthesia-free. It was noted that the battery for these devices needed to be charged more frequently; however, the benefits from the device seemed to outweigh this drawback in the opinions of the patients [53]. Additionally, 86.1% of the enrolled subjects had primary back pain versus 13.9% with leg pain [53]. Traditional SCS, in contrast, was predominantly used to treat leg pain. With such a high pain improvement rate, HF-SCS opens the door for treating a broader spectrum of chronic pain patients. Adverse events were noted to be similar to those with traditional SCS as well. Pocket pain was the leading adverse event at 8.4% [53]. It is possible that a change in the device design may lower this percentage. Given that HF-SCS is paresthesia-free, randomized, double-blinded, and more controlled study designs are possible.

The SENZA-RCT provided the first scientifically rigorous, randomized, and controlled study that demonstrated the superiority of the HF10 system over traditional SCS devices with respect to chronic back and leg pain relief [45]. Additionally, this study also corroborated previous study results. This study included 198 subjects with both leg and back pain who were trialed and, if successful, were implanted with a high-frequency (10,000 Hz) system or with a low-frequency (50 Hz) system. At 3 months, there was a statistically significant and clinically meaningful benefit seen with patients using the high-frequency system. For back pain, the responder rate was 84.5% for the HF10 therapy group versus 43.8% for the traditional SCS group. For leg pain, the responder rate was 83.1% for the HF10 group versus 55.1% for the traditional SCS group. Although not the primary measurement, there was a 35.5% reduction in pain medication use with the HF10 therapy devices versus 26.4% with the traditional SCS devices at the 12-month follow-up [45]. Using Oswestry Disability Index (ODI) for the measurement of patient disability, HF10 therapy systems had a clinically significant reduction in disability compared to traditional SCS [45]. Patient satisfaction improved with both SCS devices, but the HF10 therapy cohort had a clinically significant satisfaction rating of 55.84% versus 31.9% for traditional SCS [45]. In regards to safety, both HF10 and traditional SCS had a low incidence of adverse events ranging from 4% to 7.2% over a 12-month period, with no stimulation-related neurologic deficits [45]. Lead migration is typically the most common complication of SCS, with rates ranging from 2.1% to 23% [54]. In the SENZA-RCT trial, lead migration was comparatively low compared with previous publications (3.0–5.2%), likely secondary to improved technique, advancement in technology, and better patient selection [45].

The DRG is a readily accessible neuraxial structure that is crucial in the propagation and modulation of neuropathic painful states. The DRG stimulation system involves placement of electrical leads into the epidural space, as seen in Figure 17.5.

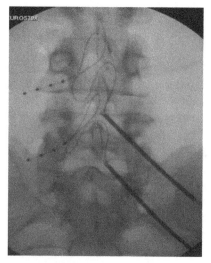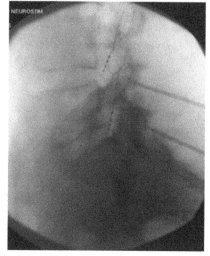

FIGURE 17.5 Anteroposterior (AP) and lateral views of dorsal root ganglion (DRG) stimulation lead placement. Image Courtesy of Maged Guirguis, MD.

Table 17.3 Common complications of spinal cord stimulation

Complications	
Mechanical	*Nonmechanical*
Lead migration	Hematoma
Lead breakage	Seroma
Connection failure	Infection
Battery depletion	CSF leak
Unwanted paresthesia	New neurological deficits
Pain at the generator incision site	

The ultimate target, the DRG, is accessed via the intervertebral foramen. The benefit of stimulation at the DRG includes selective stimulation of different nerve root fibers that traverse the DRG. Additionally, due to decreased cerebrospinal fluid present at the DRG, there is less variability of stimulation based on patient movement. The technology is also efficient, with less amplitude of stimulation required for capture, which leads to a longer generator life and solves a common complication of SCS, as noted in Table 17.3. The DRG comprises primary sensory neurons divided into type A and B neurons [55]. Type A neurons are responsible for touch, vibration, and proprioception. Type B neurons are responsible for nociception. Type B neurons are more prevalent than type A neurons, with a ratio of 71:29. The DRG is an excellent site of stimulation after nerve injury as the damaged DRG neurons become hyperexcitable. This leads to genetic changes, with increased expression of c-fos and c-jun, proto-oncogenes after injury. Additionally, there are chemical changes related to ion channels. DRG stimulation is believed to cause vasodilation of the periphery, stabilization of peripheral nociceptors, release of dorsal horn neuromodulators, and activation of wide dynamic range neurons [55]. Supraspinal centers are believed to be activated along with downregulation of ion channels. Furthermore, stimulation will stabilize the microglia involved in releasing cytokine nociceptive signaling compounds [55]. The aforementioned changes that occur with DRG stimulation result in improved pain scores compared to conventional lead placement. Finally, an unexpected effect in some patients includes improvement in mood scores as well [56].

Peripheral stimulation has a long-standing history of utility for various pain states [57]. Both peripheral nerve stimulation (PNS) and peripheral nerve field stimulation (PNFS) have proven beneficial. In PNS, a surgical incision is made and an electrode is placed directly over the nerve. In PNFS, the electrode is placed subcutaneously in the general area of pain. According to a 22-patient retrospective study done by Law et al., there was an improvement in chronic pain using PNS. They noted that the experience of the surgeon may be tied to the rate of success in PNS [58]. This process was later modified into PNFS, which was traditionally used to treat occipital neuralgia due to various cephalgias [59,60–62]. The scope of its use is growing to include well-localized areas of pain involving the abdomen, inguinal region, pelvis, occipital area, as well as postoperative orthopedic surgery and low back pain [63–66]. To widen the area of stimulation and improve pain control, multiple PNFS leads can be placed far apart from each other and still form a circuit. This cross-talk was proved by Falco in a cadaveric study [67]. The safety and accuracy of this treatment is improved with the use of ultrasound guidance. It allows the physician to use real-time imaging to differentiate the tissue layers, avoid vasculature, and visualize the targeted nerve for optimal placement of the stimulating electrode [68,69].

COMBINED SYSTEMS

As has been alluded to earlier, pain is a complex symptom that can often have multiple triggers or causes. For example, FBSS can often present with both nociceptive and neuropathic pain components, making it difficult to treat with one option alone. Chodakiewitz attempted to use two different modalities to treat the two different pain components. A case of both nociceptive axial back pain and bilateral neuropathic leg pain in a patient with past surgical history significant for 14 failed back surgeries was presented. SCS was used for the neuropathic component and deep brain stimulation of the periventricular gray for the nociceptive component. Both pain components completely resolved and have remained dormant after 22 years of follow-up [70].

One of the shortcomings of SCS is its difficulty in treating axial back pain. A new treatment approach utilizing SCS in concert with a variation to PNS has been bolstered. Instead of implanting the electrode directly over the nerve, as in PNS, it is placed subcutaneously over the painful area. This new method is termed PNFS. Mironer designed a prospective study combining SCS and PNFS with programming variables in the hopes of improved and broader low back pain coverage [71]. Twenty patients with pain secondary to FBSS and/or spinal stenosis were implanted with SCS and PNFS. The patients were asked to select the best program when tried with SCS alone, PNFS alone, or both methods together. The second group of patients were also implanted with SCS and PNFS. These patients were asked to select the best program when tried with SCS alone, PNFS alone, SCS as a cathode with PNFS as an anode, or SCS as an anode with PNFS as a cathode. Patients in the first group preferred the combined use of SCS and PNFS; in the second group, patients preferred the combined effects of SCS and PNFS via the cathode/anode communication. This latter combination has been termed *spinal-peripheral neurostimulation* (SPN) [71]. Considering the improved pain scores reported by patients, more detailed studies elucidating the mechanism of action and efficacy of SPN are needed. Finally, there appears to be a role in combining multiple treatment modalities for the certain pain syndromes.

MRI COMPATIBILITY

Since its advent in the 1980s, MRI has more frequently been turned to for visualizing soft tissues: organs, nerves, and blood vessels. The human body is mostly composed of water molecules, which are composed of hydrogen ions, or protons. An MRI uses a magnetic field and radio waves to align those protons and create an image. The static magnetic field is generated by a large superconducting magnet, which attracts metal objects to the scanner and aligns protons in the soft tissue. A strong radiofrequency pulse is then sent into the magnetic field to excite the aligned protons. The gradient magnetic field then localizes the energy signals generated by the RF pulses.

MRI has become an indispensable imaging modality in medicine. It is optimally used for the initial diagnosis of multiple sclerosis and malignant brain tumors [72].

However, with improvements in computed tomography (CT) imaging quality and reduced radiation, it is a comparable alternative to MRI in most other conditions. CT is even considered a better imaging modality for the rapid evaluation of hemorrhagic stroke. Having MRI-safe or -conditional spinal cord stimulators is the subject of debate on whether this feature of neuromodulation is essential or a useful adjunct. An "MRI-safe" item is one that poses no hazardous risk when exposed to an MR environment. "MRI-conditional" items are considered safe in an MR environment within defined parameters. Currently, only MRI-conditional spinal cord stimulators exist [72]. According to data presented by one neuromodulation company, a significant number of patients who are eligible for SCS therapy will need at least one MRI over the duration of the SCS lifetime. They further claimed that there was an extremely high proportion of SCS patients who had an MRI-requiring diagnoses [72]. Hayek felt that these claims were speculative and so analyzed data for the incidence of MRI-related explants of in situ spinal cord stimulator systems and found a range of 0.5% to 1.5%. The relative risk of explant of a system due to a required MRI study was 0.047–0.062 [73]. A case series by Moeschler from the Mayo Clinic evaluated 199 patients who were implanted with SCS from January 2001 to December 2011. Thirty-three patients were explanted, and only 4 of the 33 explants were performed due to the requirement for an MRI scan [74].

In the past, patients with SCS were unable to undergo an MRI due to adverse effects resulting therefrom. The radio frequency electrical currents generated by an MRI can heat up the SCS leads, resulting in soft tissue burns and neurologic damage. The spinal cord does not contain neural heat receptors, so the patient may not even feel the heated leads. Radiofrequency energy can be transmitted via the leads to the SCS device and potentially damage it. This can result in a loss of output, loss of communication, loss of recharging, or unintentional program changes. Ultimately, it may even require device explantation. Induced voltage can also cause changes in stimulation. Furthermore, if the device has ferromagnetic material, it can be attracted to the MRI magnet at elevated forces and become dislodged, leading to patient injury. For one reason or another, many patients with SCS require an MRI but end up receiving frequent CT scans that may not adequately visualize their condition. Due to this dilemma, companies have attempted to reconfigure their devices to make them more compatible with MRI. The Surescan by Medtronic has kept these MRI-adverse effects in mind and created a device for which MRI can safely be done in certain conditions [75]. Patients with the Precision Spectra by Boston Scientific can undergo a head MRI without complications [76]. The Protegé MRI by St. Jude Medical has upgraded its software to be compatible with head and extremity MRI [77]. The Senza SCS by Nevro has gone one step further and been approved for scans of the head and extremities with 1.5 and 3.0 Tesla MRI machines [78].

COMPLICATIONS

SCS implantation is considered a safe procedure. When puncturing the spinal canal, there is always an inherent risk of spinal bleeding and neurological deficits. However, the literature only shows six such cases [12]. Given that hundreds of thousands of implantations have been done, this appears to be a small risk.

Just as with other surgeries, there is a risk of infection with SCS implantation. The incidence is between 3.4% and 6% and generally follows an uncomplicated course with lead removal and antibiotics [12].

Unscheduled revisions due to hardware malfunction (lead dislocation, lead breakage, lead connection failures) are fairly high. A systematic review of SCS for the treatment of FBSS or chronic back/leg pain reported a 43% hardware complication rate [79]. Lead migration is the most common complication [12]. As mentioned earlier, paddle leads have a lower rate of lead migration as compared to traditional leads.

SCS malfunction can occur if there are unfavorable interactions with diathermy, cardiac pacemakers, ultrasound, or MRI. As mentioned earlier, MRI can exert forces on the implanted SCS material resulting in hardware complications [12].

CONCLUSION

SCS is a proven and effective treatment modality for neuropathic pain conditions. Initially used for the treatment of low back pain, SCS has now broadened its scope to include FBSS, CRPS I and II, diabetic neuropathy, postherpetic neuralgia, chronic angina, and visceral abdominal pain from chronic pancreatitis and other gastrointestinal entities. SCS is continuously evolving, with new device designs to maximize patient comfort and pain relief while minimizing complications. SCS is still an underutilized treatment alternative that physicians should turn to more often. With proper patient selection and diagnosis, SCS can be a useful tool in the treatment of neuropathic pain and other pain states as the technology continues to evolve.

REFERENCES

1. Deyo Rtsui-Wu Y. Descriptive Epidemiology of low-back pain and its related medical care in the United States. *Spine.* 1987;12(3):264–268.
2. Cassidy J, Carroll L, Côté P. The Saskatchewan Health and Back Pain Survey. *Spine.* 1998;23(17):1860–1866.
3. Shealy C, Mortimer J, Reswick J. Electrical inhibition of pain by stimulation of the dorsal columns. *Anesth Analg.* 1967;46(4):489–491.
4. Melzack R, Wall P. Pain mechanisms: a new theory. *Science.* 1965;150(3699):971–978.
5. Cruccu G, Aziz T, Garcia-Larrea L, et al. EFNS guidelines on neurostimulation therapy for neuropathic pain. *Eur J Neurol.* 2007;14(9):952–970.
6. Ubbink DT, Vermeulen H. Spinal cord stimulation for non-reconstructable chronic critical leg ischemia. *Cochrane Database Syst Rev* 2005;Jul 20;(3):CD004001.
7. Taylor RS, De Vries J, Buchser E, Dejongste MJ. Spinal cord stimulation in the treatment of refractory angina: systematic review and meta-analysis of randomised controlled trials. *BMC Cardiovasc Disord* 2009;9: doi:10.1186/1471-2261-9-13.
8. de Vos C, Rajan V, Steenbergen W, van der Aa H, Buschman H. Effect and safety of spinal cord stimulation for treatment of chronic pain caused by diabetic neuropathy. *J Diabetes Complications.* 2009;23(1):40–45.
9. Harke H, Gretenkort P, Ulrich Ladleif H, Koester P, Rahman S. Spinal cord stimulation in postherpetic neuralgia and in acute herpes zoster pain. *Anesth Analg.* 2002;94(3):694–700.
10. Andrell P, Ekre O, Eliasson T, et al. Cost-effectiveness of spinal cord stimulation versus coronary artery bypass grafting in patients with severe angina pectoris: long-term results from the ESBY study. *Cardiology.* 2003;99(1):20–24.

11. Kapural L, Cywinski J, Sparks D. Spinal cord stimulation for visceral pain from chronic pancreatitis. *Neuromodulation.* 2011;14(5):423–427.

12. Wolter T. Spinal cord stimulation for neuropathic pain: current perspectives. *J Pain Res.* 2014;7:651–663.

13. Shealy CN, Mortimer JT, Reswick. Electrical inhibition of pain by stimulation of the dorsal columns: preliminary clinical report. *Anesth Analg.* 1967;46(4):489–491.

14. Holsheimer J. Which neuronal elements are activated directly by spinal cord stimulation. *Neuromodulation.* 2002;5(1):25–31.

15. Levy RM. Anatomic considerations for spinal cord stimulation. *Neuromodulation.* 2014;17:2–11.

16. Struijk JJ, Holsheimer J. Transverse tripolar spinal cord stimulation: theoretical performance of a dual channel system. *Med Biol Eng Comput.* 1996;34:273–279.

17. Buvanendran A, Lubenow T. Efficacy of transverse tripolar spinal cord stimulator for the relief of chronic low back pain from failed back surgery. *Pain Physician.* 2008;11:333–338.

18. Siddall PJ, Middleton JW. A proposed algorithm for the management of pain following spinal cord injury. *Spinal Cord,* 2006;2:67–77.

19. Bockenek WL, Stewart PJB. Pain in patients with spinal cord injury. In: S. Kirshblum, D. Campagnolo, J. DeLisa (Eds.), *Spinal Cord Medicine.* Lippincott, Williams and Wilkins, Philadelphia; 2002:389–408.

20. Grider J, Manchikanti L, Caryannopoulos A, et al. Effectiveness of spinal cord stimulation in chronic spinal pain: a systematic review. *Pain Physician.* 2016;19:E33–E54.

21. North RB, Kidd DH, Farrokhi F, Piantadosi SA. Spinal cord stimulation versus repeated lumbosacral spine surgery for chronic pain: a randomized, controlled trial. *Neurosurgery.* 2005;56(1):98–106, discussion 106–107.

22. Kumar K, Taylor RS, Jacques L, et al. Spinal cord stimulation versus conventional medical management for neuropathic pain: a multicenter randomized controlled trial in patients with failed back surgery syndrome. *Pain,* 2007 Nov;132(1–2):179–188.

23. Visnjevac O, Costandi S, Patel BA, et al. A comprehensive outcome-specific review of the use of spinal cord stimulation for complex regional pain syndrome. *Pain Pract.* 2016 Oct 14;doi: 10/1111paper 12513.

24. Vergani F, Boukas A, Mukerji N, Nanavati N, Nicholson C, Jenkins A. Spinal cord stimulation for visceral pain related to pancreatitis: report of 2 cases. *World Neurosurgery.* Mar-Apr 2014;81(3–4):651.e17–9.

25. Lee KH, Lee SE, Jung JW, Jean SY. Spinal cord stimulation for intractable visceral pain due to sphincter of Oddi dysfunction. *Korean J Pain.* 2015 Jan;28(1):57–60.

26. Rana MV, Knezevic NN. Tripolar spinal cord stimulation for the treatment of abdominal pain associated with irritable bowel syndrome. *Neuromodulation.* 2013;16:73–77.

27. Lind G, Winter J, Linderoth B, Hellstrom PM. Therapeutic value of spinal cord stimulation in irritable bowel syndrome: a randomized crossover pilot study. *Am J Physiol Regul Integr Comp Physiol.* 2015;308:R887–R894.

28. Baranidharan G, Simpson KH, Dhandapani K. Spinal cord stimulation for visceral pain: a novel approach. *Neuromodulation.* 2014;17:753–758.

29. Pluijms WA, Slangen R, Joosten EA, et al. Electrical spinal cord stimulation in painful diabetic polyneuropathy, a systematic review on treatment efficacy and safety. *Eur J Pain.* 2011;15(8):783–788.

30. Hautvast RWM, DeJongste MJL, Staal MJ, van Gilst WH, Lie KI. Spinal cord stimulation in chronic intractable angina pectoris: a randomized, controlled efficacy study. *Am Heart J.* 1998;136(6):1114–1120.

31. Pan X, Bao H, Si Y, et al. Spinal cord stimulation for refractory angina pectoris: a systematic review and meta analysis. *Clin J Pain*. 2016. [https://www.ncbi.nlm.nih.gov/pmc/articles/PMC5417578/].

32. Imran TF, Malapero R, Qavi AH, et al. Efficacy of spinal cord stimulation as an adjunct therapy for chronic refractory angina pectoris. *Int J Cardiol*. 2017;227:535–542.

33. Deogaonkar M, Zibly Z, Slavin KV. Spinal cord stimulation for the treatment of vascular pathology. *Neurosurg Clin N Am*. 2014;25(1):25–31.

34. Yin D, Slavin KV. A hypothesis on possible neurochemical mechanisms of action of cervical spinal cord stimulation in prevention and treatment of cerebral arterial vasospasm after aneurysmal subarachnoid hemorrhage. *Medical Hypotheses*. 2015;85(3):355–358.

35. Loge D, De Coster O, Washburn S. Technological innovation in spinal cord stimulation: use of a newly developed delivery device for introduction of spinal cord stimulation leads. *Neuromodulation*. 2012;15: 392–401.

36. Schade CM, Schultz DM, Tamayo N, Iyer S, Panken E. Automatic adaptation of neurostimulation therapy in response to changes in patient position: results of the Posture Responsive Spinal Cord Stimulation (PRS) Research Study. *Pain Physician*. 2011;14(5):407–417.

37. Paraschiv-Ionescu A, Buchser EE, Rutschmann B, Najafi B, Aminian K. Ambulatory system for the quantitative and qualitative analysis of gait and posture in chronic pain patients treated with spinal cord stimulation. *Gait Posture*. Oct 2004;20(2):113–125.

38. Schallhorn R. Spinal cord stimulation systems with patient activity monitoring and therapy adjustments. US Patent 644090 B1. https://patents.google.com/patent/US6120467

39. Schultz DM, Webster L, Kosek P, Dar U, Tan Y, Sun M. Sensor-driven position-adaptive spinal cord stimulation for chronic pain. *Pain Physician*. 2012;15(1):1–12.

40. Perryman LT, Speck B, Garcia CM, Rashbaum R. Injectable spinal cord stimulator system: Pilot Study. *Techn Reg Anesth Pain Mgmt*. 2012;16:102–105.

41. Shellock FG, Audet-Griffin AJ. Evaluation of magnetic resonance imaging issues for a wirelessly powered lead used for epidural, spinal cord stimulation. *Neuromodulation*. 2014;17(4):334–339.

42. Washburn S, Catlin R, Bethel K, Canlas B. Patient-perceived differences between constant current and constant voltage spinal cord stimulation systems. *Neuromodulation*. 2014;17:28–36.

43. Merrill D, Bikson M, Jefferys J. Electrical stimulation of excitable tissue: design of efficacious and safe protocols. *J Neurosci Meth*. 2005;141(2):171–198.

44. Alò K, Varga C, Krames E, et al. Factors affecting impedance of percutaneous leads in spinal cord stimulation. *Neuromodulation*. 2006;9(2):128–135.

45. Kapural L, Yu C, Doust M, et al. Novel 10-kHz high-frequency therapy (HF10 therapy) is superior to traditional low-frequency spinal cord stimulation for the treatment of chronic back and leg pain. *Anesthesiology*. 2015;123(4):851–860.

46. Schade C, Sasaki J, Schultz D, Tamayo N, King G, Johanek L. Assessment of patient preference for constant voltage and constant current spinal cord stimulation. *Neuromodulation*. 2010;13(3):210–217.

47. Perruchoud C, Eldabe S, Batterham A, et al. Analgesic efficacy of high-frequency spinal cord stimulation: a randomized double-blind placebo-controlled study. *Neuromodulation*. 2013;16(4):363–369.

48. Hou A, Kemp K, Grabois M. A systematic evaluation of burst spinal cord stimulation for chronic back and limb pain. *Neuromodulation*. 2016;19:398–405.

49. De Ridder D, Vanneste S, Plazier M, van der Loo E, Menovsky T. Burst spinal cord stimulation. *Neurosurgery.* 2010;66(5):986–990.

50. De Vos CC, Bom MJ, Vanneste S, Lenders MWPM, de Ridder D. Burst spinal cord stimulation evaluated in patients with failed back surgery syndrome and painful diabetic neuropathy. *Neuromodulation.* 2014;17:152–159.

51. Gong WY, Johanek LM, Sluka KA. A comparison of the effects of burst and tonic spinal cord stimulation on hyperalgesia and physical activity in an animal model of neuropathic pain. *Anesth Analg.* Apr 2016;122(4):1178–1185.

52. Crosby ND, Janik JJ, Grill WM. Modulation of activity and conduction in single dorsal column axons by kilohertz-frequency spinal cord stimulation. *J Neurophysiology.* 2017 Jan 1;117(1):136–147.

53. Al-Kaisy A, Van Buyten J, Smet I, Palmisani S, Pang D, Smith T. Sustained effectiveness of 10 kHz high-frequency spinal cord stimulation for patients with chronic, low back pain: 24-month results of a prospective multicenter study. *Pain Med.* 2014;15(3):347–354.

54. Gazelka H, Freeman E, Hooten W, et al. Incidence of clinically significant percutaneous spinal cord stimulator lead migration. *Neuromodulation.* 2014;18(2):123–125.

55. Krames ES. The dorsal root ganglion in chronic pain and as a target for neuromodulation: a review. *Neuromodulation.* 2015;18:24–32.

56. Liem L, Russo M, Hugyen FJ, et al. *Neuromodulation.* 2015 Jan;18(1):41–48.

57. Deogaonkar M, Slavin KV. Peripheral nerve/field stimulation for neuropathic pain. *Neurosurg Clin N Am.* Jan 2014;25(1):1–10.

58. Law JD, Swett J, Kirsch WM. Retrospective analysis of 22 patients with chronic pain treated by peripheral nerve stimulation. *J Neurosurg.* 1980;52(4):482–485.

59. Weiner RL, Reed KL. Peripheral neurostimulation for control of intractable occipital neuralgia. *Neuromodulation.* 1999;2(3):217–221.

60. Burns B, Watkins L, Goadsby PJ. Treatment of intractable chronic cluster headache by occipital nerve stimulation: long-term follow-up of eight patients. *Lancet* 2007;369:(9567):1099–1106.

61. Burns B Watkins L, Goadsby PJ. Treatment of intractable chronic cluster headache by occipital nerve stimulation in 14 patients. *Neurology.* 2009;72(4):341–345.

62. Dodick DW, Silbersterin SD, Reed KL, et al. Safety and efficacy of peripheral nerve stimulation of the occipital nerves for the management of chronic migraine: long-term results from a randomized, multicenter, double-blinded, controlled study. *Cephalalgia.* 2015;35(4):344–358.

63. Paicius RM, Bernstein CA, Lempert-Cohen C. Peripheral nerve field stimulation in chronic abdominal pain. *Pain Physician.* 2006;9:261–266.

64. Rauchwerger JJ, Giordano J, Rozen D, Kent JL, Greenspan J, Closson CWF. On the therapeutic viability of peripheral nerve stimulation for ilioinguinal neuralgia: putative mechanisms and possible utility. *Pain Practice.* Mar–Apr 2008;8(2):138–143.

65. Paicius RM, Bernstein CA, Lempert-Cohen C. Peripheral nerve field stimulation for the treatment of chronic low back pain: preliminary results of long-term follow-up: a case series. *Neuromodulation.* 2007;10(3):279–290.

66. Krutsch JP, McCeney MH, Barolat G, Tamimi MA, Smolenski A. A case report of subcutaneous peripheral nerve stimulation for the treatment of axial back pain associated with post-laminectomy syndrome. *Neuromodulation.* 2008;11(2):112–115.

67. Falco FJE, Berger J, Vrable A, Onyewu O, Zhu J. Cross talk: a new method for peripheral nerve stimulation. an observational report with cadaveric verification. *Pain Physician.* 2009;12:965–983.

68. Skaribas I, Alo K. Ultrasound imaging and occipital nerve stimulation. *Neuromodulation.* Apr 2010;13(2):126–130.

69. Ilfeld BM, Gilmore CA, Grant SA, et al. Ultrasound-guided percutaneous peripheral nerve stimulation for analgesia following total knee arthroplasty: a prospective feasibility study. *J Orthop Surg Res.* 2017;12:4.

70. Chodakiewitz YG, Bicalho GVC, Chodakiewitz JW. Multi-target neurostimulation for adequate long-term relief of neuropathic and nociceptive chronic pain components. *Surg Neurol Int.* 2013;4:S170–S175.

71. Mironer YE, Hutcheson JK, Satterthwaite JR, LaTourette PC. Prospective, two-part study of the interaction between spinal cord stimulation and peripheral nerve field stimulation in patients with low back pain: development of a new spinal-peripheral neurostimulation method. *Neuromodulation.* 2011;14(2):151–155.

72. Levy RM. MRI-compatible neuromodulation devices: critical necessity or desirable adjunct? *Neuromodulation.* 2014;17:619–626.

73. Gold G, Hayek S, Mekel-Bobrov N, Cuchelkar V. Low prevalence of MRI-related SCS explants based on complaints database and Medicare claims. Paper presented at 2013 NANS 17th Annual Meeting in Las Vegas, NV.

74. Moeschler SM, Sanders RA, Hooten WM, Hoelzer BC. Spinal cord stimulator explantation for magnetic resonance imaging: a case series. *Neuromodulation.* 2014;18(4):285–288.

75. MRI Safety | MRI Safe | Safe Access to MRI Scans | Medtronic. Tamethepain. com. 2016. http://www.tamethepain.com/chronic-pain/spinal-cord-stimulation-neurostimulation/mri-safe-safety/

76. Precision Spectra Spinal Cord Stimulator System. 1st ed. Valencia: Boston Scientific Corporation; 2016:5. https://www.bostonscientific.com/content/dam/Manuals/us/current-rev-en/91008787-01RevA_Precision_Spectra_Information_for_Prescribers_DFU_en-US_S.pdf

77. St. Jude Medical. St. Jude Medical receives FDA approval for the world's smallest upgradeable MR-conditional spinal cord stimulation system. Investors.sjm.com. 2016. http://investors.sjm.com/investors/financial-news/news-release-details/2015/St-Jude-Medical-Receives-FDA-Approval-for-the-Worlds-Smallest-Upgradeable-MR-Conditional-Spinal-Cord-Stimulation-System/default.aspx

78. Nevro Corp—Physicians—MRI. Nevro.com. 2016. http://www.nevro.com/English/Physicians/MRI/default.aspx

79. Taylor RS, Van Buyten JP, Buchser E. Spinal cord stimulation for chronic back and leg pain and failed back surgery syndrome: a systematic review and analysis of prognostic factors. *Spine (Phila Pa 1976).* 2005;30(1):152–160.

18 Advances in Intrathecal Drug Delivery

Impact on Orthopedic Practice

Jay S. Grider, Michael E. Harned, and Vital Nagar

OVERVIEW OF INTRATHECAL DRUG DELIVERY: CURRENT PRACTICE

Intrathecal drug delivery became commonplace more than 40 years ago as a means to treat recalcitrant chronic pain of malignant and nonmalignant origin [1,2]. Although the concept was rooted in the techniques and applied pharmacology of modern anesthesia and obstetric anesthesia practice, the pioneering practitioners in chronic pain medicine (most of whom were anesthesiologists by training) quickly adopted the intrathecal route as a known and effective method of administering analgesics to improve the quality of life of patients suffering from chronic pain [2]. Within short order, external and eventually fully implantable systems were developed that could deliver intrathecal medications over extended periods of time, thus allowing outpatient and ambulatory applications of intrathecal medications to become commonplace. These intrathecal drug delivery systems (IDDS) and intrathecal drug delivery (IDD) itself rapidly established themselves in the treatment of malignant pain at the end of life. These therapies were also utilized for treatment of pain of nonmalignant origin, but this application of the therapy was slower to be adopted [2].

With the advent of fully implantable systems with reservoirs that could extend the refill interval to several months, pain practitioners began to see utility in the treatment of chronic nonmalignant pain with IDD [2]. This greater acceptance of IDD, coupled with liberalized systemic opioid prescribing, led to the common practice in the late 1990s and early 2000s of high-dose systemic opioids coupled with IDD. This practice was based on the concept that opioids have no ceiling effect, and, as such, theoretically doses could be titrated ad infinitum [2–4]. Later in that decade, it became clear that liberalized opioid prescribing had significant deleterious effects and in fact led to greater risk when coupled with IDD. Many practitioners began focusing on patient selection, best practices with dosing, trialing, and maintenance management of patients with an IDDS [3,4]. This focus eventually led to the establishment of the Polyanalgesic Consensus Committee (PACC), which worked to establish best practices and standardization of treatment in patients treated with IDD [5–8]. Although IDD was part of the clinical armamentarium for more than 30 years, little work had been done from a formal research standpoint concerning best practices and patient selection. Most of the work regarding IDD consisted of case reports, observational studies, and retrospective reviews concerning efficacy of IDD. With the first PACC publications, work began rapidly coalescing around "filling in the gaps" with regard to knowledge base and best practices concerning IDD—which leads us to the current state. While the only US Food and Drug Administration (FDA)-approved medications for use in the intrathecal space are morphine, baclofen, and ziconotide, this chapter will also address commonly used medications such as clonidine and local anesthetics such as bupivacaine as well [2–8].

Device-Related Information

IDD, regardless of manufacturer, utilizes a pump reservoir connected to a flexible section of catheter that links the device to the intrathecal space [8]. The catheter is anchored to the prevertebral fascia of the lumbar spine and enters the interlaminar space typically below the level of L2 with the L4–L5 and L3–L4 interlaminar spaces being most common [8]. The rate of infusion of the IDDS is very slow, with 20 mL of solution lasting 80–180 days depending on flow rate and concentration of medication [8]. The drug delivery can be programmed via an external programing system that communicates with the implanted device. Flow rate can be programmed in varying ways, from continuous slow infusion to complex blousing and can average 50–200 µL/day delivered over a 24-hour period. Intrathecal opioids are cleared from the intrathecal space at a rate of 30% of total daily dose per day, with ultimate clearance from the body being via renal excretion [3–8]. Therefore, a patient receiving 1 mg of intrathecal morphine per day (over a 24-hour period) would have at most 12.5 µg of morphine systemically per hour. At lower doses (such as 1 mg of morphine or less), there is virtually no systemic opioid detectable, and often the medication will not show on a test of opioid administration (urine or blood drug screening). As the doses increase, obviously more medication is present systemically as it is cleared from the cerebrospinal fluid (CSF), but the amount is usually miniscule compared to oral or transdermal administration [3–8]. This low systemic exposure to the medication is a major advantage of IDD because the medication is delivered at its site of action at the dorsal horn of the spinal cord with few systemic side effects that limit the effectiveness of opioid therapy orally or transdermally. Since CSF motion in the spinal canal is oscillatory in nature and only has flow with complex eddy currents, mixing of medication in the CSF is somewhat limited and tends to localize near the area of the catheter tip with some degree of diffusion away from the catheter tip site [8]. While CSF fluid dynamics is in and of itself a complex issue, it is sufficient to understand that medication localization away from the catheter tip will not be extensive, and therefore any procedure which potentially dislodges the catheter tip may result in a pronounced change in the efficacy of the IDDS [8–11]. It is important that the orthopedic practitioner dealing with an IDDS understand the basic pharmacodynamics of IDD in the patient she is

considering surgical treatment for [3–8]. The perioperative management of the orthopedic patient with an IDDS will be discussed later in the chapter.

The most common site of implantation—and in fact the FDA-approved site—is in
the abdominal fat external to the rectus sheath between the ribs and anterior superior
iliac spine. Alternatively, many practitioners will implant the device in the buttock or
lateral low back. Given the proximity of the device and catheter to many structures
that are potential targets for orthopedic intervention and orthopedic trauma, the device placement and medications in the therapy will likely at some point be an issue in
treatment. At a minimum, it is possible that patients with an IDDS may be referred
for evaluation. It is important that the practitioner understand that the presence of
an IDDS does not indicate that the patient has "overblown pain complaints" or was
"difficult" as many patients find systemic and oral opioids effective but the side effects
intolerable. The focus of this chapter will be around the aspects and application of IDD
as it pertains to the orthopedic and potentially neurosurgical spine practitioner [8].

ASPECTS OF IDD FOR THE ORTHOPEDIC PRACTITIONER

Perioperative

Perhaps the most common scenario in which an orthopedic colleague will interact with
a patient with an IDDS in a way that will directly impact clinical decision-making is
the management of the patient in the perioperative period. Our group has written what
may be the only treatise to guide the practitioner on the perioperative management of
subjects with an intrathecal pump, and we will summarize the recommendations here
for the treatment of chronic pain as well as spasticity with an IDDS [11].

Chronic Pain IDD Issues

Chronic pain of either malignant or nonmalignant origin will involve the application
of opioids, local anesthetics, ziconotide, or adjunctive medications such as clonidine
[8]. As with systemic application, sudden cessation of opioids will result in acute opioid
withdrawal which, though unpleasant, is not life-threatening. Sudden cessation of intrathecal clonidine can lead to severe rebound hypertension [11]. Local anesthetics,
when given intrathecally, have little impact if delivery is suddenly disrupted, whereas
ziconotide, an N-type calcium channel blocker used for severe, refractory neuropathic
pain, can be stopped without withdrawal sequela. The point of this information is to
convey to the surgeon that sudden cessation of opioids and clonidine can have effects
on the patient ranging from unpleasant to deleterious, whereas local anesthetics and
ziconotide could be interrupted without major effect other than loss of pain control.
We know of situations where catheter disruption was treated lightly in the face of spine
surgery, with significant effects on perioperative physiology [11]. If the possibility of
catheter disruption is considered and planned for, then, obviously, the impact of this
event can be lessened.

Perioperative pain management is also a major concern of the surgeon when treating
a patient with an IDDS [11]. There is often the mistaken idea that the pump will be sufficient to manage acute postoperative pain or that the pump should be stopped prior to
the surgery. Both approaches are categorically poor ideas, though they have been tried
to our knowledge numerous times. The reason these approaches do not work well lies

in the fact that the pump delivers a slow infusion of medication for a chronic condition, which becomes a baseline level of analgesia for the patient. The introduction of acute surgical or trauma pain on top of the preexisting chronic pain will require management beyond the baseline analgesia provided by the pump. Careful application of intravenous patient-controlled analgesia (IVPCA) with standard monitoring presents little additional risk with IDD versus patients on systemic opioids [11–13]. If the patient is not taking systemic opioids for chronic pain in addition to the IDDS, they may in fact behave more like an opioid-naïve patient [12]. Stopping the intrathecal infusion is not an option perioperatively because the sudden withdrawal would complicate postoperative analgesia [11]. Even a low dose of 1 mg of intrathecal morphine per day is the equivalent of 300 mg of oral morphine, demonstrating the power of small doses of intrathecal opioid and showing why this route of administration is often so effective when used as solo therapy [12].

Our recommendations:

1. Have the IDDS-managing physician outline the medication being administered via the IDDS. If surgery has little chance of disrupting infusion use IVPCA or intermittent oral opioids and adjuncts as normal. Do not stop or slow the current infusion
2. Monitor systemic perioperative opioids with pulse oximetry or carbon dioxide monitoring. Risk is, however, low.
3. Regional anesthesia is recommended, although neuraxial analgesia is usually contraindicated.
4. If catheter disruption occurs, consult with the IDDS-managing physician to determine how to mitigate the effects of disruption of therapy. Do not assume that disruption of therapy will be benign.

Spasticity Managed with IDDS

It is common for spasticity from spinal cord injury or central nervous system disease to be managed with baclofen via the intrathecal route. Give the widespread use of baclofen for spasticity, it is likely that an orthopedic provider in a large medical center will encounter a patient receiving these drug via an IDDS. The most important factor to understand is that sudden intrathecal baclofen cessation can be *life-threatening*, and, as such, any planned procedure which could disrupt the delivery of medication should be accounted for prior to the procedure [5]. In a trauma situation with a patient with an IDDS in which vital signs are erratic and unstable, the possibility of intrathecal baclofen delivery should be considered in the differential diagnosis of metabolic instability. While opioid withdrawal could increase heart rate and blood pressure, baclofen withdrawal can have diverse effects from hypertension to hypotension and is closely related to scenarios such as neuroleptic malignant syndrome and anesthesia-induced malignant hyperthermia. On occasion, the chronic pain patient will have baclofen added to the admixture of his or her treatment protocol [5]. The absence of a spasticity diagnosis does not exclude the possible presence of baclofen in an IDD regimen.

Treatment for baclofen withdrawal is replacement of intrathecal baclofen in an expeditious manner, although there are protocols that describe stabilization with oral or systemic baclofen. It should be noted that oral or systemic baclofen administration may not reverse the metabolic decline of acute intrathecal baclofen withdrawal. Placement of an intrathecal catheter as a temporizing measure to deliver baclofen until a permanent solution is created has been described as a bridge to therapy [5]. The final point is, again, acute baclofen withdrawal can be *life-threatening*: do not overlook this factor.

Our recommendations:

1. Always inquire about baclofen in any patient with IDDS.
2. If baclofen is present and there is a possibility of disruption of administration, create a plan for assessing and treating acute baclofen withdrawal.
3. In a trauma patient with IDDS and unstable metabolic symptoms, always consider the possibility of acute baclofen withdrawal.
4. Treatment of acute baclofen withdrawal can be undertaken with oral/systemic baclofen replacement, although intrathecal replacement is the only sure method to lessen the impact.

PAIN CONDITIONS COMMONLY TREATED WITH IDDS

IDD has been utilized for a variety of chronic pain syndromes such as complex regional pain syndrome, failed back surgery syndrome, spinal stenosis, scoliosis, degenerative disc disease, and many others [15]. Essentially, any chronic pain condition that has been previously responsive to systemic opioids could be trialed and treated with IDD. Despite this wide category of potential subjects, recent data suggest that certain patient populations will respond to certain applications of IDD better than others.

Chronic Pain of Mechanical and Neuropathic Origin

For example, recent studies of monotherapy opioid have suggested that this treatment paradigm is more likely to help patient with mechanical pain syndromes (lumbar/cervical spondylosis, stenosis, spondylolisthesis) than purely neuropathic syndromes (complex regional pain syndrome or diabetic peripheral neuropathy) [3–15]. Conversely, ziconotide, a relatively new and novel N-type calcium channel blocker derived from snail toxin, has been shown to be very effective in the treatment of neuropathic pain and many mixed mechanical/neuropathic pain syndromes, albeit with a significantly narrow therapeutic window and distinct side-effect profile. Ziconotide does have the advantage that sudden cessation does not produce any withdrawal effect. As such, if side effects do occur, the medication can be abruptly discontinued. Side effects of this medication include severe neural impact such as dizziness, nausea, memory loss, vivid dreams, and potentially worsening of anxiety and depression leading to suicidal ideation in some instances [3].

Cancer-Related Pain

While all cancer-related pain is of neuropathic or mechanical origin in many regards, the mindset and approaches to dosing can be very different in patients with cancer.

First, cancer patients are much more likely to be on high-dose systemic opioids with IDD added later. This combination can lead to dramatic opioid tolerance complicating postoperative pain management for the orthopedic oncologist. Second, given the nature of the disease process, aggressive treatment with higher dose local anesthetic may be utilized to create not only analgesia but in some cases anesthesia [16]. Neurologic monitoring postprocedure in patients on high-dose intrathecal local anesthetics can be challenging. Most of the medications used for cancer-related pain will be identical to those mentioned in previous sections. The difference will be, in some cases, significantly higher doses of medication with less emphasis on function and greater emphasis on analgesia despite their impact on cognition or mobility. In other words, comfort measures may take precedent over function, and disruption or alteration of this therapy may have disconcerting effects on the patient and family [16].

ADVANCES IN IDD

The field of neuromodulation has recently experienced significant growth in new technologies and the application of these new technologies to increase the number of patients who may be assisted with improved pain control and function [5–8]. The spinal cord stimulation side of neuromodulation has seen the bulk of this growth in treatment options, but important advances have taken place in the area of IDD with regard to patient selection, medication selection, trialing, and patient management after implant. Although basic technology has remained unchanged (i.e., the basic components of an infusion device and catheter with anchoring to the fascia are still in place), there have been alternative devices introduced to market with important patient management considerations, as well as new research on patient management. This section will focus on each in a concise manner germane to orthopedic practice, with additional resources for further study if desired [3–8].

Devices

There are two major manufacturers in the IDDS space with important differences in approach to IDD. Medtronic Corp (Minneapolis, MN). has long been the only player in the IDDS market with a rotary delivery system that incrementally delivers medication through a roller pump system. This system has a long history of reasonable clinical outcomes, but Medtronic has recently issued an advisory bulletin notifying clinicians that drug delivery may be variable when medications other than morphine, baclofen, and ziconotide are placed within the pump. This has led to an FDA black-box warning and quality improvements from Medtronic [8]. These issues include over- and underinfusion of medication. Although few patient issues have been reported nationally, an increase in the number of rotor stalls have been reported. Currently, Medtronic reports that the issues have been identified and improvements placed within current generations of the Synchromed II IDDS. The information is being assessed by the FDA. Magnetic resonance imaging (MRI) compatibility and safety with the Synchromed II system is established with the proviso that the system must be checked after MRI for rotor stall and to ensure restart and reinfusion of medication [8].

The Synchromed II device has a feature called the "patient therapy manager," which allows the clinician to program "on-demand" boluses of a prescribed amount of medication that the patient can utilize. This feature has a lock-out and cannot be altered by the patient and is programmed by the clinician with limits on the percentage of daily dose and frequency of boluses allowed. This feature allows the device to have improved acceptance by the patient, who is given a degree of control over his or her therapy, and it has been associated with improved outcomes in industry-sponsored studies [8].

The Prometra IDDS by Flowonix (Mt. Olive, NJ), in contrast, operates by a piston injection system with very accurate delivery of medication and reliable dosing. The issue of safety concern with the current generation of the Flowonix device centers around the need to drain the device of medication before MRI scans are performed. There have been reports of device failure leading to delivery of the entire contents of the device to the patient during MRI [6,8]. This potential obviously could have devastating consequences. There has been confusion surrounding this issue in some settings, as previously the Medtronic system (as the only device in the marketplace) was MRI-compatible with a check for stall required after the scan. The arrival of the Prometra has required vigilance on the part of radiology staff and managing physicians because the procedures for preparation and management during MRI scanning for these two devices are very different. Removal of medication from the Flowonix system is essential. Clearly, if the protocol is followed, Flowonix IDDS safety is maintained, but knowing the type of device implanted is of paramount importance. The Prometra manufacturer is working on improved MRI compatibility, but, at present, the medication draining protocol must be followed. Also it must be noted that the Flowonix device is not FDA-approved for baclofen administration. Clearly, there is no reason why it would not be suitable for this medication, but the device has not undergone FDA testing for this indication.

Device-Related Complications

As noted in the previous section, rotor stall is a potential issue with the Medtronic device in the MRI setting but has also been reported outside of this scenario. Loss of efficacy should trigger a rotor study and a possible pump myelogram to determine if there is loss of patency of the catheter system and to ensure a continuity to the intrathecal space. Catheter-related issues include kinking of the catheter or breaking and/or dislodgment of the catheter from the anchor and intrathecal space. All of these scenarios can lead to sudden loss of efficacy [6,8].

Chronic infusion of opioids can lead to the formation of an inflammatory mass at the catheter tip. This granuloma formation can lead to the mass attaching to the spinal cord, with resultant neuropathy and possibly spinal cord compromise. Any patient doing well for an extended period of time who suddenly presents with neurologic decline (weakness, cauda equina syndrome, etc.). should have an immediate MRI to assess the catheter tip for inflammatory mass formation [6]. If a granuloma is noted, neurosurgical evaluation should be obtained with possible decompression verses cessation of infusion. There are reports in the literature that granulomas will resorb with cessation of infusion in 4–6 weeks [6]. If neurologic function is not in rapid decline, this approach can resolve the issue with careful neurologic monitoring. The risk factors for granuloma formation are high hydrophilic opioid concentration and low flow rate. Because hydrophilic opioid doses increase the risk of granuloma formation, these should create a high index of suspicion in clinicians managing IDDS.

Our device-related management recommendations:

1. Prior to MRI scanning of patients with an IDDS, determine the manufacturer:
   a. If Medtronic, the managing physician must be alerted to perform a rotor check after the scan.
   b. If a Flowonix system is implanted, at present the managing physician must drain the device and replace medication thereafter.
2. Sudden loss of efficacy could be a result of catheter malfunction, but rotor stall must considered in a Medtronic system.
3. Progressive neurologic decline in the form of weakness, cauda equina syndrome, sensory loss, and/or loss of bowel and bladder function should trigger an evaluation for granuloma formation.

MEDICATIONS

Opioids

The most common medication class used in IDD are opioids. Opioids may be classified as either hydrophilic or lipophilic. Commonly used hydrophilic opioids for IDD are morphine and hydromorphone, with fentanyl and, rarely, sufentanil being the lipophilic opioids used. Morphine represents the only FDA-approved opioid for use in IDD, but the PACC recognizes a long history of clinical use of all the medications listed, and the consensus statements acknowledge morphine, hydromorphone, and fentanyl as first- or second-line agents in the treatment of chronic pain [4–8,13,14]. Common side effects of pruritus and urinary retention occur perhaps more frequently with the hydrophilic opioids. Common systemic side effects of nausea, constipation, and sedation are lessened with IDD and lipophilic opioid administration. All intrathecal opioids have been shown to stay relatively close to the catheter tip at the infusion site, with hydrophilic opioids spreading more extensively than lipophilic opioids [10]. If lipophilic opioids are employed, they must be delivered at a very precise target zone in order to determine efficacy [5]. Recent epidemiologic studies have suggested that opioid monotherapy is effective for mechanical pain syndromes and may be effective for mixed mechanical and neuropathic pain syndromes, whereas opioids alone may not be as effective for pure neuropathic pain syndromes [6]. There is no recommendation on which trialing method (single-shot intrathecal vs. continuous inpatient catheter trial) is superior for identifying patients for opioid therapy.

Baclofen

Baclofen is a γ-aminobutyric acid (GABA-A) agonist used for spasticity management and, on occasion, as an adjunct for chronic pain of neuropathic origin or severe muscle spasm. As discuss previously, it has a wide therapeutic window, but sudden cessation of infusion can be life-threatening and should be considered in any patient with an IDDS and metabolic instability of cognition or blood pressure accompanied by neurologic decline [5]. Baclofen is a well-tolerated and well-studied medication for IDD. Titration of initial dose should be done slowly in an outpatient setting or more rapidly in a monitored setting as baclofen can cause flaccidity and respiratory compromise if dosed too aggressively [5].

Ziconotide

Ziconotide is an FDA-approved N-type calcium channel blocker utilized as a PACC-recommended first-line agent for chronic pain of mixed and neuropathic origin. It has found particular utility in chronic pain syndromes recalcitrant to other intrathecal medications [17–21]. It has a very narrow therapeutic window, with severe neurologic and psychiatric side effects possible with titration that is too rapid. Interested readers are directed to the work of Deer and Pope as a new, modified, gradual outpatient trialing method has been developed and has been shown to be highly effective in predicting success and those patients likely to experience adverse events with ziconotide [21]. Ziconotide also has several efficacy studies that are among the best in the IDD literature. Orthopedic specialists should be aware of the narrow therapeutic window, the risk of psychiatric side effects with the medication (though once on established dosing this becomes rare and is a phenomena mostly associated with dose establishment or titration), and the fact that the medication can be discontinued without fear of withdrawal [3].

Local Anesthetics

Local anesthetics (LA), mainly bupivacaine alone or in combination with opioids, have been shown to be effective in decreasing pain via the intrathecal route [22,23]. Studies have shown effectiveness of bupivacaine alone or of synergistic combinations of bupivacaine and opioid being effective for neuropathic and nociceptive pain [6]. Bupivacaine is a highly lipid-soluble amide local anesthetic that is often used off-label in intrathecal therapy. The intrathecal medications such as bupivacaine target pain-generating spinal segments [24], whereas opioid medications target drug receptors located in the dorsal horn of spinal cord or substantia gelatinosa [25]. Thus, the location of the catheter close to the pain-processing segment is important in the delivery of LA into the intrathecal space; however, CSF volume and flow will determine the final concentration of LA and opioid medication dose [5]. Bupivacaine at low concentrations alters sensory processing but spares motor functioning and has not been known to cause tachyphylaxis in patients with neuropathic or nociceptive pain [5].

Some animal studies have shown bupivacaine to cause modest neuronal vacuolation with continuous infusion and minor leptomeningeal cellular infiltration with bolus delivery [6]. Human cancer patient autopsies have not shown any significant histopathologic changes in patients on intrathecal bupivacaine [26]. A combination of bupivacaine with opioids has been shown to be effective for pain reduction in acute postoperative and labor pain studies [27,28]. A retrospective study involving 109 intrathecal drug delivery patients who were managed with a mixture of intrathecal bupivacaine and opioid after an initial period of opioid only intrathecal therapy showed decreased utilization of oral opioid and effective pain control with the combination therapy [5]. Another study involving non–cancer pain patients revealed blunting of intrathecal opioid dose escalation when patients received bupivacaine in addition to intrathecal opioid [29–31]. Another study which compared epidural with intrathecal drug delivery showed higher pain relief and patient satisfaction and lesser catheter complications along with better sleep in the intrathecal group [24]. Lethal cardiac toxic side effects can occur when significant amounts of bupivacaine reach the bloodstream; this should not be of concern with the intrathecal bupivacaine infusion. One limiting factor for bupivacaine infusion is sensorimotor loss; however, catheter tip placement, CSF dynamics, and patient mobility will play a major role in sensorimotor loss [27]. Even though bupivacaine is not FDA-approved for continuous intrathecal use, it is the most common local anesthetic used in spinal anesthesia and has been considered safe and efficacious when used alone or in combination with opioids [27].

Bupivacaine's high lipid solubility limits its spread intrathecally, and the implanting physician should place the catheter close to the pain pathology-processing site [24]. One recent study that used a hydromorphone and bupivacaine combination optimized with a personal therapy manager device found that the average intrathecal bupivacaine doses were 5.8 ± 0.3 mg/day (implant), 9.5 ± 0.6 mg/day (6 months), 12.2 ± 0.7 mg/day (12 months), and 12.6 ± 0.9 mg/day (24 months) [32]. The most recent PACC guidelines have suggested a maximal concentration of 30 mg/mL, with a starting dose of 1–4 mg/day and maximal daily dose of 10 mg [6]. The maximal dose is the average dose noted to be effective in some of the previous studies [29]. Additional bupivacaine is sometimes self-administered in boluses by patients through a personal therapy manager device. The recent PACC guidelines have suggested utilizing bupivacaine in combination with morphine for neuropathic pain (first-line therapy) and as second-line therapy for nociceptive pain when used in combination with fentanyl or hydromorphone [29].

There have been reports of tachyphylaxis with LAs in general and bupivacaine specifically. Despite data suggesting that LAs in high doses are neurotoxic, bupivacaine has a long safety history for use in IDD even though it is not FDA-approved for intrathecal use. The medication can be stopped without concern for withdrawal [3,12]. At infusion rates common with IDDS, little motor weakness even at relatively high doses (8–10 mg/day) is seen. With bolus dosing through a patient therapy manager, patients with higher doses of bupivacaine (>16 mg/day) may experience some transient weakness [30, 31].

Clonidine

Clonidine is an α_2 adrenergic agonist used as a second-line medication in the treatment of nociceptive, neuropathic, and mixed pain syndromes. While clonidine can be used as a standalone agent, it is most often used in combination with an opioid or ziconotide. Intrathecal clonidine is especially beneficial in the treatment of CRPS, where level I evidence supports improvement in pain, allodynia, and hyperalgesia [5–8]. Clonidine can precipitously drop arterial blood pressure, therefore small starting doses and vigilant patient monitoring are recommended during initiation. Moreover, clonidine may not be abruptly stopped because rebound hypertension and accompanying sequela may occur. While clonidine has been proved to improve pain and reduce opioid requirements, it is not a currently FDA-approved for intrathecal use. Despite this, clonidine is not associated with a risk of neurotoxicity during extended use in the intrathecal space [5–8]. Orthopedic providers should be aware that interruption of clonidine intrathecal infusion may result in unpredictable swings in blood pressure and that restoration of intrathecal delivery of clonidine may be required to stabilize blood pressure because the increased arterial pressures may be quite refractory to treatment.

Our recommendation:

1. If an IDDS contains clonidine and disruption of infusion during surgery may be possible, the anesthesia care team should be alerted. Discontinuation of infusion prior to surgery is not recommended because this would almost certainly increase the risk of poorly controlled blood pressure in the perioperative period

CONCLUSION

While IDD is a common practice in the setting of interventional pain, it may be rarely seen by the orthopedic provider but may manifest itself in orthopedic trauma or perhaps in the setting of joint replacement or spinal surgery. Understanding the basics of treatment and when to be alert to issues that may impact patient safety and outcomes is important. While this chapter serves as general overview of a topic with long history and a rapidly developing literature, a basic understanding of the modality and medications is important. The interested reader is directed toward many of the recent papers published by the PACC.

REFERENCES

1. Onofrio BM, Yaksh TL, Arnold PG. Continuous low-dose intrathecal morphine administration in the treatment of chronic pain of malignant origin. *Mayo Clin Proc.* 1981 Aug;56(8):516–520.
2. Krames E. A history of intraspinal analgesia: a small and personal journey. *Neuromodulation.* (2012)15(3):172–193.
3. Yaksh TL, Fisher C, Hockman T, Wiese A. Current and future issues in the development of spinal agents for the management of pain. *Curr Neuropharmacol.* 2017;15(2):232–259.
4. Wallace M, Yaksh TL. Long-term spinal analgesic delivery: a review of the preclinical and clinical literature. *Reg Anesth Pain Med.* 2000 Mar–Apr;25(2):117–157.
5. Deer TR, Prager J, Levy R, et al. Polyanalgesic Consensus Conference, 2012: recommendations on trialing for intrathecal (intraspinal) drug delivery: report of an interdisciplinary expert panel. *Neuromodulation.* 2012 Sep–Oct;15(5):420–435; discussion 435.
6. Deer TR., Pope JE, Hayek SM, et al. The Polyanalgesic Consensus Conference (PACC): recommendations on intrathecal drug infusion systems best practices and guidelines. *Neuromodulation.* 2017a; doi: 10.1111/ner.12538.
7. Deer TR., Hayek SM, Pope JE, et al. The Polyanalgesic Consensus Conference (PACC): recommendations for trialing of intrathecal drug delivery infusion therapy. *Neuromodulation.* 2017b; doi:10.1111/ner.12543.
8. Deer TR, Pope JE, Hayek SM, et al. The Polyanalgesic Consensus Conference (PACC): recommendations for intrathecal drug delivery: guidance for improving safety and mitigating risks. *Neuromodulation.* 2017c; doi:10.1111/ner.12579.
9. Bernards CM. Understanding the physiology and pharmacology of epidural and intrathecal opioids. *Best Pract Res Clin Anaesthesiol.* 2002 Dec;16(4):489–505.

10. Bernards CM. Cerebrospinal fluid and spinal cord distribution of baclofen and bupivacaine during slow intrathecal infusion in pigs. *Anesthesiology.* 2006 Jul;105(1):169–178.

11. Grider JS, Brown RE, Colclough GW. Perioperative management of patient with an intrathecal drug delivery system. *Anesth Analg.* 2006;107(4):1393–1396.

12. Coffey RJ, Owens ML, Broste SK, et al. Mortality associated with implantation and management of intrathecal opioid drug infusion systems to treat noncancer pain. *Anesthesiology.* 2009 Oct;111(4):881–891.

13. Prager J, Deer T, Levy R, et al. Best practices for intrathecal drug delivery for pain. *Neuromodulation.* 2014 Jun;17(4):354–372; discussion 372.

14. Grider JS, Etscheidt MA, Harned ME, et al. Trialing and maintenance dosing using a low-dose intrathecal opioid method for chronic nonmalignant pain: a prospective 36-month study. *Neuromodulation.* 2016 Feb;19(2):206–219.

15. Hayek SM, Deer TR, Pope JE, Panchal SJ, Patel VB. Intrathecal therapy for cancer and non-cancer pain. *Pain Physician.* 2011 May–Jun;14(3):219–248.

16. Medtronic Bulletin, MRI Guidelines. http://professional.medtronic.com/pt/neuro/idd/ind/mri-guidelines/index.htm?fgm=mri:isomed#.WJs2CPLpw-Y.

17. Pope JE, Deer TR. Ziconotide: a clinical update and pharmacologic review. *Expert Opin Pharmacother.* 2013 May;14(7):957–966.

18. Rauck RL, Wallace MS, Leong MS, et al.; Ziconotide 301 Study Group. A randomized, double-blind, placebo-controlled study of intrathecal ziconotide in adults with severe chronic pain. *J Pain Symptom Mgmt.* 2006 May;31(5):393–406.

19. Staats PS, Yearwood T, Charapata SG, et al. Intrathecal ziconotide in the treatment of refractory pain in patients with cancer or AIDS: a randomized controlled trial. *JAMA.* 2004 Jan 7;291(1):63–70.

20. Wallace MS, Charapata SG, Fisher R, et al.; Ziconotide Nonmalignant Pain Study 96-002 Group. Intrathecal ziconotide in the treatment of chronic nonmalignant pain: a randomized, double-blind, placebo-controlled clinical trial. *Neuromodulation.* 2006 Apr;9(2):75–86.

21. Pope JE, Deer TR. Intrathecal pharmacology update: novel dosing strategy for intrathecal monotherapy ziconotide on efficacy and sustainability. *Neuromodulation.* 2015 Jul;18(5):414–420.

22. Maves TJ, Gebhart GF. Antinociceptive synergy between intrathecal morphine and lidocaine during visceral and somatic nociception in the rat. *Anesthesiology.* 1992;76:91–99.

23. Penning JP, Yaksh TL. Interaction of intrathecal morphine with bupivacaine and lidocaine in the rat. *Anesthesiology.* 1992;77:1186–2000.

24. Dahm PO, Nitescu PV, Appelgren LK, Curelaru ID. Intrathecal infusion of bupivacaine with or without buprenorphine relieved intractable pain in three patients with vertebral compression fractures caused by osteoporosis. *Reg Anesth Pain Med.* 1999;24:352–357.

25. Yaksh TL, Woller SA, Ramachandran R, Sorkin LS. The search for novel analgesics: targets and mechanisms. *F1000 Prime Rep.* 2015;26:7–56.

26. Wagemans MF, van der Valk P, Spoelder EM, Zuurmond WW, de Lange JJ. Neurohistopathological findings after continuous intrathecal administration of morphine or a morphine/bupivacaine mixture in cancer pain patients. *Acta Anaesthesiol Scand.* 1997;41:1033–1038.

27. Ortner CM, Posch M, Roessler B, et al. On the ropivacaine-reducing effect of low-dose sufentanil in intrathecal labor analgesia. *Acta Anaesthesiol Scand* 2010;54: 1000–1006.

28. Parpaglioni R, Baldassini B, Barbati G, Celleno D. Adding sufentanil to levobupivacaine or ropivacaine intrathecal anaesthesia affects the minimum local anaesthetic dose required. *Acta Anaesthesiol Scand.* 2009;53:1214–1220.

29. Deer TR, Caraway DL, Kim CK, Dempsey CD, Stewart CD, McNeil KF. Clinical experience with intrathecal bupivacaine in combination with opioid for the treatment of chronic pain related to failed back surgery syndrome and metastatic cancer pain of the spine. *Spine J.* 2002;2:274–278.

30. Veizi IE, Hayek SM, Narouze S, Pope JE, Mekhail N. Combination of intrathecal opioids with bupivacaine attenuates opioid dose escalation in chronic noncancer pain patients. *Pain Med.* 2011;12:1481–1489.

31. Dahm PO, Nitescu PV, Appelgren LK, Curelaru ID. Intrathecal infusion of bupivacaine with or without buprenorphine relieved intractable pain in three patients with vertebral compression fractures caused by osteoporosis. *Reg Anesth Pain Med.* 1999;24:352–357.

32. Hayek SM, Veizi E, Hanes M. Intrathecal hydromorphone and bupivacaine combination therapy for post-laminectomy syndrome optimized with patient-activated bolus device. *Pain Med.* 2016 Mar;17(3):561–571.

19 Neuromodulation and Spinal Cord Stimulators

A Long Overdue Paradigm Disruption with the Interventional Pain Management Ladder

Anh L. Ngo, Bruce A. Piszel,
Mark R. Jones, Hector J. Cases,
Alan D. Kaye, and Mark V. Boswell

INTRODUCTION

Neuromodulation with spinal cord stimulation (SCS) is an effective, reversible, and minimally invasive interventional therapy for many types of chronic and difficult-to-treat pain. Introduced in 1967, SCS involves placing stimulator leads into the epidural space at affected levels and then subcutaneously implanting a small programmable pulse generator [1–3]. This procedure, initiated with a brief temporary trial of lead placement to prove efficacy prior to permanent implantation, can result in significant pain relief and reduced use of healthcare resources and costs, while increasing patient satisfaction and neurologic and cognitive function [4–11]. In a competitive marketplace, SCS manufacturers have developed devices that can provide single-source current, single-source voltage, multiple independent source current control, burst currents, and high-frequency currents.

In the United States, the present standard of practice for treatment of chronic pain consists of first pharmacotherapy with nonsteroidal anti-inflammatory drugs (NSAIDs), opioids, and calcium membrane channel stabilizers by a primary care physician (as described by the World Health Organization [WHO] Pain Ladder), then spine surgery by an orthopedic surgeon or neurosurgeon [12,13]. Often as a modality of last resort when others have failed, patients are referred to interventional pain specialists for long-term management. Given the option of less-invasive interventional spine

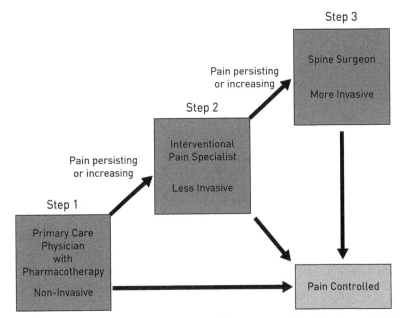

FIGURE 19.1 Paradigm disruption with introduction of the Interventional Pain Management Ladder.

procedures, reduced costs to patient and healthcare systems, and high rates of success, a paradigm shift is occurring in which interventional pain management is becoming the second line of treatment before open back surgery. This philosophical approach of patient management with least invasive therapies prior to more tissue disruptive measures is seen in the care pathways of other serious medical conditions, such as myocardial infarction and intracranial aneurysms [14,15]. This chapter discusses the history of SCS, technological advances in SCS devices, current practice standards, and the new paradigm disruption of using first minimally invasive SCS for neuromodulation in chronic pain control as the preferred treatment prior to open-back spine surgery. We propose this change in chronic pain management as the new Interventional Pain Management Ladder (Figure 19.1).

HISTORY OF NEUROMODULATION AND SCS

Electrical stimulation of the spinal cord is a pain relief technique that traces its roots back 4,000 years to the ancient Egyptians [16]. In a book published in 43 AD, called the *Compositiones*, Scribonius Largus, a physician and pharmacologist, reported the use of a torpedo fish, a type of electric ray, as a treatment for both gout and headaches. On a moist shore, the patient would stand on the torpedo fish until the foot and leg were numb up to the knee; as a result, the pain associated with gout and headaches was largely relieved [17–19]. In current medical practice, there are two clinical applications for electrical stimulation to nerves. The first is designed to treat motor disorders such as tremors caused by advanced Parkinson's disease. The more common use for electrical stimulation uses focused electrical treatment to neural targets that results in analgesia. Current targets for stimulation include the spinal cord, dorsal root ganglia (DRG), and peripheral nerve tracts [20].

Introduced in 1967, SCS was created as a less invasive and less anatomically disruptive surgical treatment for untreatable pain. Norman Shealy, a Harvard-trained neurosurgeon at Case Western Reserve University, implanted the first unipolar SCS device [21]. This first device, modified from preexisting cardiovascular devices that stimulated the carotid sinus and nerve to treat hypertension and angina, effectively relieved cancer-derived pain during a patient's final months. SCS systems primarily indicated for chronic pain became commercially available soon thereafter from Medtronic, Inc. in 1968 [22]. The 1970s ushered in physician-developed methods of minimally invasive percutaneous insertion of temporary catheter electrodes for SCS screening trials [2,3]. Fully implantable SCS systems were released in 1981, with rechargeable devices in production by 2004 [6]. In a short time, this percutaneous approach for permanent implantation had achieved results of pain control close to those of open spine surgery [23].

An alternative to open spine surgery for chronic pain control, SCS is reversible and offers patients the experience of a screening trial with temporary SCS before proceeding to permanent implantation of the device. SCS, where direct electrical stimuli is applied to the spinal cord to produce an analgesic effect, was based on the gate control theory formulated by Melzack and Wall [24]. This theory dictates that the stimulation of large β fibers closes the gate on small fiber transmission, resulting in perceived analgesia through its association with the inhibitory and excitatory relationships in pain pathways. Current understanding suggests that an inhibitory process occurs in the dorsal horn [25,26]. Nociceptive and somatosensory fibers synapse with second-order neurons of the substantia gelatinosa as they enter the dorsal horn. SCS, by a mechanism that remains elusive, prevents the nociceptive signal from propagating further to the sensory cortex. Theories on the mechanism range from signal inhibition via interneurons to modulation of neuroactive mediators [27]. Regardless of the mechanism, SCS remains a proven and effective method of treatment for chronic pain.

Many different types of pain may be treated with SCS. The chronic refractory neuropathic pain resulting from failed back surgery syndrome (FBSS) affects 25,000–50,000 new patients each year and is the most common indication for SCS [28]. Complex regional pain syndrome (CRPS), characterized by intractable pain of one or more extremities, is the second most common indication for SCS with an incidence of 5.6–26.2 per 100,000 person-years [29–31]. Other common indications for SCS include peripheral vascular disease (PVD), diabetic neuropathy, refractory angina, and visceral abdominal pain [32–36]. A complete list of accepted indications for use of SCS in pain control can be found in the US Centers for Medicare and Medicaid Services (CMS) ICD-9, ICD-10 Clinical Modification (ICD-10-CM), and ICD-10-Procedure Classification System (ICD-10-PCS) code sets [37].

In 1989, the first SCS device from Medtronic was approved by the US Food and Drug Administration (FDA) to relieve pain from nerve damage in the trunk, arms, or legs, and it now accounts for about 90% of all neuromodulation treatments, with more clinical scenarios being approved annually.

Many studies show that SCS is superior to repeated surgeries in FBSS and to physical therapy in CRPS [38–40]. On average, approximately 50% of patients see at least a 50% reduction in pain scores and a significant and persistent decrease in narcotic use [41]. Proper patient selection based on psychological evaluation results in markedly improved success rates because psychological factors are the most common reason for SCS failure [42–44]. As is the case with any type of spinal surgery, the most serious complications involve paralysis or severe neurological deficits. Fortunately, permanent complications are rare; less than 1% of SCS implants result in neurological injury [45]. Hardware complications such as electrode migration, lead breakage, and battery failure have become less common as technology improves, with rates presently varying between 1% and 4% [46]. Other potential complications include infection, cerebrospinal fluid (CSF) leak, and persistent pain at the implant site [46].

CURRENT TECHNOLOGY IN IMPLANTABLE PULSE GENERATORS FOR SPINAL CORD STIMULATION

Technological advances for SCS have been rapidly introduced in the clinical environment. Through percutaneously placed electrodes or via a surgical paddle lead inserted by laminotomy, traditional SCS therapies apply electrical current in the dorsal column to alter pain processing and mask the sensation of pain [47]. Although traditional SCS therapies, built on single-source current or voltage administration, demonstrate safety, efficacy, and cost-effectiveness in treating chronic refractory low back pain, newer versions of SCS systems include DRG SCS, innovative advances in stimulation frequency application through high-frequency 10 (HF10) SCS, burst SCS, and neural targeting SCS or multi-independent source control with three-dimensional imaging [47–54]. These newer modalities have improved efficacy and individualization of treatment for patients while providing the possibility of recapturing those who have previously failed neuromodulation.

Neuromodulation implantable pulse generator (IPG) delivery systems for pain control vary in size, specifications, and administration of electrical current or voltage therapy (Figure 19.2). All devices are remotely programmable and are rechargeable transcutaneously. At present, the major manufacturers in the SCS market are Medtronic (NYSE: MDT), Nevro Corporation (NYSE: NVRO), Boston Scientific Corporation (NYSE: BSX), and St. Jude Medical (formerly NYSE: SJM), which was purchased by Abbott Laboratories (NYSE: ABT) in January 2017 [55]. Earlier entrants, such as Medtronic and St. Jude Medical, developed SCS pulse generators based on existing cardiovascular and pacemaker technology that provided a single current or single voltage source [56,57]. Boston Scientific, which acquired hearing aid manufacturer Advanced Bionics Corporation in 2004, developed its SCS implantable pulse generators with multiple independent current source control from cochlear implant

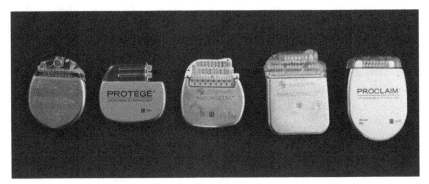

FIGURE 19.2 Implantable pulse generators from various manufacturers including Medtronic, Boston Scientific, and St. Jude Medical. A Nevro device is not shown here.

technology and incorporated three-dimensional modeling for ease and accuracy of lead placement [56–60]. Nevro, the most recent entrant in the marketplace, was founded in 2006 and provides a device with a high-frequency single-current source that can function up to 10,000 Hz [49].

Single-source current and single-source voltage IPGs are similar in construction, with two electrode leads of 8 individual contacts for a total of 16 application areas. The majority of IPG delivery systems are manufactured on this standard. Although many studies document the effectiveness of SCS in treating chronic spinal pain, tolerance to single-source current and single-source voltage SCS has been observed in some patients, in whom it has become necessary to increase pulse amplitude to achieve the same analgesic results and efficacy over time [61,62]. One study presented a tolerance rate of 29% with possible causes including patients redefining their pain, neuroplasticity of pain transmission pathways, psychiatric affective disorders, and, most likely, fibrotic tissue formation around the electrodes impeding effectiveness of electrical current delivery [61,63–67].

To help address tolerance from tissue fibrosis at lead sites, DRG SCS provides a highly targeted form of neuromodulation therapy [68]. Fine electrodes with four contacts are placed via percutaneous needle insertion in the epidural space through the intervertebral foramen and against the DRG [69]. Electrical current application with low amplitudes can selectively affect different parts of the DRG, thus providing stimulation to specific nerve roots or parts of the nerve [69]. This characteristic makes DRG SCS particularly useful in the treatment of focal areas of pain, specifically difficult-to-target locations such as groin and foot pain, by applying stimulation around the DRG [51,61,70]. However, lead placement into the DRG is technically more challenging than electrode installation in the dorsal column and requires advanced provider skill and more time [69].

HF10 single source current SCS (HF10) is an innovative upgrade in SCS system technology [49]. As most patients prefer uncomplicated therapy, HF10 systems deliver electrical waveforms up to 10,000 Hz at a subthreshold level for patients' pain relief without the annoyance of paresthesias [50,71]. Since 2011, HF10 has been approved for clinical use in Europe and Australia and has received FDA approval in 2015 for patients with chronic refractory pain of the limbs and trunk [4,71].

Another advance in IPG technology is *burst SCS*, in which a conventional frequency of 500 Hz is delivered in intervals of five burst pulses at 40 Hz. Specifically, burst technology delivers bundles of pulses, called *burst trains*, which are separated by pauses, called *interburst intervals*. Each burst train consists of a string of pulses at set pulse amplitude, pulse width, and interpulse frequency provided in an arrangement comparable to that of the burst firing neurons that exist, alongside tonic firing neurons, in some pain paths [72,73]. With the goal of reduced to no paresthesia, burst SCS amplitudes are decreased to achieve subthreshold stimulation [52,53,74]. Although this approach does not prevent long-term development of tissue resistance, burst SCS may possibly prolong original permanent lead placement utilization through the intermittent application of stimulation [52,53].

Neural targeting SCS, also known as *multiple independent current source control*, provides excellent potential for wider and more specific application of stimuli while delaying the detrimental effects of fibrotic tissue formation from electrical current in the spine, thus improving pain control with lower explantation rates. With 32 contacts and 32 individually dedicated power sources, the multiple independent current source control system allows for the separate delivery of electrical current in small increments to each of the 32 independent electrical leads in the dorsal column [54]. This division of separate power sources enables more focused pain targeting and provides patients with stimuli in only specific areas needed for pain control [54,75]. With many independent dedicated power sources, multiple independent current source control SCS can avoid unnecessary stimulation and development of tissue fibrosis in areas requiring lesser therapy [54]. By contrast, single-source current or voltage SCS systems have only one power source that provides equal intensity of stimulation to all 16 stimulation points, regardless of medical necessity [54,75]. With the integration of three-dimensional modeling to accurately select the correct neural target and position for optimal anatomical lead placement, neural targeting SCS can significantly decrease intraoperative time of IPG implantation while allowing a highly significant improvement in patient control of pain that is twofold greater than with non–neural targeting spine stimulation [54].

SCS pain control is not indicated for all patients. General contraindications for SCS system implantation include poor surgical candidates; those who fail to receive effective pain relief during trial stimulation; patients who are unable to operate an SCS system; untreated severe psychiatric or psychological disorders, including somatization; nonorganic etiologies of pain; unwillingness to stop improper drug use; and patients unable to give informed consent [48]. Certain medical conditions also exclude SCS, including severe coagulopathy, site infection, sepsis, central canal stenosis, neurogenic claudication, and cauda equina syndrome [48].

PARADIGM DISRUPTION AND THE INTERVENTIONAL PAIN MANAGEMENT LADDER

As with many care pathways for major medical conditions, such as heart attack and stroke, the order of treatment starts with less-invasive modalities and progresses to more-invasive procedures [14,15]. In 2012, under current standards for stroke management by the American Heart Association and American Stroke Association, a patient with an aneurysmal subarachnoid hemorrhage would undergo pharmacotherapy prior to occlusion of the aneurysm by an interventional endovascular approach with electrolytically detachable coils, and then, if appropriate, with open cranial microsurgical clip obliteration for treatment by neurosurgery [14,76]. This convention of first less-invasive to more disruptive intervention is also established in present guidelines for myocardial infarction management by the American College of Cardiology and the American Heart Association [15]. In a heart attack scenario, protocol for care begins with medication treatment and then progresses to less-invasive endovascular procedures, only to follow with open cardiac surgery if necessary [15]. This practice of least invasive prior to engaging in more tissue disruptive measures has been a common standard of practice among many major medical condition algorithms.

However, for the past several decades, the spine-mediated pain treatment algorithm has started with a visit to the primary care physician, internist, chiropractor, physical therapist, acupuncturist, or emergency department. If superficial, manipulative and then pharmacologic management of a patient's pain fails with NSAIDs to opioids, anticonvulsants, and steroids, as reminiscent of the WHO Pain Relief Ladder (also known as Conventional Medical Management [CMM]), the patient is referred to

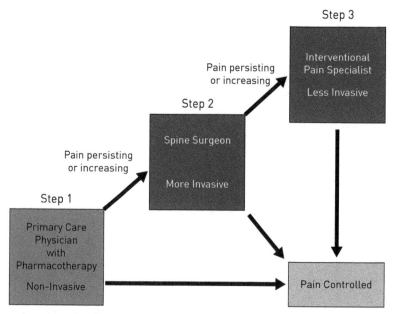

an orthopedic spine surgeon or a spinal neurosurgeon (Figure 19.3) [12,77,78]. This chapter questions the order of treatment for spine-mediated pain. In the same way that the WHO Pain Relief Ladder prioritizes treatment progression, we believe that more conservative, less-invasive treatments should be used before spine surgery is contemplated, with the exception of diagnoses of severe central canal stenosis, neurogenic claudication, cauda equina syndrome, or new neurologic deficit [48]. Instead of immediate referral to a surgeon first from the primary care provider, the patient should be evaluated by an interventional spine specialist.

In this new paradigm of first involving an interventional spine specialist prior to a spine surgeon, a diagnosis is established, and, if symptoms are amenable, an interventional procedure (including, but not limited to medial branch blocks, epidurals, stellate ganglion blocks, and lumbar sympathetic blocks) is performed for pain control. Effectiveness is established with a positive result defined as greater than 50% pain relief [5,41,79,80]. If a response of 50% or greater pain relief is not achieved, then neuromodulation should be considered prior to surgery [80]. A neuromodulatory trial is completely reversible, and a positive result is defined as greater than 50% reported relief of the primary pain complaint [48]. Only if a trial failure results should SCS be avoided and a referral to a spinal surgeon considered. This argument is especially valid due to multiple studies that show SCS to be a successfully viable treatment for FBSS and that it is more effective, both medically and cost-wise, than reoperation as a treatment for persistent radicular pain after lumbosacral spine surgery, where, in the large majority of patients, it avoids the necessity for reoperation [5–11,81,82].

Using the WHO Pain Ladder as a template, we recommend adoption of the Interventional Pain Management Ladder (Figure 19.1). Our Interventional Pain Management Ladder uses WHO recommendations as the first step and incorporates advanced procedures for pain management. This approach to care of spine-mediated pain embraces the concept of beginning with the least invasive modality first (with the

FIGURE 19.3 Current paradigm in medical and surgical management of chronic pain.

exception again of aforementioned diagnoses of central canal syndrome, cauda equina syndrome, neurogenic claudication, or new neurological deficit) and moving to more invasive treatment if the patient fails to respond to neuromodulation. Being similar to standard practice in many surgical subspecialties, this least-invasive-first approach will result in fewer postprocedural and postoperative complications and limit high costs to payors [5–11].

The incidence of FBSS is high, as documented in the literature on the management of chronic pain. Several studies present FBSS as being around 40%, with one 2015 study listing FBSS as the primary cause for 76.8% of failure in patients with workers' compensation claims to return to work and regular function [81–85]. In FBSS, patient treatment options are limited to continued pharmacologics and neuromodulatory trials. Given this, why not begin with a less-invasive, minimally tissue disruptive, fully reversible SCS trial first?

Finally, SCS is specifically designed to modulate and reduce a patient's pain, whereas spine surgery is designed to repair a spinal pathologic injury or defect [86–88]. Currently, both state and federal regulatory agencies are compelling physicians to minimize opioid utilization. According to data reported from the Centers of Disease Control, in the United States alone, deaths from prescribed opioids exceeded 183,000 from 1999 to 2014 [89,90]. Given the negative societal impact of opioid abuse, neuromodulation through decreased reported pain by patients allows for reduction and weaning of opioids. Additionally, offering patients a SCS trial assists in differentiating patients who desire potential pain resolution using pharmacologics from any associated euphoric effects they experience [91]. Inherent in this approach, there is a need for noninterventionalists to manage pain. This should improve outcomes, as it is widely accepted that singularly managing pain with opioids fails over the long term due to downregulation of opioid receptors [92]. This in turn requires never-ending elevations in frequency and dosages, which regulatory agencies want practitioners to avoid. In essence, neuromodulation gives patients the option for nonopioid-based pain control while reducing the risk of narcotic abuse and death, it may reduce the need for spine surgery, and it will facilitate greater compliance with governmental rules limiting opioid prescribing.

CONCLUSION

The Interventional Pain Management Ladder reflects a possible paradigm disruption in chronic pain management. For treatment of chronic pain after failure of pharmacotherapy, the standard of care should shift to less-invasive interventional pain management as the preferred second-line treatment prior to more tissue-disruptive spine surgery. This approach is in line with the care pathways of other major medical conditions, such as heart attack and stroke. SCS with neuromodulation is an effective, reversible, and minimally invasive interventional therapy for many types of chronic and difficult-to-treat pain. Introduced in 1967, SCS involves placing electrodes into the epidural space at affected levels and then subcutaneously implanting a small programmable pulse generator. This procedure, first with a brief trial to prove efficacy prior to permanent implantation, can result in satisfactory pain relief and reduced use of healthcare resources and costs, while improving outcomes.

SCS manufacturers have developed devices that can provide single-source current, single-source voltage, multiple independent source current control, burst currents, and high-frequency currents. In the United States, present approaches for chronic pain management consist of first pharmacotherapy by a primary care physician and then spine surgery by an orthopedic surgeon or neurosurgeon. Often as a treatment of last resort, patients are referred to interventional pain specialists for long-term management. This chapter presents a modern approach of least invasive therapies first prior to more tissue-disruptive measures and aligns chronic pain care with treatment of other serious medical conditions. Our hope is that a new Interventional Pain Management Ladder would help shift spinal pain management to less-invasive treatment first, prior to more tissue-disruptive open-back surgery.

ACKNOWLEDGMENTS

The authors wish to thank Edwin Delfin and Justice Rosario for their invaluable input. Bruce Piszel is a consultant for Boston Scientific and peer-to-peer teaching. The other authors (ALN, MJ, HJC, and MVB) declare no conflicts of interest.

REFERENCES

1. Shealy CN, Mortimer IT, Reswick JB. Electrical inhibition of pain by stimulation of the dorsal columns: preliminary clinical report. *Anesth Analg.* 1967;46(4):489–491.
2. Erickson, DL. Percutaneous trial of stimulation for patient selection for implantable stimulating devices. *J Neurosurg.* 1975;34:440–444.
3. Hosobushi Y, Adams JE, Weinstein PR. Preliminary percutaneous dorsal column stimulation prior to permanent implantation. *J Neurosurg.* 1972;17:242–245.
4. Grider JS, Manchikanti L, Carayannopoulos A, Lal Sharma M. Effectiveness of spinal cord stimulation in chronic spinal pain: a systematic review. *Pain Physician.* 2016;19:33–54.
5. Jeon YH. Spinal cord stimulation in pain management: a review. *Korean J Pain.* 2012 Jul;25(3):143–150.
6. Kumar K, Rizvi S. Cost-effectiveness of spinal cord stimulation therapy in management of chronic pain. *Pain Med.* 2013 Nov;14(11):1631–1649.
7. Hollingworth W, Turner JA, Welton NJ, Comstock BA, Deyo RA. Costs and cost-effectiveness of spinal cord stimulation (SCS) for failed back surgery syndrome: an observational study in a workers' compensation population. *Spine (Phila Pa 1976).* 2011 Nov 15;36(24):2076–2083.
8. Kemler MA, Raphael JH, Bentley A, Taylor RS. The cost-effectiveness of spinal cord stimulation for complex regional pain syndrome. *Value Health.* 2010 Sep–Oct;13(6):735–742.
9. Taylor RS, Taylor RJ, Van Buyten JP, Buchser E, North R, Bayliss S. The cost effectiveness of spinal cord stimulation in the treatment of pain: a systematic review of the literature. *J Pain Symptom Mgmt.* 2004 Apr;27(4):370–378.
10. Taylor RS, Ryan J, O'Donnell R, Eldabe S, Kumar K, North RB. The cost-effectiveness of spinal cord stimulation in the treatment of failed back surgery syndrome. *Clin J Pain.* 2010 Jul-Aug;26(6):463–469.
11. *Economic Aspects of Spinal Cord Stimulation* (SCS). Boston: Boston Scientific; 2013.
12. World Health Organization (1996). *Cancer Pain Relief. With a Guide to Opioid Availability,* 2nd ed. Geneva: WHO.
13. World Health Organization (1998). *Cancer Pain Relief and Palliative Care in Children.* Geneva: WHO.

14. Connolly ES, Rabinstein AA, Carhuapoma JR, et al. Guidelines for the management of aneurysmal subarachnoid hemorrhage: a guideline for healthcare professionals from the American Heart Association/American Stroke Association. *Stroke.* 2012;43:1711–1737.

15. Ryan TJ, Anderson JL, Antman EM, et al. ACC/AHA guidelines for the management of patients with acute myocardial infarction: executive summary. A report of the American College of Cardiology/American Heart Association Task Force on Practice Guidelines (Committee on Management of Acute Myocardial Infarction). *Circulation.* 1996;94:2341–2350.

16. Kane K, Taub A. A history of local electrical analgesia. *Pain.* 1975;1:25–138.

17. Nutton, V. Scribonius Largus, the unknown pharmacologist. *Pharmaceutical History.* 1995;25:5–8.

18. Hamilton JS. Scribonius Largus on the medical profession. *Bulletin of the History of Medicine. 1986;60:209–216.*

19. Pellegrino ED, Pellegrino AA. Humanism and ethics in Roman medicine: translation and commentary on a text of Scribonius Largus. *Literature and Medicine.* 1988;7:22–38.

20. Benjamin R, Grider JS, Vallejo R, Tilley DM, Kaye AD. Spinal cord stimulation: principles and applications. In: Kaye AD, S Davis S, eds., *Principles of Neurophysiological Assessment, Mapping, and Monitoring.* New York: Springer; 2014:245–258.

21. Rossi U. The history of electrical stimulation of the nervous system for the control of pain. In: Simpson BA, ed., *Electrical Stimulation and the Relief of Pain: Pain Research and Clinical Management.* Vol. 15. New York: Elsevier Science; 2003:5–16.

22. Gildenberg PL. History of electrical neuromodulation for chronic pain. *Pain Med.* 2006;7:7–13.

23. North RB, Fischell TA, Long DM. Chronic stimulation via percutaneously inserted epidural electrodes. *Neurosurgery.* 1977;1(2):215–218.

24. Melzack R, Wall PD. Pain mechanisms: a new theory. *Science* 1965;150:171–179.

25. Linderoth B, Foreman RD. Physiology of spinal cord stimulation: review and update. *Neuromodulation.* 1999;2:150–164.

26. Oakley JC, Prager JP. Spinal cord stimulation: mechanisms of action. *Spine.* 2002;27:2574–2583.

27. Bengt L, Robert DF. Mechanisms of spinal cord stimulation in painful syndromes: role of animal models. *Pain Med.* 2006;7:S14–S26.

28. Heithoff KB, Burton CV. CT evaluation of the failed back surgery syndrome. *Orthop Clin North Am.* 1985;16:417–444.

29. Harden RN, Bruel S, Stanton-Hicks M, Wilson PR. Proposed new diagnostic criteria for complex regional pain syndrome. *Pain Med.* 2007;8:326–331.

30. Sandroni P, Benrud-Larson LM, McClelland RL, Low PA. Complex regional pain syndrome type I: incidence and prevalence in Olmsted county, a population-based study. *Pain.* 2003;103:199–207.

31. De Mos M, Huygen, FJ, van der Hoeven-Borgman M, Dieleman JP, Stricker BHC, Sturkenboom MC. Outcome of the complex regional pain syndrome. *Pain.* 2009;25:590–597.

32. Cook AW, Oygar A, Baggenstos P, Pacheco S, Kleriga E. Vascular disease of extremities: electric stimulation of spinal cord and posterior roots. *NY State J Med.* 1976;76:366–368.

33. De Vos CC, Vinayakrishnan R, Wiendelt S, Hans E, van der AA, Hendrik PJ, Buschman HP. Effect and safety of spinal cord stimulation for treatment of chronic pain caused by diabetic neuropathy. *J Diabetes Complications.* 2009;23:40–45.

34. Sanderson JE, Brooksby P, Waterhouse D, Palmer RGB, Neubauer K. Epidural spinal electrical stimulation for severe angina: a study of its effects on symptoms, exercise tolerance and degree of ischaemia. *Eur Heart J.* 1992;13:628–633.

35. Ceballos A, Cabezudo L, Bovaira M, Fenollosa P, Moro B. Spinal cord stimulation: a possible therapeutic alternative for chronic mesenteric ischaemia. *Pain.* 2000;87:99–101.

36. Vallejo R, Benyamin RM, Kramer J, Bounds D. Spinal cord stimulation. In: Manchikanti L, Singh V, eds., *Interventional Techniques in Chronic Spinal Pain.* Paducah, KY: American Society of Interventional Pain Physicians; 2007:655–661.

37. Centers for Medicare and Medicaid Services (CMS). *ICD-10-PCS Official Guidelines for Coding and Reporting 2016.* Washington D.C.: United States Government.

38. Turner JA, Loeser JD, and Bell KG. Spinal cord stimulation for chronic low back pain: a systematic literature synthesis. *Neurosurgery.* 1995;37:1088–1095.

39. Burchiel KJ, Anderson VC, Brown FD. Prospective, multicenter study of spinal cord stimulation for relief of chronic back and extremity pain. *Spine.* 1996;21:2786–2794.

40. Kemler MA, Barendse GAM, Van Kleef M. Spinal cord stimulation in patients with chronic reflex sympathetic dystrophy. *N Engl J Med.* 2000;343:618–624.

41. Rauck RL, Nagel S, North JL, Machado AG, Hayek SM. *Neurostimulation for the Treatment of Chronic Pain.* New York: Saunders; 2012.

42. Shealy CN. Dorsal column stimulation: optimizing of application. *Surg Neurol.* 1975;4:142–145.

43. Long D. Psychological factors and outcomes of electrode implantation for chronic pain. *Neurosurgery.* 1980;7:225–229.

44. North R, Shipley J. Practice parameters for the use of spinal cord stimulation in the treatment of chronic neuropathic pain. *Pain Med.* 2007;8:S200–S275.

45. Jacobs MJ, Jorning P, Joshi S. Epidural spinal cord electrical stimulation improves microvascular blood flow in severe limb ischemia. *Ann Surg.* 1988;207:179–183.

46. Rosenow JM, Stanton-Hicks M, Rezai AR, Henderson JM. Failure modes of spinal cord stimulation hardware. *J Neurosurg Spine.* 2006;5:183–190.

47. Deer TR, Krames E, Mekhail N, et al. The appropriate use of neurostimulation: new and evolving neurostimulation therapies and applicable treatment for chronic pain and selected disease states. *Neuromodulation.* 2014;17(6):599–615.

48. Verrills P, Sinclair C, Barnard A. A review of spinal cord stimulation systems for chronic pain. *J Pain Res.* 2016;9:481–492.

49. Tiede J, Brown L, Gekht G, Vallejo R, Yearwood T, Morgan D. Novel spinal cord stimulation parameters in patients with predominant back pain. *Neuromodulation.* 2013;16(4):370–375.

50. Van Buyten JP, Al-Kaisy A, Smet I, Palmisani S, Smith T. High-frequency spinal cord stimulation for the treatment of chronic back pain patients: results of a prospective multicenter European clinical study. *Neuromodulation.* 2013;16(1):59–65.

51. Liem L, Russo M, Huygen FJ, et al. One-year outcomes of spinal cord stimulation of the dorsal root ganglion in the treatment of chronic neuropathic pain. *Neuromodulation.* 2015;18(1):41–48.

52. De Ridder D, Plazier M, Kamerling N, Menovsky T, Vanneste S. Burst spinal cord stimulation for limb and back pain. *World Neurosurg.* 2013;80(5):642–649.

53. De Ridder D, Vanneste S, Plazier M, van der Loo E, Menovsky T. Burst spinal cord stimulation: toward paresthesia-free pain suppression. *Neurosurgery.* 2010;66(5):986–990.

54. Mekel-Bobrov N, Hayek S, Veizi E, et al. Long-term clinical outcomes of neural targeting spinal cord stimulation (SCS): final results of the LUMINA clinical study.

Presented at the Annual Meeting of the American Academy of Pain Medicine, Jul 31–Aug 4 2016. Washington, DC.

55. Yahoo Finance. https://finance.yahoo.com/

56. St. Jude Medical. *St. Jude Medical™ Proclaim™ Neurostimulation System Clinician's Manual*. Plano, TX: St. Jude Medical; 2016.

57. *Medtronic RestoreSensor SureScan® Implant Manual*, M940100A004. 2013:12. Medtronic Corporation.

58. PR Newswire. June 1, 2004. http://www.prnewswire.com/news-releases/boston-scientific-announces-acquisition-of-advanced-bionics-corporation-74277207.html

59. *Boston Scientific Precision Spectra ImageReady™ MRI Guidelines*, 90829497-02 Rev B, 2014. Boston Scientific Corporation.

60. *ImageReady™ MRI Full Body Guidelines for Precision™ Montage™ MRI Spinal Cord Stimulator System*, 91035972-01 Rev C, 2016.

61. Deer TR, Mekhail N, Provenzano D, et al. The appropriate use of neurostimulation: avoidance and treatment of complications of neurostimulation therapies for the treatment of chronic pain. *Neuromodulation*. 2014;17(6):571–598.

62. Hayek SM, Veizi E, Hanes M. Treatment-limiting complications of percutaneous spinal cord stimulator implants: a review of eight years of experience from an academic center database. *Neuromodulation*. 2015;18(7):603–608.

63. Kumar K, Wilson JR, Taylor RS, Gupta S. Complications of spinal cord stimulation, suggestions to improve outcome, and financial impact. *J Neurosurg Spine*. 2006;5(3):191–203.

64. Gibson-Corley KN, Flouty O, Oya H, Gillies GT, Howard MA. Postsurgical pathologies associated with intradural electrical stimulation in the central nervous system: design implications for a new clinical device. *BioMed Research International*. 2014;Article ID 989175.

65. Hurlbert RJ, Tator CH, Theriault E. Dose-response study of the pathological effects of chronically applied direct current stimulation on the normal rat spinal cord. *J Neurosurg*. 1993;9(6):905–916.

66. Brown WJ, Babb TL, Soper HV, Lieb JP, Ottino CA, Crandall PH. Tissue reactions to long term electrical stimulation of the cerebellum in monkeys. *J Neurosurg*. 1977;47(3):366–379.

67. Yuen TGH, Agnew WF, Bullara LA. Histological evaluation of neural damage from electrical stimulation: considerations for the selection of parameters for clinical application. *Neurosurgery*. 1981;9,(3):92–299.

68. Shanthanna H, Chan P, McChesney J, Paul J, Thabane L. Assessing the effectiveness of "pulse radiofrequency treatment of dorsal root ganglion" in patients with chronic lumbar radicular pain: study protocol for a randomized control trial. *Trials*. 2012;13:52.

69. Kramer J, Draper CE, Deer TR, Pope JE, Levy R, Grigsby EJ. Dorsal root ganglion stimulation: anatomy, physiology, and potential for therapeutic targeting in chronic pain. In: *Atlas of Pain Medicine Procedures*. Sudhir Diwan, Peter Staats. McGraw-Hill Education; 2015:73:626–631.

70. Song JJ, Popescu A, Bell RL. Present and potential use of spinal cord stimulation to control chronic pain. *Pain Physician*. 2014;17(3):235–246.

71. Kapural L, Yu C, Doust MW, et al. Novel 10-kHz High-frequency therapy (HF10 therapy) is superior to traditional low-frequency spinal cord stimulation for the treatment of chronic back and leg pain: the SENZA-RCT randomized controlled trial. *Anesthesiology*. 2015;123(4):851–860.

72. Lopez-Garcia JA, King AE. Membrane properties of physiologically classified rat dorsal horn neurons in vitro: correlation with cutaneous sensory afferent input. *Eur J Neurosci*. 1994;6:998–1007.

73. Courtney P, Espinet A, Mitchell B, Russo M, Muir A, Verrills P, Davis K. Improved pain relief with burst spinal cord stimulation for two weeks in patients using tonic stimulation: results from a small clinical study. *Neuromodulation.* 2015 Jul;18(5): 361–366.

74. de Vos CC, Bom MJ, Vanneste S, Lenders MW, de Ridder D. Burst spinal cord stimulation evaluated in patients with failed back surgery syndrome and painful diabetic neuropathy. *Neuromodulation.* 2014;17(2):152–159.

75. *Precision Spectra Spinal Cord Stimulator System: Information for Prescribers.* Boston: Boston Scientific; 2015.

76. Murayama Y, Nien YL, Duckwiler G, et al. Guglielmi detachable coil embolization of cerebral aneurysms: 11 years' experience. *J Neurosurg.* 2003;98:959–966.

77. World Health Organization. *WHO's Pain Relief Ladder.* 1986. www.who.int/cancer/palliative/painladder/en/

79. WebMD. *Understanding Back Pain.* 2015. www.webmd.com/back-pain

80. Practice guidelines for chronic pain management. A report by the American Society of Anesthesiologists Task Force on Pain Management, Chronic Pain Section. *Anesthesiology.* 1997 Apr;86(4):995–1004.

81. North RB, Kidd DH, Zahurak M, James CS, Long DM. Spinal cord stimulation for chronic, intractable pain: experience over two decades. *Neurosurgery.* 1993 Mar;32(3):384–394.

82. North RB, Kidd DH, Farrokhi F, Piantadosi SA. Spinal cord stimulation vs repeated lumbosacral spine surgery for chronic pain: a randomized trial. *Neurosurgery.* 2005;56:98–106.

83. Eldabe S, Kumar K, Buchser E, Taylor RS. An analysis of the components of pain, function, and health-related quality of life in patients with failed back surgery syndrome treated with spinal cord stimulation or conventional medical management. *Neuromodulation.* 2010;13:201.

84. Thomson S. Failed back surgery syndrome: definition, epidemiology and demographics. *Br J Pain.* 2013. Feb;7(1):56–59.

85. Wilkinson HA. *The Failed Back Syndrome: Etiology and Therapy.* Philadelphia: Harper & Row, 1991.

86. Anderson JT, Haas AR, Percy R, Woods ST, Ahn UM, Ahn NU. Return to work after diskogenic fusion in workers' compensation subjects. *Orthopedics.* 2015 Dec;38(12):e1065–e1072.

87. Wikipedia. Laminectomy. https://en.wikipedia.org/wiki/Laminectomy

88. Wikipedia. Spinal decompression. https://en.wikipedia.org/wiki/Spinal_decompression

89. Wikipedia. Foraminotomy. https://en.wikipedia.org/wiki/Foraminotomy

90. CDC. Wide-ranging online data for epidemiologic research (WONDER). Atlanta, GA: CDC, National Center for Health Statistics, 2016. http://wonder.cdc.gov

91. Rudd RA, Seth P, David F, Scholl L. Increases in drug and opioid-involved overdose deaths: United States, 2010–2015. *MMWR Morb Mortal Wkly Rep.* ePub: 16 Dec 2016; doi: http://dx.doi.org/10.15585/mmwr.mm6550e1.

92. Chang YP, Compton P. Management of chronic pain with chronic opioid therapy in patients with substance use disorders. *Addiction Sci Clin Pract.* 2013;8:21. doi: 10.1186/1940-0640-8-21.

93. Al-Hasani R, Bruchas MR. Molecular mechanisms of opioid receptor-dependent signaling and behavior. *Anesthesiology.* 2011 Dec;115(6):1363–1381.

Index

Page numbers followed by *f*, *t*, and *b* refer to figures, tables, and boxes respectively.